Healthwise® Handbook

Take Charge of Your Health

18th Edition

Donald W. Kemper, MPH

Eileen Ellig, Editor

Adam Husney, MD, Medical Editor

Kathleen Romito, MD, Medical Editor

Take Control, Live Better
First Aid and Emergencies
Common Health Problems
Living Better With Chronic Disease
Staying Healthy

Healthwise
P.O. Box 1989
Boise, Idaho 83701

for every health decision®

A mother's use of the *Healthwise® Handbook* may have helped save her child's life.

Lauren's Story

Children get sick. It's a reality all parents face. But how do you know when to treat your child's symptoms at home or when to take your child to the doctor?

Lauren's mom faced this question when Lauren was just 4 years old. Not many things would slow down her daughter, so when Lauren got sick, Lauren's mom knew something was wrong. Over the phone, Lauren's pediatrician assured Lauren's mom that it was flu season and she shouldn't worry.

When she saw Lauren rubbing her neck, Lauren's mom looked up the symptoms herself in the *Healthwise Handbook*. She read that fever, aches, pains, and a stiff neck can be signs of meningitis.

An informed second call to the doctor sent Lauren, her mom, and Lauren's doctor straight to the emergency room for testing. Lauren had meningitis. The doctors

told Lauren's mom that her knowledge and quick action might well have saved her daughter's life.

Like Lauren's mom, you can use the *Healthwise Handbook* as a guide to making important health decisions for you and your family. Just look up your health problem to learn about home treatments you can try to relieve symptoms and when to call your doctor for help. It's that simple. For tips on how to find what you need in this book, see the next page.

Four Ways to Find What You Need in This Book

Index: Look up your health issues in the index starting on **page 337**.

Symptom Guides: Look for your symptoms in the easy-to-use charts starting on **page 61**.

Table of Contents: Check the table of contents on **pages v and vi**. It lists all the topics in the book. Each colored section has its own table of contents on the first page.

Color Bars: Use the color bars on the edge of the pages to browse for topics that interest you:

Tips for taking charge of your care

First aid and emergency topics, A to Z

Common health problems, A to Z

Major chronic diseases, plus advance directives

Healthy habits, preventive care, and safety tips

Find More Info on the Web

"Go to Web" codes make it easy to find the latest in-depth information on each topic. Go to **www.gotoweb.healthwise.net**. Then enter the code, and you'll find tools to help make a decision, master a skill, or learn more about your health.

Healthwise: Information You Can Trust

Healthwise is a nonprofit organization. Since 1975 our mission has been to help people make better health decisions. Through the years, we have been helping people do more for themselves, ask for the care they need, and say "no" to the care that may not be right for them.

People use our handbooks, online content, and nurse call center resources more than **110 million times a year**. More than **28 million copies of the** *Healthwise Handbook* are in print.

Healthwise is a top source for consumer health information for three reasons:

- ◆ **Trust.** As a nonprofit, we are driven by our mission.
- ◆ **Quality.** We keep up with the latest medical research, and medical experts review our work.
- ◆ **Plain language.** We're known for using words and images to explain complex medical issues in ways that anyone can understand.

A book, or even a Web site, cannot replace the need for good doctors—and no doctor can replace the need for people to care for themselves and be involved in their treatment decisions.

Use the book to ask good questions, but please follow the advice of your doctor. In most cases, this book will be helpful, but there is no guarantee that it will work for you in every case. Healthwise will not accept responsibility for any problems that may occur from following its guidelines. Remember to use your common sense and good judgment.

We wish you the best of health!

Learn more about who we are at **www.healthwise.org**.

We would like to thank the many people on the Healthwise staff who have contributed to this new edition of the *Healthwise Handbook*. We also would like to thank the following health professionals for the clinical wisdom and experience they shared in reviewing this book: Adam Husney, MD; Kathleen Romito, MD; Robert Kloner, MD; John McPherson, MD; Carl Orringer, MD; Anne Poinier, MD; and John Pope, MD. Special acknowledgement goes to Michael Linkinhoker, MA, CMI, at Link Studio, for creating the book's beautiful illustrations.

Table of Contents

Your Health: Take Control, Live Better

Your Health: Take Control, Live Better

Good health care doesn't just happen. It begins with you. Taking an active role in your health care is the best way to make sure you get the right care at the right time.

This means:

◆ **Do as much for yourself as you can.**

◆ **Ask for the care you need.**

◆ **Say "no" to the care that may not be right for you.**

This chapter is a practical guide to getting the care you need—no more and certainly no less. It covers 6 areas where you can have a big impact on the quality of your care:

1. Working closely with your doctor

2. Considering all your options before you decide on treatment

3. Being smart about medicines

4. Using medical tests wisely

5. Asking questions before you decide on surgery

6. Saving the emergency room for emergencies

Wellness Begins With You

A healthy lifestyle can help you feel good, stay at a healthy weight, and have plenty of energy for both work and play. It also can lower your risk for serious health problems.

Here are some things you can do to live a healthier life now.

◆ Eat a healthy, balanced diet.

◆ Get active.

◆ Get immunized.

◆ Schedule wellness visits and screening tests.

◆ Don't smoke.

◆ Limit alcohol.

◆ Manage stress.

◆ Make safety a priority.

These things can all be done, but they are not always easy to do. For more tips on how to live a healthier life, see page 299.

Work Closely With Your Doctor

A strong partnership between you and your doctor is key to getting great care and reducing costs. A doctor who not only knows your medical history but understands what's important to you may be the resource you need most when you face a major health care decision.

1. Use your doctor as a teacher and coach.

◆ Don't just ask your doctor what you should do. Ask why. Your doctor is in a unique position to help you understand your care.

◆ Always ask if you have options. Which seem best for you? What are their pros and cons? What effects might your choice have in the short term and over the long run?

◆ Learn from your doctor's experience with other patients. While every patient's situation is unique, your doctor has probably helped other patients work through the same questions and decisions that you have to deal with.

2. Tell your doctor that you care about cost. Your doctor probably won't know the exact cost of a drug or test or treatment. There are so many things that determine the cost of care—your health plan's arrangement with your doctor, how your plan bills for care, where you get the care, and others. But your doctor can give you an idea of how the cost of one choice compares to another.

Three Ways to Get Involved in Your Care

Title: Your Health

Director: You

Take: Action

1. Do as much for yourself as you can. For most common health problems, there are things you can do at home to help you feel better. Look up your health problem in this book to learn about home treatments you can try and when you should call your doctor.

2. Ask for the care you need. Learn as much as you can about the best treatments for your health problem and what the experts recommend. The more you know, the better questions you can ask about which treatment options may be right for you. If you learn about treatments that may help, but your doctor has not suggested them, ask why.

3. Say "no" to the care that may not be right for you. Often doctors offer treatment options because they think that's what you want them to do.

Always ask:

◆ What's my risk of waiting?

◆ Are there other treatment options?

◆ Where can I learn more?

◆ What do you think this treatment will cost me?

Without your input, you may get care that doesn't help you or even get care that may make your health problem worse.

3. Prepare for every doctor visit.

◆ Be ready to say what your main symptoms are, when they started, and what you have done to treat them so far. It may help to write these things down beforehand. Use the Self-Care Checklist on page 10.

◆ Write down the three questions that you most want to have answered.

◆ Bring a list of any medicines, vitamins, and herbal supplements that you are taking.

◆ Bring copies of recent test results if the tests were done by a different doctor.

4. Take an active role in every visit or call. Ask questions if you don't understand something. Write down the diagnosis, the treatment plan, and any guidelines for self-care and follow-up visits or calls.

Smart Decisions: Know Your Options

Good health decisions can help you reduce costs and get better care. A good decision takes into account:

◆ The benefits of each option.

◆ The risks of each option.

◆ The costs of each option.

◆ Your own needs and wants.

1. Always ask why. Too much care can be just as bad as—or worse than—too little. Most medicines can have side effects. Medical tests can give false results that lead to the wrong care. Surgery almost always has risks. And anytime you get care, there is a chance of error.

When your doctor suggests or orders a medicine, surgery, a test, or any other kind of care, ask why you need it and what would happen if you waited. If you don't need it now, you might want to wait.

Asking why can help you and your doctor make the decision that's right for you.

2. Know the pros and cons. Every treatment choice has pros and cons. It's up to you to know what they are. Your doctor can be a big help here, as can the Web site on the back cover.

Partner with your doctor to help you understand what a decision might mean for you now and in the long run.

Remember, the goal is to get the care you need, no more and no less, and to get it at the lowest cost you can.

3. Think about your needs and wants. People value things differently. When you have a health care decision to make, you have to balance issues like:

◆ The desire for better health versus the risks of treatment.

◆ The certainty of doing something versus the uncertainty of waiting (the known versus the unknown).

◆ Convenience versus cost.

For many decisions, these issues are just as important as the medical facts. They are part of what makes a decision right for *you*.

Stop. Think. Decide.

You'll make health decisions throughout your life. Some may be easy. And some may be so hard that you don't know how to sort through your choices.

Tools called decision aids can help you stop and think about your choices so you can decide what is best for you. Use the many "Go to Web" codes in this book to get to decision aids.

Through these decision aids, you can get facts about a problem or treatment option. Read stories of people who faced the same decision. And record your feelings and concerns.

Try them out and see how they can help you:

◆ Should you consider surgery for back pain? See page 95.

◆ What care do you want at the end of life? See page 297.

Smart Tips for Medicines

If you and your doctor have decided that you need prescription medicine, these three tips can help you get it at a lower cost:

◆ Choose generic medicines instead of brand names when you can. (Generics are the same medicine without the brand.)

◆ If there is no generic option, know whether your health plan makes you pay more for one brand name than another. Many plans do, using a list called a **drug formulary**.

◆ Compare prices and shop smart.

Generics and Brand Names

All drugs have a generic name, also known as the scientific name. For example, Glucophage is a brand name for the generic drug metformin. The generic name for Prozac is fluoxetine. Many drugs also have one or more brand names.

A generic drug has the same active ingredients as its brand-name version and almost always costs less. In many cases, generics are less than half the cost of the brands.

Are generics really as good as brand-name drugs?

◆ Yes. Generics are very carefully tested to make sure they have the same ingredients, same effects, and same safety profile as the brands. The medicines may look or taste slightly different.

◆ For a few medicines, the body does not respond to the generic drug in quite the same way as it does to the brand-name drug. Talk to your doctor or pharmacist before you switch from the brand to the generic (or vice versa).

Medicines and Your Health Plan

Most health plans use a drug formulary to help control costs. A formulary is simply a list of preferred prescription medicines. The plan may pay more of the cost of drugs on the list than other drugs that treat the same health problem.

The formulary may put drugs into three groups, or "tiers," based on how much your health plan will pay and how much you will have to pay.

◆ **Group 1: Generic drugs.** These are usually drugs that have been in use for a long time, have proven benefits, and cost less to make and sell. You pay the least for drugs in this group.

◆ **Group 2: Brand-name drugs that are on the formulary.** For the same health problem, there often are competing drugs from different companies. Your health plan may put one drug on the formulary instead of the others if the drug company agrees to reduce the price. You still pay more for the "formulary" brand-name drug than for the generic, but it costs less than the competing brand-name drugs that are not on the formulary.

◆ **Group 3: Brand-name drugs that are not on the formulary.** These drugs cost more because your health plan does not have an agreement with the drug company to reduce the price. When the health plan pays more, so do you.

The difference in cost to you between these three groups can be huge. If your doctor prescribes a medicine, make sure you know how much you will have to pay and whether a different choice would save you money without giving up quality. If he or she prescribes a medicine that is not on your health plan's preferred list, ask if there is a medicine on the list that will cost less and work just as well.

Sometimes there are good reasons to use a brand-name drug that's not on the formulary instead of one that is. The drug may have a dosing schedule that works better for you. Or it may have fewer or different side effects.

Smart Shopping for Medicines

If you pay for medicines out of your own pocket or through a health savings account (HSA), you have even more to gain from careful spending.

1. Compare prices. The speed and convenience of a local pharmacy helps in emergencies or if you're in a rush. But for medicines you take on a regular basis, mail-order or online pharmacies may be cheaper. They may be more convenient too, sending the medicines right to your mailbox.

2. Ask your doctor for free samples if you are trying a new medicine. This can let you try out the medicine for a couple of weeks without buying a full prescription. But beware—often the samples doctors get are for newer, more expensive drugs.

3. Buy in bulk. Once you know you will be using a medicine for a long time, you can often save money and time by ordering a large supply (90 days' worth, for example). Ask your doctor to write a prescription that covers a few months.

4. Ask your doctor or pharmacist about pill splitting. You can buy some pills at twice the dose you need (100 mg instead of 50 mg, for instance) for the same or nearly the same cost as the lower dose. By splitting the larger dose, you can get two doses for the price of one.

It is not safe to split all medicines this way. Capsules and time-release pills should never be split. With many medicines, the dose needs to be extremely precise. So be sure to check with your doctor or pharmacist about whether splitting your pills is safe.

5. Find out about discounts and patient assistance programs. Some drug companies offer free or discounted drugs for people who need help paying for medicine. To learn more about these programs, look online at RxAssist (www.rxassist.org) or at the Partnership for Prescription Assistance (www.pparx.org).

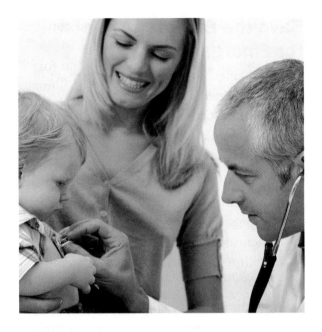

Help may also be available through your state, your community, or the Veterans Administration. Some drugstores and organizations, such as AARP, may offer discounts for older adults.

Smart Tips for Medical Tests

If you need a test, do your part to make sure that you do not have to repeat it. The tips below can make a big difference:

1. Follow instructions about how to prepare. Are you supposed to stop eating the night before? Not drink alcohol? Stop taking medicines, or take a special medicine? Get written instructions from your doctor or nurse, and follow them. This reduces the chance of error and the need to repeat the test.

Before you have a medical test, look it up at the Web site on the back cover so you know more about the test and what you need to do.

2. Keep a copy of the results. Get a copy of the full test results, even if they're normal. Do not assume that no news is good news. If you do not hear from your doctor, call to get your written test results. This helps in three ways:

- ◆ It makes sure you have the results if you later need to compare them to past or future tests.

- ◆ You have a backup record in case you see a different doctor who does not get your test results from your previous doctor. If you can provide a copy, he or she may not have to repeat the test.

- ◆ Having the results helps you better understand what's going on with your health.

3. Do not check into the hospital just for tests unless you have to. Sometimes a hospital stay is necessary, but often the point is just to better control what you eat, drink, and do before the test.

Talk to your doctor. He or she may be fine with your having the tests as an outpatient (which means not staying in the hospital overnight) as long as you agree to follow instructions for before and after the test.

4. Don't have tests more often than you need to. If you have a health problem that requires frequent tests and you are worried about the cost, tell your doctor. Maybe you can go a little longer between tests. Maybe you can have a less costly test some of the time and the more expensive one less often.

5. Ask about options, and shop around. The cost of some testing can vary widely without any difference in how reliable the results are. For expensive tests, it may pay to compare the costs of your best options.

Smart Tips for Surgery

If surgery is a possibility, get the facts about the surgery and consider your options. Tools called decision aids (see page 5) can help you make a decision. Use the many "Go to Web" codes in this book to get to decision aids.

If you can't find a decision aid for your surgery, ask your health care team to answer the questions below. Often it is up to you to say "no" to risky, unneeded, and unwanted surgery.

- ◆ How might surgery help you?
- ◆ What results would you have to get from the surgery for you to consider it a success? How likely are those results?
- ◆ What could go wrong if you have surgery?
- ◆ How long would it take to recover from surgery? How much time off would you have to take? What kind of rehab would you need?
- ◆ What happens in the short term if you don't have surgery? What might happen over the long run if you don't have it?
- ◆ Are there other treatments you could try first?
- ◆ Could the problem come back after surgery?
- ◆ If you need surgery, where should you have it? How can you reduce the chance of an error?

You will probably have other questions unique to your health problem and situation. Use the "Go to Web" codes in this book to get information that can help you work through these decisions.

Save the Emergency Room for Emergencies

Hospital emergency rooms (ERs) are set up to focus on medical emergencies. They are not set up to focus on routine health care. If you go to the ER for a problem that is not an emergency:

- ◆ It will cost a lot more than it would at a doctor's office or "walk-in" clinic (see page 9). A trip to the ER for an earache, for example, may cost three or four times as much as it would at your doctor's office.
- ◆ You will probably spend a lot more time there than you would at a walk-in clinic or doctor's office.
- ◆ You will get care from a doctor who has probably never seen you before. It's always best to get as much of your care as you can from a doctor who knows and understands you.

Go to the ER if you think you are having a medical emergency. That's what the ER is for. Otherwise, call your doctor's office first, or go to a walk-in clinic.

How Do You Know When It's an Emergency?

There are few clear rules about what is an emergency and what isn't. Most doctors would agree on a short list of problems that should always be treated as emergencies— chest pain that could be a heart attack, not being able to breathe, severe and uncontrolled bleeding, stroke symptoms, and a few others.

Most health problems are *not* emergencies. You may want to take care of the problem right away because you feel sick or uncomfortable, but nothing bad is going to happen to you if you wait a bit. Then again, you don't always know that for sure. Some problems that seem minor can become serious if you ignore them. And it may be even harder to know what to do when a child is sick.

One good question to ask yourself is, "Am I thinking about going to the ER because it's *convenient* or because it's *necessary*?" If you are choosing the ER because you can get in without an appointment, keep in mind the high price you will pay for that convenience. You may have to wait a long time to be seen. And you may have other options.

You can always call your doctor's office or a nurse line for help. You can also look for information about your problem in this book or at the Web site on the back cover to help you decide what to do.

What's a "Walk-In" Clinic?

Walk-in clinics are often called "minor emergency," "urgent care," or "immediate care" centers. They deal with all kinds of health problems and are often open in the evenings and on weekends. You do not need an appointment.

These types of clinics can be a great option when:

◆ You can't or don't want to wait for an appointment at your doctor's office.

◆ You don't need the level of care an ER provides.

What If a Problem Happens on a Weekend or at Night?

If you think you are having a medical emergency, go to the ER.

If you don't think the problem is an emergency:

◆ Look up your problem in this book or at the Web site on the back cover, and read the information about when to call a doctor. See if there is home treatment you can try.

◆ Call your doctor's office and see if there is a number to call for after-hours service.

◆ Call a nurse line for advice. The nurse can help you decide whether you need to get help now or whether it is safe to wait.

◆ Go to a walk-in clinic (if one is open).

◆ Go to the ER if you feel the problem cannot wait until your doctor's office or a walk-in clinic is open.

Take Charge

When it comes to staying healthy and getting good care, you are in charge. Stay healthy by eating a well-balanced diet, getting plenty of exercise, and keeping up with recommended health screenings. When you do get sick, take charge by learning about your health problem and working with your doctor to make the decision that is right for you. Let this book be your guide.

And remember to:

◆ Do as much for yourself as you can.

◆ Ask for the care you need.

◆ Say "no" to the care that may not be right for you.

The Healthwise® Self-Care Checklist

Step 1. Know the problem.

☐ When did it start? What are the symptoms? _____
_____

☐ Do you have pain? Is it a dull ache or stabbing pain? _____
_____

☐ Write down your vital signs:
- ▶ Temperature _____
- ▶ Blood pressure _____ / _____
- ▶ Pulse _____ beats per minute
- ▶ Breaths _____ per minute

☐ Have you had this problem before? What did you do for it? _____
_____
_____

☐ Have you had any changes in your life, such as new stress, medicines or supplements, food, or exercise? _____
_____

☐ Does anyone else at home or work have these symptoms? _____
_____

Step 2. Learn more about the problem.

☐ *Healthwise Handbook* (note page number) _____

☐ Advice from family, friends, or your doctor _____

☐ The Internet _____

Step 3. Make an action plan.

☐ Your home care plan _____

☐ When to call your doctor _____

Step 4. Check your progress.

☐ Are your actions working? _____

Go to Web   Get forms to help prepare for a doctor visit. Go to the Web site on the back cover and enter **f830** in the search box.

First Aid and Emergencies

Abdominal Injury

When to Call a Doctor

Call 911 if:

◆ The person has severe belly pain after an injury.

◆ The belly is swollen and hard all over, or pressing anywhere on the belly causes severe pain.

◆ The person faints.

◆ The person vomits a lot of blood or what looks like coffee grounds.

◆ The person has severe rectal bleeding. Severe means that the person is passing a lot of stool that is maroon or mostly blood.

◆ You can clearly see that the person has blood in his or her urine.

Call a doctor if:

◆ There is any bleeding from the rectum, blood in the stools or urine, or unexpected vaginal bleeding.

◆ The injury causes nausea, vomiting, heartburn, or loss of appetite.

◆ Constant mild or moderate pain gets worse or does not start to feel better after 12 hours.

For a cut or puncture to the belly, also see page 29.

A blow to the belly (abdomen) can cause severe bruising and bleeding inside the body. Such injuries are often caused by car, bike, sledding, or skiing accidents, when the person is thrown into an object or to the ground.

If there is internal bleeding or organ damage, the person may go into shock (see page 47). This can be life-threatening.

Home Treatment

◆ Have the person lie down with the feet higher than the heart. Loosen the person's clothes, and cover him or her with a blanket for warmth.

◆ Do not give the person anything to eat or drink until a medical evaluation has been done and you are sure the person is okay.

◆ Watch the person for the next few days. Signs of serious internal bleeding may not show up right away.

Bites From Animals and Humans

When to Call a Doctor

◆ The wound is severe and may need stitches, or it is on your face, hand, or foot, or over a joint. If the wound needs stitches, you should get them within 6 to 8 hours. See page 30.

◆ The bite or scratch is from a bat or other wild animal.

◆ The bite is from a human or a cat. These bites get infected quickly and easily.

◆ The animal that bit you foams at the mouth, acts strangely, or attacked for no clear reason. Also call the local animal control or public health office.

◆ You can't find the owner of a pet that bit you, or the owner can't confirm that the pet's rabies vaccine is up to date.

◆ You lose feeling or movement below the wound.

◆ You have signs of infection. These may include increased pain, swelling, warmth, or redness; red streaks leading from the wound; pus; and fever.

◆ You have not had a tetanus shot in the past 5 years or don't know when your last shot was. If you need a shot, you should get it as soon as possible.

Infection and scarring are the main concerns with bites and scratches that break the skin. You can also get tetanus if your shots are not up to date. See page 326.

After an animal bite, you may want to know if you need a rabies shot. Rabies is quite rare, but it is deadly if you are not vaccinated soon after a bite from an infected animal.

◆ The main carriers of rabies in North America are bats, raccoons, skunks, foxes, and coyotes.

◆ Vaccinated pets, such as dogs, cats, and ferrets, rarely have rabies.

◆ Many stray animals have not been vaccinated.

Home Treatment

If you are bleeding a lot, see Stopping Severe Bleeding on page 17.

◆ Scrub the wound with soap and water. Do not use alcohol, iodine, or any other cleansers.

◆ Call the local animal control or public health office for advice on what to do. In general:

  ❖ If a pet dog, cat, or ferret bites you, find out whether the animal has a current rabies vaccine. A healthy pet that does not have a current vaccine should be confined and watched for up to 10 days by a veterinarian.

  ❖ If a wild animal bites or scratches you, the animal control or public health office can tell you whether you need to worry about rabies.

13

Bites and Stings—Insects, Spiders, and Ticks

When to Call a Doctor

Call 911 if:

◆ You have signs of a severe allergic reaction soon after a bite or sting. These may include:

  ❖ Wheezing or trouble breathing.

  ❖ Swelling around the lips, tongue, or face.

  ❖ Severe swelling around the bite or sting (for example, your entire arm or leg is swollen).

  ❖ Fainting or other signs of shock. See page 47.

◆ You have just been bitten or stung by something that caused a serious reaction in the past.

Call a doctor if:

◆ You get a spreading skin rash, itching, a feeling of warmth, or hives.

◆ You get a blister at the site of a spider bite, or the skin around it changes color.

◆ A black widow or brown recluse spider bites you.

◆ Symptoms are not better in 2 to 3 days.

◆ You have signs of infection. These may include increased pain, swelling, warmth, or redness; red streaks leading from the bite; pus; and fever.

◆ A tick is attached to you and you cannot remove the whole tick.

◆ You were recently exposed to ticks and have a rash.

◆ You want to talk about allergy kits or allergy shots because you have had a serious allergic reaction in the past.

Insects and Spiders

Bites and stings from insects (bees, wasps, yellow jackets) and spiders usually cause pain, swelling, redness, and itching at the site of the sting or bite. In some people, especially children, the redness and swelling may be worse and last up to a few days.

A few people have severe allergic reactions that affect the whole body. This type of reaction can be deadly. If you have had a severe allergic reaction to a past sting or bite, you may want to keep an allergy kit with an epinephrine syringe (such as an EpiPen) with you at all times. Ask your doctor or pharmacist how and when to use it.

Spider bites are rarely serious. But any bite can be serious if it causes a person to have an allergic reaction.

A single bite from a poisonous spider, such as a black widow or brown recluse spider, may cause a severe reaction and needs medical care right away.

◆ A bite from a female black widow spider may cause chills, fever, nausea, and severe belly cramps.

◆ A bite from a brown recluse spider causes intense pain, and you may get a blister that turns into a large, open sore. The bite may also cause nausea, vomiting, headaches, and chills.

Black widow spiders can be up to 2 inches across and are shiny black with a red or yellow hourglass mark on their undersides.

Brown recluse (fiddler) spiders are about ½ inch long and have long legs. They are brown with a violin-shaped mark on their heads. (This picture is enlarged.)

Ticks

Ticks are small bugs that bite into the skin and feed on blood. They live in bird feathers and animal fur. Tick bites occur more often from early spring to late summer.

◆ Most ticks do not carry diseases, and most tick bites do not cause serious health problems. Still, it is best to remove a tick as soon as you find one.

◆ Many of the diseases that ticks may pass to humans (such as Lyme disease, Rocky Mountain spotted fever, relapsing fever, and Colorado tick fever) have the same flu-like symptoms: fever, headache, body aches, and fatigue.

◆ Sometimes a rash or sore may occur with the flu-like symptoms. A red rash that gets bigger is a classic early sign of Lyme disease. It may appear 1 day to 1 month after a tick bite.

Home Treatment

For insect and spider bites and stings:

◆ Remove a bee stinger by scraping or flicking it out. Do not squeeze it; you may release more venom into the skin. If you can't see the stinger, assume it's not there.

◆ If a black widow or brown recluse spider bites you, put ice on the bite and call a doctor. Do not use a tourniquet.

◆ Put ice or a cold pack on the bite or sting. For some people, a paste of baking soda or unseasoned meat tenderizer mixed with a little water helps relieve pain and decrease the reaction.

◆ Take an antihistamine (such as Benadryl or Chlor-Trimeton) to relieve pain, swelling, and itching. Some antihistamines (Alavert, Claritin, Zyrtec) are less likely to make you sleepy. Before you use these medicines, check the label. They may not be safe for young children or for people with certain health problems. Calamine lotion or hydrocortisone cream may also help.

◆ Wash the area with soap and water.

◆ Trim your fingernails so you don't scratch too hard.

◆ Do not break any blisters that develop. They could get infected.

More

For ticks:

◆ Check your body often for ticks when you are out in the woods. Closely check your clothes, skin, and scalp when you get home. Check your pets for ticks too. The sooner you remove ticks, the less likely they are to spread infection.

◆ If you find a tick, try to remove it. Use tweezers to gently pull on it as close to the skin (where its mouth is) as you can get. Fine-tipped tweezers may work best. Pull straight out, and try not to crush the tick's body. Do not try to "unscrew" the tick.

◆ Do not try to burn off the tick or smother it with petroleum jelly, nail polish, gasoline, or rubbing alcohol.

Use tweezers to pull the tick straight out.

◆ Save the tick in a jar for tests in case you get flu-like symptoms after the bite.

◆ Wash the area with soap and water.

Mosquitoes and West Nile Virus

West Nile virus is an infection spread to humans by mosquitoes. Most people who get the virus do not get sick.

When symptoms do occur, they appear 3 to 14 days after the bite and include fever, headache, body aches, and sometimes a skin rash. This is called West Nile fever. It is usually a mild illness.

Rarely, West Nile virus may affect the brain, causing serious illness that can lead to long-lasting problems or even death. Older adults are most likely to have serious illness from the West Nile virus.

When to Call a Doctor

Call a doctor if you were exposed to mosquitoes in the past 2 weeks and have any of these symptoms:

◆ Fever, headache, stiff neck, and confusion.

◆ Muscle weakness or loss of movement.

◆ Mild fever, rash, body aches, or swollen lymph nodes in the neck, armpits, or groin that last more than 2 or 3 days.

How to Avoid West Nile Virus

◆ Stay indoors at dawn, at dusk, and in the early evening. Mosquitoes are most active at these times.

◆ Wear long-sleeved shirts and pants made of thick fabric.

◆ Use an insect repellent that contains DEET, picaridin, or oil of lemon eucalyptus. For the best protection, apply and reapply as the label says.

◆ Don't keep open containers of water near your home. Mosquitoes can breed in even a small amount of standing water.

Bleeding Emergencies

When to Call a Doctor

Call 911 if:

◆ You have severe bleeding that you cannot stop.

◆ You are bleeding and you faint or feel lightheaded.

◆ You vomit a lot of blood or what looks like coffee grounds.

◆ You have severe rectal bleeding. Severe means that you are passing a lot of stool that is maroon or mostly blood.

◆ You have heavy vaginal bleeding, and you are in your second or third trimester of pregnancy.

Call a doctor if:

◆ Bleeding has slowed but not stopped after 45 minutes of direct pressure.

Stopping Severe Bleeding From a Wound

◆ Raise the area that is bleeding—higher than your heart if you can.

◆ Wash your hands well with soap and water. Put on medical gloves or place several layers of fabric or plastic bags between your hands and the wound.

◆ Remove any objects you can see on the surface of the wound. Do not try to clean out the wound.

◆ Press firmly on the wound with a clean cloth or the cleanest material you can find. If there is an object deep in the wound, put pressure around the object but not directly over it. Do not try to remove the object.

◆ If bleeding from a large or deep wound does not stop or slow down after applying direct pressure, or blood quickly soaks through several bandages, continue to put pressure on the wound and **call 911**.

◆ If bleeding slows or stops with pressure but starts again if you remove the pressure, apply pressure to the wound for a full 15 minutes. Do not lift your hands to see if the bleeding has stopped before 15 minutes have passed. If blood soaks through the cloth, put another cloth on top of the first one.

◆ For light bleeding, you can apply pressure for up to three 15-minute periods (total of 45 minutes). If any bleeding continues after 45 minutes of direct pressure, call a doctor.

Elevate the area and apply pressure with a clean cloth.

Blood Under a Nail

When to Call a Doctor

- The pain is severe, and you do not want to drain the blood from the nail yourself.

- You drained the blood from under the nail, but your finger or toe still hurts a lot.

- You have diabetes, blood flow problems, or a weak immune system (from HIV, steroid use, cancer treatment, or organ transplant) and need help with blood under a nail.

- You have signs of infection. These may include increased pain, swelling, warmth, or redness; red streaks leading from the nail; pus draining from the hole; and fever.

- You need help removing a nail that has torn or separated from the nail bed.

When a fingernail or toenail gets banged or smashed, blood may build up under the nail. The pressure can hurt a lot. Ice may help with pain and swelling. You can also take an over-the-counter medicine like acetaminophen (Tylenol) or ibuprofen (Advil, Motrin) for pain. Read and follow all instructions on the label.

If the pain is severe and throbbing, the only way to relieve it is to make a hole in the nail to drain the blood. Do not try this unless you have severe pain. If you have diabetes, blood flow problems, or a weak immune system, don't try it at all.

To drain the blood:

- Straighten a paper clip. Then heat the tip in a flame until it is red-hot.

- Place the tip of the paper clip over the area with blood and let it melt through the nail. Do not push. This should not hurt, because the nail has no nerves. Go slowly and reheat the clip as needed. A thick nail may take a few tries.

- As soon as there is a hole, blood will drain out and the pain should not be as bad. If the pain does not get better, you may have a more serious injury, such as a broken bone or a deep cut. In this case, you should see a doctor.

- Soak the finger or toe twice a day for 10 minutes in warm, soapy water. Apply an antibiotic ointment and a bandage.

- If the pressure builds up again in a few days and you do not have any signs of an infection, repeat the process. Use the same hole.

Breathing Emergencies

When to Call a Doctor

Call 911 if:

◆ The person stops breathing.

◆ An adult or older child has severe trouble breathing. A person with this problem may:

❖ Have chest tightness so severe that the person is worried he or she can't keep breathing.

❖ Be so short of breath that he or she can't speak.

❖ Gasp for breath or have severe wheezing.

❖ Feel very anxious, afraid, or restless.

❖ Respond slowly or have trouble waking up or staying awake.

◆ A child has severe trouble breathing. Look for these signs:

❖ Breathing very fast.

❖ Drooling or grunting with each breath.

❖ Not being able to speak, cry, or make sounds.

❖ Using the neck, chest, and belly muscles to breathe. The skin may "suck in" between the ribs with each breath, and the child may need to sit up and lean forward or tilt the nose up.

❖ Flaring the nostrils with each breath.

❖ Having a gray, blotchy, or blue color to the skin. Look for color changes in the nail beds, lips, and earlobes.

For less severe breathing problems, see When to Call a Doctor on page 107.

CPR

CPR (cardiopulmonary resuscitation) is pushing down on a person's chest and breathing into his or her mouth. It is used in emergencies when someone's heart stops beating, or when he or she is not breathing normally (may be gasping for breath) or is not breathing at all.

The chart on the next page has the basic steps for CPR. Use it for quick reference. The rest of this topic explains each step in more detail and with pictures. It is best to take a class on how to give CPR and then use this book as a reference.

Automated External Defibrillators

Automated external defibrillators (AEDs) are in many public places. Before you use an AED, follow all the steps for CPR.

To use an AED, place it next to the person and turn it on. The AED will tell you what to do next.

More

CPR Basics

What to do	Recommendations for:		
	Adults and older children (who have reached puberty)	**Young children (who have not reached puberty)**	**Babies younger than 1 year**
If the person is not breathing normally or is gasping, find the spot to do chest compressions.	Place two fingers on the spot where the ribs come together. Put the heel of your other hand just above your fingers on the breastbone.	Place two fingers on the spot where the ribs come together. Put the heel of your other hand just above your fingers on the breastbone.	Place two fingers on the breastbone just below the nipple line.
How do you give chest compressions?	Use the heel of one hand with the other hand stacked on top of it. Lace your fingers together.	Use the heel of one hand. If you need more force for a larger child, use both hands as you would for an adult.	Use two fingers.
How fast should you do compressions?	Do at least 100 compressions per minute.	Do at least 100 compressions per minute.	Do at least 100 compressions per minute.
How far down should you press the chest?	Press chest down at least 2 inches.	Press chest down at least 1/3 its depth (about 2 inches).	Press chest down at least 1/3 its depth (about 1.5 inches).
If you are trained in CPR, how many compressions and breaths do you give? (See "Step 3: Start rescue breaths" on page 22.) **Note:** Rescue breathing may be more important to do for children and babies than adults.	**30 compressions, 2 breaths.** Repeat this 30/2 cycle until help arrives or person breathes on his or her own.	**30 compressions, 2 breaths.** Repeat this 30/2 cycle until help arrives or child breathes on his or her own.	**30 compressions, 2 breaths.** Repeat this 30/2 cycle until help arrives or baby breathes on his or her own.

Step 1: Check to see if the person is conscious.

Tap or gently shake the person and shout, "Are you okay?" But do not shake someone who might have a neck or back injury. That could make the injury worse.

If the person does not respond, follow these steps.

◆ For an adult or older child who has reached puberty, **call 911** and then get an AED if there is one nearby. Then start CPR. (A child who has reached puberty has breasts or body hair.)

◆ For a baby or young child who has not reached puberty, start CPR. Do CPR for 2 minutes. Then **call 911** and get an AED if there is one nearby. **Note:** If there is another person with you, one person should call 911 while the other starts CPR.

Step 2: Start chest compressions.
For an adult or child older than 1 year:

◆ Kneel next to the person. Use your fingers to locate the end of the person's breastbone, where the ribs come together. Place two fingers at the tip of the breastbone.

◆ Place the heel of the other hand just above your fingers (on the side closest to the person's face).

Breastbone (sternum)

Place two fingers at the tip of the breastbone. Then put the heel of the other hand just above your fingers.

◆ For adults and larger children, use both hands to give compressions. Stack your other hand on top of the one that you just put in position. Lace the fingers of both hands together, and raise your fingers so they do not touch the chest.

◆ For smaller children, use the heel of one hand to give compressions.

◆ Straighten your arms, lock your elbows, and center your shoulders directly over your hands.

Keep your shoulders directly over your hands with your elbows straight as you push on the chest.

◆ Press down in a steady rhythm, using your body weight. The force from each thrust should go straight down onto the breastbone, pressing it down at least 2 inches for an adult or older child who has reached puberty. For a young child who has not reached puberty, press down at least one-third of the depth of the child's chest (about 2 inches).

◆ If you are not trained in CPR, **give at least 100 chest compressions a minute. Push hard and push fast.** If you are trained in CPR, see Step 3: Start rescue breaths.

◆ Keep giving at least 100 chest compressions a minute until help arrives or the person is breathing normally.

More

For a baby under 1 year:

◆ Picture a line connecting the nipples, and place two fingers on the baby's breastbone just below that line. Press the chest down at least one-third of the depth of the baby's chest (about 1.5 inches).

◆ If you are not trained in CPR, **give at least 100 chest compressions a minute. Push hard and push fast.** If you are trained in CPR, see Step 3: Start rescue breaths.

◆ Keep giving at least 100 chest compressions a minute until help arrives or the baby is breathing normally.

Step 3: Start rescue breaths.

Note: If you are not trained in CPR, it's okay to only give chest compressions. (See Step 2: Start chest compressions.) But rescue breathing may be more important to do for children and babies than adults.

If you are trained in CPR, give 30 compressions, then 2 rescue breaths. Repeat the cycle of 30 compressions and 2 rescue breaths until help arrives or the person is breathing normally.

To give rescue breaths:

◆ Put one hand on the person's forehead, and pinch the person's nostrils shut with your thumb and finger. Put the fingers of your other hand under the bony part of the lower jaw near the chin. Then tilt the chin up to keep the airway open.

Tilt the chin up to open the airway.

◆ Take a normal breath (not a deep one), and place your mouth over the person's mouth, making a tight seal. For a baby, place your mouth over the baby's mouth and nose. Blow into the person's mouth for 1 second, and watch to see if the person's chest rises.

◆ If the chest does not rise, tilt the person's head again, and give another breath.

◆ Between rescue breaths, remove your mouth from the person's mouth and take a normal breath. Let his or her chest fall, and feel the air escape.

When you give a breath, watch to see if the chest rises.

Breathing Too Fast

When to Call a Doctor

◆ You cannot get your breathing under control.

◆ You often have problems with fast breathing and anxiety (see page 80).

◆ You don't know why you're breathing too fast.

When you breathe very fast and deep (hyperventilate), the carbon dioxide level in your blood can drop too low. This can cause:

◆ Numbness or tingling in your hands and feet or around your mouth or tongue.

◆ Anxiety and a fast, pounding heartbeat.

◆ A feeling that you cannot get enough air.

◆ Lightheadedness or fainting.

◆ Muscle cramps or spasms, often in the hands.

◆ Chest pain.

Home Treatment

◆ Sit down and focus on slowing your breathing. Try breathing through pursed lips or through your nose. Try for 1 breath every 5 seconds.

◆ Try a relaxation technique. See page 320.

◆ Hold a paper bag over your nose and mouth, and take 6 to 12 easy, natural breaths. Keep doing this on and off for 5 to 15 minutes. Do not breathe continuously into the bag. Do not use this technique at all if you are ill, have heart or lung problems, or are at an altitude above 6,000 feet.

Breathing into a paper bag on and off for a few minutes may help slow your breathing.

Bruises

When to Call a Doctor

- The pain is severe.
- You can't use or move the bruised body part.
- You have signs of infection. These may include increased pain, swelling, warmth, or redness; red streaks leading from the bruise; and fever.
- You suddenly start to bruise easily, or you have lots of bruises for no clear reason.

- After a blow to the eye:
  - ❖ You have blood in the colored part of your eye or blood in the white part of your eye.
  - ❖ You have vision changes.
  - ❖ You can't move your eye normally in all directions.
  - ❖ You have severe pain.

Bruises occur when small blood vessels under the skin break or tear after a bump or fall. Older adults and people who take aspirin or blood thinners may bruise easily.

A **black eye** is a type of bruise. If you get a black eye, use the home treatment for a bruise, and check the eye for blood.

Home Treatment

- Put ice or cold packs on the bruise for 10 to 15 minutes several times a day for the first 2 to 3 days. Always put a thin cloth between the ice and your skin. The sooner you use ice, the less bleeding and swelling there will be.

- Take an over-the-counter medicine like acetaminophen (Tylenol) or ibuprofen (Advil, Motrin) for pain. Read and follow all instructions on the label.

- Keep the bruised area at or above the level of your heart when you can. (For example, if you bruise your foot, prop it up on a pillow when you are sitting or lying down.) This helps keep the swelling down.

- Rest the area so you don't hurt it more.

- If the area still hurts after 2 days, put a warm towel or heating pad on it.

Burns

More ▶

When to Call a Doctor

Call 911 if:

◆ You have a third-degree or worse burn. The burned skin may be dry, pale white or charred black, and swollen, or it may have broken open.

◆ The burn encircles an arm or leg, or it covers more than one-fourth of any body part.

Call a doctor if:

◆ You have severe pain.

◆ You are not sure how serious the burn is.

◆ You have a burn worse than a mild sunburn on your face, ears, eyes, hands, feet, genitals, or a joint.

◆ Pain from the burn lasts longer than 48 hours.

◆ You have signs of infection. These may include increased pain, swelling, warmth, or redness; red streaks leading from the burn; pus; and fever.

◆ A child younger than 5, an older adult, or a person with a weak immune system or a chronic health problem (such as cancer, heart disease, or diabetes) is burned.

◆ There is a chance the burn was caused on purpose.

The degree of a burn is based on how deep it is, not on how much pain it causes.

◆ A **first-degree burn** involves only the outer layer of skin. The skin is dry and painful and hurts when you touch it. A mild sunburn is a first-degree burn.

◆ A **second-degree burn** involves several layers of skin. The skin may be swollen, puffy, weepy, or blistered.

First-degree burn

Second-degree burn

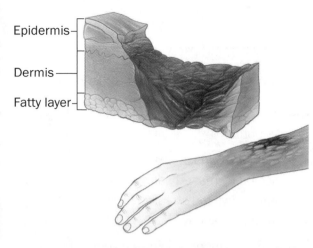

Epidermis

Dermis

Fatty layer

Third-degree burn

◆ A **third-degree burn** involves all layers of skin and may include tissue beneath the skin. The skin is dry, pale white or charred black, and swollen. It sometimes breaks open. This kind of burn destroys the nerves, so it may not hurt except on the edges.

◆ A **fourth-degree burn** extends through the skin to muscle and bone.

Home Treatment

For third- and fourth-degree burns:

These burns need medical care right away. **Call 911**, and then:

◆ Make sure the fire that caused the burn has been put out.

◆ Have the person lie down to prevent shock (see page 47).

◆ Cover the burned area with a clean sheet.

◆ Do not put any ice, salve, or medicine on the burn.

For first- and second-degree burns:

You can treat most of these burns at home.

◆ Run cool water over the burn until the pain stops (15 to 30 minutes). Do not use ice or ice water, because it may further damage the skin.

◆ Remove rings, jewelry, or clothing from the burned limb. Swelling may make these items hard to remove later. And if they are left on, they may damage nerves or blood vessels.

◆ Clean the burn with mild soap and water.

◆ Use an antibiotic ointment such as bacitracin, Polysporin, or Silvadene. Do not use butter, grease, or oil. They increase the risk of infection and do not help the burn heal.

◆ If the skin breaks open, use a bandage. Otherwise, don't cover the burn unless clothing rubs on it. If you need to cover the burn:

❖ Use a nonstick gauze pad. Make sure the tape is well away from the burn.

❖ Do not wrap tape all the way around a hand, arm, or leg.

❖ Keep the bandage clean and dry. If it gets wet, replace it.

❖ Remove the bandage once a day, clean the burn, and put on a new bandage.

◆ If blisters form, do not break them. If they break on their own, use water and mild soap to clean the area. Don't cut off the flap over a blister; it's a natural bandage. Apply an antibiotic ointment, and cover the burn with a nonstick gauze pad.

◆ Do not touch the burned area with your hands or any unclean objects. Burns get infected easily.

◆ Take an over-the-counter medicine like acetaminophen (Tylenol) or ibuprofen (Advil, Motrin) for pain. Read and follow all instructions on the label.

◆ After 2 to 3 days, use aloe to soothe the burn.

Chemical Burns

When to Call a Doctor

Call 911 if:

◆ A strong chemical such as acid or lye splashes into your eye.

◆ You have swallowed a chemical that may cause burning or be poisonous.

◆ A large area of skin (more than one-fourth of any body part) or any part of the face is exposed to a strong acid, such as battery acid, or to a caustic substance, such as lye or Drano.

Call a doctor or Poison Control at 1-800-222-1222 if:

◆ A burned eye still hurts after rinsing it with water for 30 minutes.

◆ Your eye is very red; has yellow, green, bloody, or watery discharge; or has a gray or white discolored area.

◆ You have vision problems that do not clear when you blink.

◆ Your skin is red, blistered, or blackened.

Burns can occur when a harmful chemical, such as a cleaning product, gasoline, or turpentine, splashes into an eye or onto the skin. Fumes can also burn the eyes, the skin, and the airways and lungs.

A burned eye may be red and watery and may be sensitive to light. If the damage is severe, the eye may look white.

Chemically burned skin may be red, blistered, or blackened. It depends on how strong the chemical was.

Home Treatment

◆ Call Poison Control for specific advice. Have the chemical's container or label nearby.

◆ Right away, flush your eye or skin with a lot of water. Use a cold shower for skin burns. For eye burns, fill a sink or bowl with water, put your face in the water, and open and close your eyelids with your fingers to force the water to all parts of the eye. Or rinse your eye under a faucet or shower. A sink with a sprayer also works well.

◆ Keep rinsing with water for 30 minutes or until the pain stops, whichever takes longer.

Be Safe With Chemicals

◆ Wear safety glasses, goggles, or a face shield when working with chemicals.

◆ Follow the product label's advice about wearing gloves.

◆ Know where the nearest sink or shower is.

◆ Store chemicals where children and pets can't reach them.

Choking

Choking is usually caused by food or an object stuck in the windpipe. A person who is choking cannot talk, cough, or breathe, and may turn gray or blue. The Heimlich maneuver can help get the food or object out.

WARNING: Do not try the Heimlich maneuver unless you are sure the person is choking. It is best to take a class on the Heimlich maneuver and CPR and then use this book as a reference.

A person older than 1 year is choking

If the person can cough or make sounds, let him or her cough to try to get the object out. If you are worried about the person's breathing, **call 911**.

If the person can't breathe, cough, or make sounds, then:

◆ Stand behind the person, and wrap your arms around his or her waist. If the person is standing, place one of your feet between his or her legs so you can support the person if he or she faints.

◆ Make a fist with one hand. Place the thumb side of your fist against the person's belly, just above the belly button but well below the breastbone.

Give quick upward thrusts.

◆ Grasp your fist with your other hand. Give a quick upward thrust into the belly. This may cause the object to pop out. You may need to use more force for a large person and less for a child or small adult.

◆ Repeat thrusts until the object pops out or the person faints.

Call 911 if the person faints (if you haven't called already). Then:

◆ Start CPR. See page 19. If you are giving rescue breaths, look for an object in the mouth each time you open the airway. If you see an object, remove it.

◆ Do not do any more Heimlich thrusts.

◆ Keep doing CPR until the person is breathing on his or her own or until help arrives.

You are choking

If you choke while you are alone, use your fists to do thrusts on yourself. Or lean over the back of a chair and press hard to pop out the object.

A baby younger than 1 year is choking

If the baby can cough loudly or make sounds, let him or her cough to try to get the object out. If you are worried about the baby's breathing, **call 911**.

If the baby can't breathe, cough, or make sounds, then:

◆ Put the baby facedown on your forearm so the baby's head is lower than his or her chest. Support the baby's head in your palm, against your thigh. Do not cover the baby's mouth or twist his or her neck.

◆ Use the heel of one hand to give up to 5 firm thumps (back slaps) between the baby's shoulder blades.

Give up to 5 firm thumps between the baby's shoulder blades.

- If the object does not pop out, support the baby's head and turn him or her faceup on your thigh. The baby's head should point toward the floor.

- Place two or three fingers on the lower part of the baby's breastbone, and give up to 5 quick chest thrusts straight down.

- Keep giving 5 back slaps and 5 chest thrusts until the object comes out or the baby faints.

If the baby faints, call 911 (if you haven't called already). Then:

- Do not do any more back slaps or chest thrusts.

- Start CPR (see page 19). If you are giving rescue breaths, look for an object in the baby's mouth each time you open the airway. If you see the object, take it out. If you can't see it, don't stick your finger down the baby's throat to feel for it.

- Do CPR until the baby breathes and responds on his or her own or until help arrives.

Cuts and Punctures

When to Call a Doctor

Call 911 if:

- The person faints or has other signs of shock (see page 47), even if the bleeding has stopped.

- Bleeding from a large or deep cut does not stop or slow down after applying direct pressure, or blood quickly soaks through several bandages. See page 17.

Call a doctor if:

- The skin near the wound is blue, white, or cold.

- You have numbness, tingling, or loss of feeling or movement below the wound.

- You have a puncture wound to the head, neck, chest, or belly, unless you know it is minor.

- Bleeding has slowed but has not stopped after 45 minutes of direct pressure.

- You cannot remove an object from the wound, or you think part of the object may still be in the wound.

- A cut has removed all the layers of skin.

- The cut needs stitches. See page 30. Stitches usually need to be done within 6 to 8 hours.

- A deep puncture to the foot occurred through a shoe.

- A cat or human bite punctured the skin.

- You have not had a tetanus shot in the past 5 years or don't know when your last shot was. If you need a shot, you should get it as soon as possible.

- You have signs of infection. These may include increased pain, swelling, warmth, or redness; red streaks leading from the wound; pus; and fever.

More

Cuts

When you get a cut, the first steps are to stop the bleeding and decide whether to see a doctor. Bleeding from a minor cut will usually stop on its own or after you apply a little pressure.

If the cut is bleeding heavily or spurting blood, raise the area above the level of your heart and apply firm pressure with a clean cloth. Then **call 911**. See Stopping Severe Bleeding on page 17.

Home Treatment

◆ Wash the cut well with soap and water. Do not use any other cleanser.

◆ If you think the cut may need stitches, see a doctor right away. If the cut does not need stitches, proceed with home treatment. (See Do You Need Stitches? on this page.)

◆ Bandage the cut if it is large or in an area that may get dirty or irritated.

❖ Use antibiotic ointment, such as bacitracin or Polysporin, to keep the cut from sticking to the bandage.

❖ Use an adhesive strip (such as a Band-Aid) to put pressure on the cut and protect it. Always put the bandage across a cut rather than lengthwise. Butterfly bandages can help hold the edges of the cut together.

❖ Replace the bandage once a day and anytime it gets wet or dirty.

Punctures

Punctures are caused by sharp, pointed objects (nails, tacks, knives, needles, teeth) that go through the skin. Puncture wounds get infected easily because they are hard to clean and are a warm, moist place for bacteria to grow.

Do You Need Stitches?

For best results, cuts that need stitches should get them within 6 to 8 hours. Stitches can help some cuts heal with less scarring. Glue or staples may also be used.

After you have washed the cut and the bleeding has stopped, pinch the sides of the cut together. If it looks better that way, you may want to get stitches. If you think you need stitches, do not use an antibiotic ointment until after a doctor has looked at the cut.

If the cut does not need stitches, you can clean and bandage it at home.

You may need stitches for:

◆ Deep cuts (more than ¼ inch deep) that have jagged edges or gape open.

◆ Deep cuts on a joint, such as an elbow, knuckle, or knee.

◆ Deep cuts on the hands or fingers.

◆ Cuts on the face, eyelids, or lips.

◆ Cuts in any area where you are worried about scarring.

◆ Cuts that go down to the muscle or bone.

◆ Cuts that keep bleeding after you have applied direct pressure for 15 minutes.

Home Treatment

◆ If the object that caused the wound is small, such as a tack or a sewing needle, remove it. Be careful not to break it off in the wound. If the object is large or caused a deep wound, leave it in place and call a doctor right away.

◆ If bleeding is heavy, raise the area above the level of your heart and apply firm pressure with a clean cloth. Then **call 911**. If there is an object in the wound, press around it, not directly on it. See Stopping Severe Bleeding on page 17.

◆ Clean the wound with soap and water twice a day. Do not use any other cleanser.

◆ Put antibiotic ointment on the wound, and cover it with a nonstick bandage. Replace the bandage when you clean the wound and whenever the bandage gets wet or dirty.

◆ Watch for signs of infection. If the wound closes, an infection under the skin may be hidden for several days.

Dehydration

When to Call a Doctor

Call 911 if there are signs of severe dehydration. These include:

◆ Feeling very dizzy or lightheaded.

◆ Fast breathing and heartbeat.

◆ Not feeling or acting alert, or having trouble waking up.

Call a doctor if:

◆ There are signs of moderate dehydration. These include:

❖ Sunken eyes, no tears, and a dry mouth and tongue.

❖ A sunken soft spot on a baby's head.

❖ Little or no urine for 8 hours.

❖ Skin that sags when you pinch it.

◆ You are sick to your stomach and cannot keep down even small sips of fluid.

◆ Symptoms of mild dehydration (dry mouth, dark urine, not much urine) get worse even with home treatment.

One of these topics may be helpful as well:

❖ Diarrhea, Age 11 and Younger, page 136

❖ Diarrhea, Age 12 and Older, page 138

❖ Vomiting and Nausea, Age 11 and Younger, page 258

❖ Vomiting and Nausea, Age 12 and Older, page 260

Dehydration means that your body has lost too much fluid. When you stop drinking water or lose a lot of fluids through diarrhea, vomiting, sweating, or exercise, your body's cells take fluid from blood and tissues. Severe dehydration can be life-threatening.

More

Dehydration

Dehydration is harmful for everyone, but it is most dangerous for babies, small children, and older adults. Watch closely for its early signs anytime you have high fever, vomiting, or diarrhea. The early symptoms are:

◆ A dry, sticky mouth.

◆ Dark yellow urine, and not much of it.

◆ Having no energy, or acting fussy or edgy.

Home Treatment

Age 12 years and older

◆ To stop vomiting or diarrhea, do not eat any solid foods for several hours or until you feel better. During the first 24 hours, take small, frequent sips of water or a rehydration drink.

◆ After the vomiting or diarrhea is controlled, sip water, weak broth, or sports drinks until your stomach can handle larger amounts. Drinking too much fluid too soon can make you vomit again.

◆ If vomiting or diarrhea lasts longer than 24 hours, take frequent sips of a rehydration drink to replace lost fluids and minerals. See page 33.

Age 1 through 11 years

◆ Treat diarrhea or vomiting promptly. See Diarrhea on page 137 and Vomiting on pages 259 and 261.

◆ Make sure your child is drinking often. Small, frequent amounts work best.

◆ Give your child a rehydration drink. See page 33.

◆ Let your child drink as much as he or she wants if the fluids are not making your child vomit. Let him or her drink extra fluids or suck on Popsicles.

◆ Cereals mixed with water can also help.

Babies younger than 1 year

◆ Treat diarrhea or vomiting promptly. See Diarrhea on page 137 and Vomiting on page 259.

◆ Give your baby a rehydration drink. See page 33.

◆ Feed your baby more often than usual and in small amounts, whether you breast-feed or use a bottle.

◆ If your baby has started eating cereal, you may replace lost fluids with cereal.

If You Exercise or Work in the Heat

◆ Drink water before, during, and after exercise or work.

◆ Use a sports drink if you will be working or exercising for more than an hour and will be sweating a lot.

◆ Don't take salt tablets. Most people already have enough salt in their diets. Use sports drinks instead.

◆ Avoid caffeine. It makes you urinate more often, which makes you dehydrate faster.

◆ Do not drink alcohol.

◆ Wear one layer of lightweight, light-colored clothes. Change into dry clothes if your clothes are soaked with sweat.

◆ If you start to feel dehydrated, stop what you are doing. Try to find a cool spot to rest in, and drink plenty of fluids.

Rehydration Drinks

Diarrhea, vomiting, and sweating can cause you to lose large amounts of water and important minerals called electrolytes. If you are too sick to eat for a few days, you also lose nutrients.

Rehydration drinks (such as Pedialyte) and sports drinks (such as Gatorade or Powerade) replace fluids and electrolytes in amounts your body can use. These drinks won't make diarrhea or vomiting go away faster, but they will help prevent serious dehydration.

Plain water replaces fluids only and has no nutrition. If you have diarrhea, your body may not absorb the water anyway.

For children under 12 years, buy rehydration drinks at a drugstore or grocery store. The amount you should give depends on the child's weight. Ask your doctor for advice. Do not give sports drinks to babies and young children who are dehydrated.

For people over 12, you can make a cheap drink at home. Measure everything exactly. Small changes can make the drink less effective or even harmful. Mix:

◆ 1 quart water

◆ ½ teaspoon baking soda

◆ ½ teaspoon table salt

◆ ¼ teaspoon salt substitute

◆ 2 tablespoons sugar

Ear (Object in)

When to Call a Doctor

◆ You cannot remove the insect or object, or it does not fall out on its own within 24 hours.

◆ Pain, fever, swelling, bleeding, or drainage develops.

◆ You feel dizzy or have any new hearing problems.

Children sometimes place food or other small objects in their ears. A piece of cotton from a swab or cotton ball may get stuck in the ear canal. An insect may crawl into the ear.

These objects usually cause only mild symptoms, such as slight pain or strange noises in the ear. But if an object stays in the ear too long, it can lead to infection.

Home Treatment

◆ Do not try to kill an insect in your ear. Pull the ear up and back, and let the sun or a bright light shine into it. The insect may crawl out toward the light.

◆ If the insect does not crawl out, fill the ear canal with warm mineral, olive, or baby oil. The insect may float out.

More

Ear (Object in)

◆ To remove an object other than an insect from the ear, tilt the head to the side and shake it gently. (Never shake a baby.) Gently pulling the ear up and back may help the object fall out.

◆ If you can see the object, try to remove it gently with tweezers. Don't try this if the person will not hold very still or if the object is in the ear so far that you can't see the tips of the tweezers. Use care not to push the object farther in.

Electrical Shocks and Burns

When to Call a Doctor

Call 911 if a person has been electrocuted, especially if he or she has stopped breathing, has no pulse, or has fainted.

Call a doctor for any electrical burn you can see, even if it looks minor.

Sometimes when you touch a light switch or outlet, you get a small shock. It may tingle for a few minutes. But if the shock does not cause skin damage or other problems, you don't need to worry.

A shock that burns your skin is more serious. Electrical burns may look minor at first, with the damage not showing up for several days. You may have burns where the current entered and left your body.

Electricity can cause severe damage inside your body, including internal burns and heart rhythm problems. It can cause your throat and lungs to swell quickly, making it hard for you to breathe.

For a minor burn

Rinse the burn with water, and apply a nonstick bandage.

If someone has been electrocuted or struck by lightning

◆ **Call 911.**

◆ Do not approach the person until you are sure the area is safe. If you feel tingling in your lower body, turn around and hop to a safe place.

◆ Unplug or turn off the power if you can.

◆ If you can't turn off the power, try to remove the person from the electrical source if you can do it safely.

  ❖ Do not touch the person with your hands until you have removed him or her from the electrical source.

  ❖ Stand on a dry, nonmetal surface, like a rubber doormat or a pile of papers or books. Make sure you are not standing in or near water.

  ❖ Use a dry piece of wood, like a broom handle, to push the person away from the electrical source. Do not use anything wet or made of metal.

◆ Once the power is off or you have removed the person from the source, check for breathing. If needed, start CPR while you wait for help to arrive. See page 19.

Eye (Object in)

When to Call a Doctor

Call 911 if the eyeball seems to be punctured.

Call a doctor if:

◆ The object is over the colored part of the eye or is stuck in the eye. Do not try to remove the object.

◆ There is blood over or in front of the colored part of the eye.

◆ You can't remove an object from the eye.

◆ You have removed the object but:

  ❖ The pain is severe or does not go away.

  ❖ It feels like there is still something in your eye.

  ❖ Light hurts your eye.

  ❖ Your vision is blurred.

  Your cornea may be scratched. Keep your eye closed as much as you can until you visit the doctor.

A speck of dirt or a small object in the eye will often wash out with your tears. If the object does not come out, it may scratch the surface of the eye (the cornea). Most corneal scratches will heal on their own in 1 to 2 days.

If an object is thrown forcefully into the eye (from a machine, for example), it may puncture the eyeball. This needs emergency care.

Always wear safety glasses or other protective eyewear when you work with machines or tools, mow the lawn, or ride a bike or motorcycle.

Home Treatment

◆ Wash your hands before you touch the eye.

◆ Do not rub the eye. You might scratch the cornea.

◆ Do not try to remove an object that is over the colored part of the eye or stuck in the white of the eye. Try flushing it out with water or saline.

◆ If the object is at the side of the eye or on the lower lid, moisten a cotton swab or the tip of a twisted piece of tissue and touch the end to the object. The object should cling to the swab or tissue. Your eye may be a little irritated afterward.

Use a moist cotton swab.

◆ Gently wash the eye with cool water. An eyedropper helps.

◆ Never use tweezers, toothpicks, or other hard items to remove an object from the eye.

Frostbite

When to Call a Doctor

◆ The skin is white or blue, and hard, rubbery, and cold. These are signs of severe frostbite. You need careful rewarming and antibiotics to prevent permanent tissue damage and infection.

◆ Blisters form. Do not break them. The risk of infection is very high.

◆ You have signs of infection. These may include increased pain, swelling, warmth, or redness; red streaks leading from the area; pus; and fever.

Frostbite is freezing of the skin and, if it is severe, the tissues beneath it. Frostbite is most likely to occur on the feet, hands, ears, nose, and face.

How severe the frostbite is depends on how long you were in the cold and how cold it was. Wind and damp air can make things worse.

With mild frostbite (sometimes called frostnip):

◆ The skin may be pale or red and may tingle or burn.

◆ If you rewarm the area soon, it will probably not blister or get worse.

As frostbite gets worse:

◆ The skin may feel hard, frozen, and numb. Later you may feel burning, throbbing, or shooting pain.

◆ Blisters may form as the skin warms. In severe cases, blisters may appear as small bloody spots under the skin.

◆ The tissue beneath the skin may freeze and harden.

◆ At its worst, the skin may turn dry, black, and rubbery. You may also have deep, aching joint pain.

Home Treatment

◆ Get inside, or take shelter from the wind.

◆ Check for signs of hypothermia (see page 41), such as violent shivering, clumsy movement and speech, and confusion. Treat those before treating frostbite.

◆ Protect the frozen body part from further cold.

◆ To warm small areas (ears, face, nose, fingers, toes), breathe on them or tuck them inside warm clothing next to bare skin.

◆ Do not rub or massage the frozen area. This can further damage the skin and tissue beneath it. Do not walk on frostbitten feet unless you have no choice.

◆ Keep the area warm, and prop it up at or above the level of your heart. Wrap it with blankets or soft clothing to prevent bruising. If possible, soak it in warm water (104°F to 108°F) for 15 to 30 minutes.

◆ If blisters form, do not break them.

◆ Take an over-the-counter medicine like acetaminophen (Tylenol) or ibuprofen (Advil, Motrin) for pain. Read and follow all instructions on the label.

Head Injury

When to Call a Doctor

Call 911 if:

- The person is unconscious for more than a few seconds.

- Severe bleeding does not stop or slow down after applying direct pressure, or blood quickly soaks through several bandages. See page 17.

- The person has a seizure.

- The person feels weak or numb on one side of the body.

- Double vision or trouble speaking lasts more than a minute or two.

- The person seems confused, does not remember being hurt, or keeps asking the same questions.

- You have trouble waking the person anytime in the next 24 hours.

Call a doctor if:

- The person fainted for a second or two and is now awake.

- Vomiting occurs more than once after the injury.

- The person has a severe headache.

- Blood or clear fluid drains from the ears or nose.

- There is bruising around both eyes or behind one ear.

- There is a new "dent" or deformity in the skull.

- The wound needs stitches. See page 30.

Most bumps on the head are minor and heal as easily as bumps anywhere else.

Minor cuts on the head often bleed a lot because the blood vessels of the scalp are so close to the skin's surface. In these cases, the injury may look worse than it is. (In children, though, blood loss from a scalp injury may be enough to cause shock.)

But a head injury may also be worse than it looks. An injury that doesn't bleed on the outside may still have caused dangerous bleeding and swelling inside the skull. The more force involved in the injury, the more likely it is serious.

Anyone who has had a head injury should be watched carefully for 24 hours for signs of a serious problem.

Home Treatment

- If the person is unconscious, assume he or she has a spinal injury. Do not move the person without first protecting the neck from movement. See page 49.

- If there is bleeding, put firm pressure directly over the wound with a clean cloth. If the blood soaks through, put another cloth over the first one. See page 17.

- Check for injuries to other parts of the body. The panic from seeing a head injury may cause you to miss other injuries that need attention.

- Use ice or cold packs to reduce the swelling. A "goose egg" may appear anyway, but ice will help ease the pain.

More

◆ For the first 24 hours after a head injury, watch the person closely for signs of a severe head injury. Every 2 hours, check for the symptoms listed in When to Call a Doctor on page 37.

◆ The person should avoid any sport or activity until cleared by a doctor.

Protect Children From Head Injuries

◆ Make sure all family members wear their seat belts every time they are in the car. Use child car seats. See page 333.

◆ Make sure your child wears a properly fitted helmet when biking, skating, snowboarding, riding a scooter, and doing other activities like these. Parents can set a good example by wearing helmets of their own.

◆ Teach your children never to dive into shallow or unfamiliar water.

◆ If you keep guns in your home, store them unloaded and locked up. Store and lock ammunition in a separate place.

Heart Attack

Signs of a Heart Attack

◆ Chest pain or pressure, or a strange feeling in your chest. Chest pain or pressure is the most common symptom. Some people—especially women—may not have chest pain but may have some other symptoms.

◆ Sweating.

◆ Shortness of breath.

◆ Nausea or vomiting.

◆ Pain, pressure, or a strange feeling in your back, neck, jaw, upper belly, or one or both shoulders or arms.

◆ Lightheadedness or sudden weakness.

◆ Fast or irregular heartbeat.

The symptoms of a heart attack usually last longer than 5 minutes and do not go away with rest.

When to Call a Doctor

Call 911 if you think you may be having a heart attack. Do not wait to see if you will feel better.

After you call 911, the operator may tell you to chew 1 adult-strength aspirin or 2 to 4 low-dose aspirin (unless you are allergic to it).

If you can't get an ambulance, have someone drive you to the hospital. Do not drive yourself.

Call a doctor if you have mild chest pain that does not stop or keeps coming back, and there is no clear cause. See Chest Pain on page 119.

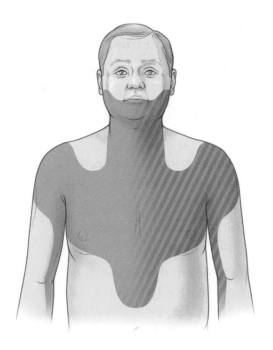

A heart attack may cause discomfort in any of the shaded areas as well as the upper back.

A heart attack occurs when one or more of the coronary arteries are blocked and blood cannot flow through. The coronary arteries carry blood to the heart (see the picture on page 275). They can get blocked when a fatty substance called plaque inside the artery breaks open and a blood clot forms.

Many people mistake a heart attack for another problem, such as heartburn or a pulled muscle. It is important to recognize the signals your body sends during the early stages of a heart attack and get help. Quick treatment may reduce the damage caused by a heart attack and may save your life.

Heat Sickness

When to Call a Doctor

Call 911 if:

◆ Body temperature reaches 102°F and keeps rising.

◆ A person has signs of heatstroke, such as:

❖ Confusion, fainting, or seizure.

❖ Skin that is red, hot, and dry, even in the armpits.

❖ Sweating may be heavy or may have stopped.

Call a doctor if you still have symptoms of heat exhaustion (headache, fatigue, dizziness, or nausea) after you have cooled off.

Heat sickness occurs when your body does not stay cool enough in hot temperatures.

Heat exhaustion usually occurs when you are sweating a lot and do not drink enough to replace lost fluids. It often happens when you are working or exercising in hot weather.

Heatstroke can quickly follow if you don't correct the problem. It occurs when your body cannot control its own temperature and your temperature keeps rising, often to 105°F or higher. This can lead to death.

More ➤

Symptoms of heat exhaustion	Symptoms of heatstroke
◆ Sweating a lot	◆ Sweating that may be heavy or may have stopped
◆ Skin that is cool, moist, pale, or red	◆ Skin that may be red, hot, and dry, even in the armpits
◆ Fatigue, weakness, headache, dizziness, or nausea	◆ Confusion, fainting, or seizure
◆ Muscle cramps	

Home Treatment

◆ Have the person stop and rest.

◆ Help the person get out of the sun to a cool spot and drink lots of cool water, a little at a time. If the person is nauseated or dizzy, have him or her lie down.

◆ Take the person's temperature. If it is 102°F or higher (or if you don't have a thermometer but think the person may have a high temperature), **call 911** and try to lower the temperature quickly:

  ❖ Remove the person's clothing.

  ❖ Apply cool (not cold) water to the person's whole body. Then fan the person.

  ❖ Put ice packs on the groin, neck, and armpits.

  ❖ Do not put the person in an ice-water bath.

  ❖ Once the temperature is below 102°F, take care to avoid overcooling. Stop cooling the person once his or her body temperature is back to normal or the person's skin feels the same temperature as yours.

  ❖ Do not take any medicine to reduce the temperature.

◆ Watch for signs of heatstroke (confusion or unconsciousness; red, hot, dry skin).

◆ If the person stops breathing, start CPR. See page 19.

Put ice packs on the groin, neck, and armpits.

Hypothermia

When to Call a Doctor

Call 911 if a person is very confused, stumbles a lot, or faints, and you suspect hypothermia.

Call a doctor if:

- The person's temperature is still below 96°F after 2 hours of warming.

- The victim is a child or an older adult. It is a good idea to call even if the symptoms seem mild.

Hypothermia is below-normal body temperature that happens when the body loses heat faster than it can produce heat. It is an emergency that can quickly lead to death.

It does not have to be that cold for a person to get hypothermia.

- You can get it at temperatures of 50°F or even higher in wet and windy weather.

- It can happen in water that is 60°F to 70°F.

- Frail and inactive people can get hypothermia indoors if they are not dressed warmly enough.

Do not ignore early warning signs. Often a hiker or skier will lose a lot of heat before you notice something is wrong. If someone starts to shiver fiercely, stumble, or respond strangely to questions, suspect hypothermia and warm the person quickly.

Home Treatment

The goal of home or "in-the-field" treatment is to stop heat loss and safely rewarm the person.

- Get the person out of the cold and wind.

- Remove cold, wet clothes first, and give the person dry or wool clothing to wear. Or warm the person with your own body heat by wrapping a blanket or sleeping bag around both of you.

- Give the person warm fluids and high-energy foods, such as candy. Do not give food or drink if the person is confused or has fainted. Do not give the person alcohol or caffeine.

- If home treatment is not working and you cannot get help, put the person in a warm (100°F to 105°F) bath. This can cause shock or heart attack, so do it only as a last resort.

Early warning signs	Advanced warning signs
- Shivering	- A cold belly
- Cold, pale skin	- Stiff, hard muscles. Shivering may stop if the person's temperature drops below 90°F.
- Lack of interest or concern	- Slow pulse and breathing
- Poor judgment	- Weakness or drowsiness
- Clumsy movement and speech	- Confusion

More

Stay Warm

Protect yourself whenever you plan to be out in cold weather.

◆ Dress warmly, and wear windproof, waterproof clothing. Wear fabrics that stay warm even when wet, such as wool or polypropylene.

◆ Wear a warm hat.

◆ Keep your hands and feet dry.

◆ Find shelter if you get wet or cold.

◆ Eat well before you go out, and carry extra food.

◆ Do not drink alcohol while in the cold. It makes your body lose heat faster.

Older or less active people should keep indoor temperatures above 65°F and dress warmly.

Nose (Object in)

When to Call a Doctor

◆ A disc battery is stuck in the nose. The moist tissue in the nose can cause the battery to release harmful chemicals, often in less than an hour.

◆ You cannot remove the object after several tries.

◆ Removing the object causes a severe nosebleed. See page 43.

Children sometimes put small objects, like beads, popcorn, or small batteries, up their nose. If the child does not tell you about it, your first clue may be a smelly, green or yellow discharge from just one nostril. The nose may also be tender and swollen.

Home Treatment

◆ Have the child pinch the other nostril closed and try to blow the object out.

◆ If you can see the object, try to remove it with blunt-nosed tweezers. Hold the child's head still, and use care not to push the object farther in. If the child resists, do not try tweezers. Minor bleeding from the nostril is not serious.

◆ **Unless you think the object is a disc battery**, spray a nasal decongestant like Neo-Synephrine in the nostril to reduce the swelling.

Nosebleeds

When to Call a Doctor

◆ Your nose is still bleeding after pinching it for 30 minutes.

◆ Blood runs down the back of your throat even when you pinch your nose.

◆ Your nose looks or feels broken.

◆ You get lots of nosebleeds—four or more a week, for instance.

◆ You take blood thinners (such as warfarin or Coumadin) or high doses of aspirin and have more than one nosebleed in a day.

Most nosebleeds are not serious. You may get one because of dry air or high altitude, an injury to the nose, or medicines (especially aspirin). Blowing or picking your nose can also cause a nosebleed.

People who have allergy problems may get nosebleeds a lot because the inside of the nose is irritated. Some allergy medicines may help with this, but they can make the problem worse if you use them too often. Talk to your doctor about how best to use these medicines.

Home Treatment

◆ Sit up straight and tip your head slightly forward. Tilting your head back may cause blood to run down your throat, which may make you vomit.

◆ Pinch your nose shut with your thumb and index finger for 10 minutes.

◆ After 10 minutes, check to see if your nose is still bleeding. If it is, pinch it shut for 10 more minutes. Most nosebleeds will stop after doing this for 10 to 30 minutes.

◆ Do not blow your nose for at least 12 hours after the bleeding has stopped.

◆ If your nose is very dry, breathe moist air for a while (such as in the shower). Then put a little petroleum jelly on the inside of your nose. A saline nose spray may also help. See page 234.

To stop a nosebleed, tip your head forward and pinch your nose shut.

Poisoning

Call 911 or Poison Control at 1-800-222-1222 for any poisoning. Have the poison's container or label near you so you can describe it. The medical staff will tell you what to do.

Do not use syrup of ipecac or activated charcoal unless Poison Control staff tells you to.

Kids will swallow just about anything. When in doubt, assume the worst. Always trust a child who says that he or she swallowed poison, no matter what it is.

Common Poisons in Homes

Make sure you keep these kinds of items where children and pets can't get to them:

◆ Drugs and vitamins

◆ Makeup, nail polish, and perfumes

◆ Bleach, drain cleaners, and toilet bowl cleaners

◆ Dishwasher soap

◆ Arts and crafts products like glue and paint

◆ Plant food and bug killer

◆ Some houseplants

◆ Windshield washer fluid and antifreeze

◆ Batteries

◆ Mothballs

For more tips on how to protect your child from poisons, see page 332.

Scrapes

When to Call a Doctor

◆ The scrape is still bleeding after 30 minutes of pressure.

◆ You cannot clean the scrape well because it is too large, deep, or painful, or because dirt and other matter is stuck under the skin.

◆ You have not had a tetanus shot in the past 5 years or don't know when you last had one. If you need a shot, you should get it as soon as possible.

◆ You have signs of infection. These may include increased pain, swelling, warmth, or redness; red streaks leading from the scrape; pus; or fever.

Home Treatment

Good home treatment may help reduce scarring and prevent an infection.

◆ Scrapes are usually very dirty. Remove large pieces of dirt and gravel with tweezers. Then scrub well with soap and water and a washcloth. Scrubbing may cause some minor bleeding. Using a water sprayer from a sink is a good way to wash a scrape.

◆ Apply steady pressure with a clean cloth to stop any bleeding.

◆ Use ice or a cold pack to reduce swelling and bruising. Put a thin cloth between the ice and your skin.

◆ If the scrape is large or in an area where clothing may rub on it, apply an antibiotic ointment (such as bacitracin or Polysporin) and cover the scrape with a nonstick bandage. Change the bandage once a day and anytime it gets wet.

Seizures

When to Call a Doctor

If you think your child has had a fever seizure, see page 161.

Call 911 if:

◆ A person has a seizure for the first time.

◆ A person having a seizure stops breathing for longer than 30 seconds.

◆ A seizure lasts longer than 3 minutes.

◆ More than one seizure occurs within 24 hours.

◆ A seizure occurs with any signs of a stroke. These may include sudden numbness, paralysis, or weakness; sudden problems with walking or balance; sudden vision changes; sudden problems speaking to or understanding others; and sudden, severe headache.

◆ A seizure occurs with signs of serious illness, such as fever, severe headache, stiff neck, trouble breathing, or an unexplained rash.

◆ A seizure follows a head injury.

◆ A person has a seizure after using illegal drugs or drinking a lot of alcohol.

◆ A pregnant woman has a seizure.

◆ A person with diabetes has a seizure.

Call a doctor if you have been diagnosed with epilepsy, and you notice a change in your seizures (for instance, they happen more often or are worse than they used to be).

More

The brain controls how the body moves by sending electrical signals through the nerves to the muscles. You can have a seizure if the normal signals from the brain change.

◆ Your whole body may stiffen or jerk violently, or you may have only slight shaking of a hand or other body part.

◆ You may briefly lose touch with your surroundings and appear to stare into space.

◆ You may or may not faint.

◆ You may not remember the seizure afterward.

A single seizure usually lasts less than 3 minutes and is not followed by a second one.

Any normally healthy person can have a single seizure under certain conditions. For instance, being hit in the head may cause a seizure. But a seizure may also be a sign of a more serious problem, so see a doctor to find the cause.

A quickly rising fever is a common cause of seizures in children up to 5 years old. Fever seizures are scary but usually harmless. To learn more, see Fever Seizures on page 161.

Home Treatment

No matter what causes the seizure, there are things you can do to help a person during and after a seizure.

During a seizure:

◆ Protect the person from injury. If you can, keep him or her from falling. Try to move furniture or other objects out of the way.

◆ Don't force your fingers or anything else into the person's mouth.

◆ Don't try to hold down or move the person.

◆ Try to stay calm.

◆ Pay close attention to what the person is doing so you can describe the seizure to doctors.

◆ Time the seizure if you can.

After a seizure:

◆ Check for injuries.

◆ Turn the person onto his or her side once he or she is more relaxed.

◆ If the person has trouble breathing, use your finger to gently clear the mouth of any vomit or saliva.

◆ Loosen tight clothing around the person's neck and waist.

◆ Provide a safe area where the person can rest.

◆ Do not give the person anything to eat or drink until he or she is fully awake and alert.

◆ Stay with the person until he or she is awake and aware of the surroundings. Most people will be sleepy or confused after a seizure.

Shock

When to Call a Doctor

Call 911 if you think someone is in shock. Signs of shock include:

◆ Passing out (losing consciousness).

◆ Feeling very dizzy or lightheaded, like you might pass out. A child may be very sleepy or hard to wake up.

◆ Breathing fast.

◆ Feeling very weak or having trouble standing.

◆ Being less alert. The person may suddenly be unable to respond to questions or be confused, restless, or fearful. A child may not know who people are or where he or she is at.

Shock means that your body and its functions are shutting down. The body goes into shock when it cannot get enough blood to vital organs like your heart or brain. This may be caused by a sudden illness, an injury, or bleeding. Sometimes even a mild injury will lead to shock.

Prompt home treatment of shock can save the person's life.

Home Treatment

◆ **Call 911.**

◆ Have the person lie down. If there is an injury to the head, neck, or chest, keep the legs flat. Otherwise, raise the person's legs at least 12 inches.

◆ If the person vomits, roll him or her to one side to let fluids drain from the mouth. If there could be an injury to the back or neck, move the head, neck, and shoulders together as a unit. See page 49.

◆ Stop any bleeding (see page 17) and splint any broken bones (see page 52).

◆ Keep the person warm but not hot. Put a blanket under the person, and cover him or her with a sheet or blanket, depending on the weather. If the person is in a hot place, try to keep the person cool.

◆ Take the person's pulse in case medical staff on the phone need to know how fast or slow it is. See page 48. Take it again if the person's condition changes.

◆ Try to keep the person calm.

12 inches

Raise the legs, and keep the person warm but not hot.

More

Taking a Pulse

Your pulse is the rate at which your heart beats. It is measured in beats per minute.

As the heart pumps blood through the arteries to the rest of the body, you can feel a throbbing wherever the arteries come close to the skin's surface. Most of the time, you can take a pulse at the wrist, neck, or groin.

◆ Place two fingers gently against the wrist to find the heartbeat. Do not use your thumb. Or find the heartbeat in the neck, on either side of the windpipe. Press gently with two fingers.

◆ Count the beats for 30 seconds. Then double the result to know beats per minute.

Carotid artery

Taking a pulse at the neck

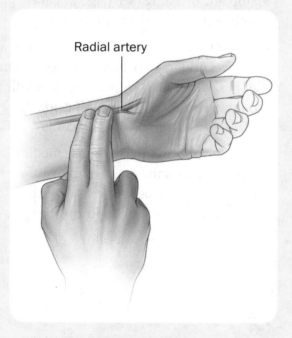

Radial artery

Taking a pulse at the wrist

Resting pulse

To get a resting pulse, take the pulse after you have been resting quietly for at least 10 minutes. Certain illnesses can raise your pulse, so it helps to know what your resting pulse rate is when you are well. The pulse rate rises about 10 beats per minute for every degree of fever.

Normal resting pulse:

◆ Up to age 12 months: 100–160 beats/minute

◆ 1 to 6 years: 65–140 beats/minute

◆ 7 to 10 years: 60–110 beats/minute

◆ 11 years and up: 50–100 beats/minute

Spinal Injury

When to Call a Doctor

Call 911 if you think a person has a spinal injury after a fall or an accident. Symptoms include:

◆ Severe pain in the neck or back.

◆ Bruises on the head, neck, shoulders, or back.

◆ Weakness, tingling, or numbness in the arms or legs.

◆ Loss of bowel or bladder control.

◆ Fainting.

Any accident, injury, or fall that affects the back or neck can damage the spine. It is important to keep the spine from moving and transport the person the right way to prevent permanent loss of movement and feeling (paralysis).

If you suspect a spinal injury:

◆ Do not move the person unless there is an immediate threat to life, such as fire. Do not drag victims from car accidents unless you have no choice.

◆ If you must move the person to safety, try to move the head, neck, and shoulders together as a unit.

◆ If the person was hurt in a diving accident, do not pull him or her from the water. Float the person faceup in the water until help arrives. The water will act as a splint and keep the person's spine from moving.

Splinters

When to Call a Doctor

◆ A splinter is very large or deep in the skin, and you cannot easily remove it.

◆ The splinter is in the eye.

◆ You have signs of infection. These may include increased pain, swelling, warmth, or redness; red streaks leading from the wound; pus; and fever.

Home Treatment

To remove a splinter:

◆ Try Scotch tape first. Put a piece of tape over the splinter and pull it up.

◆ If that doesn't work, grip the end of the splinter with tweezers and try to gently pull it out.

◆ If the splinter is not sticking out where you can reach it, clean a needle with alcohol and make a small hole in the skin over the end of the splinter. Then lift the splinter with the tip of the needle until you can grab it with the tweezers.

After you have removed the splinter, wash the area with soap and water. Use a bandage if the wound is in an area that might get dirty. Otherwise, leave the wound open to the air.

Strains, Sprains, and Broken Bones

When to Call a Doctor

Call 911 if a bone is poking through the skin.

Call a doctor if:

◆ The hurt limb or joint looks odd, is a strange shape, or is out of its normal position.

◆ The skin over the site of an injury is broken.

◆ You have signs of nerve or blood vessel damage, such as:

  ❖ Numbness, tingling, or a pins-and-needles feeling.

  ❖ Skin that is pale, white, or blue, or feels colder than the skin on the limb that is not hurt.

❖ Not being able to move the limb normally because of weakness, not just pain.

◆ You cannot put weight on or straighten a hurt limb, or a joint wobbles or feels unstable.

◆ You have severe pain.

◆ You have a lot of swelling within 30 minutes of the injury.

◆ Swelling and pain do not improve after 2 days of home treatment.

◆ You have signs of infection after an injury. These may include increased pain, swelling, warmth, and redness; red streaks leading from the area; and fever.

A **strain** is caused by overstretching or tearing a muscle or tendon. Tendons connect muscle and bone.

A **sprain** is an injury to the ligaments or soft tissues around a joint. Ligaments connect one bone to another.

A broken bone is called a **fracture**.

A **dislocation** occurs when one end of a bone is pulled or pushed out of its normal position.

All of these injuries cause pain and swelling. Unless a broken bone is obvious, it may be hard to tell whether you have a strain, sprain, break, or dislocation. Rapid swelling often means you have a more serious injury.

Stress Fractures

A stress fracture is a weak spot or small crack in a bone caused by overuse. For example, stress fractures in the small bones of the foot may occur during heavy training for basketball, running, and other sports.

The usual sign of a stress fracture is pain in one spot that keeps coming back or will not go away. The pain may get better while you exercise but will be worse before and after activity. There may not be any swelling you can see.

Stress fractures need 2 to 4 months of rest to heal.

You can treat most minor strains and sprains at home. Bad sprains, broken bones, and dislocations need medical care. Do home treatment while you wait to see your doctor.

Home Treatment

The first steps in home treatment are usually the same no matter what the injury. They are known as "RICE," which stands for rest, ice, compression, and elevation. Start the RICE process right away.

1. Rest (RICE)

◆ Do not put weight on the injury for at least 24 to 48 hours.

◆ Use crutches for a badly sprained knee or ankle.

◆ Support a sprained wrist, elbow, or shoulder with a sling. See page 52.

◆ Rest a sprained finger by taping it to the healthy finger next to it. This works for toes too. Always put padding between the two fingers or toes that you tape together. See page 52.

2. Ice (RICE)

◆ Put ice or cold packs on the injury right away to reduce pain and swelling. For the first 48 to 72 hours, use ice for 10 to 15 minutes at a time once an hour (or as often as you can). For hard-to-reach injuries, a cold pack or a bag of frozen vegetables works better than ice. Put a thin cloth between the ice and your skin. See Ice and Cold Packs on page 243.

◆ You may use heat (warm towel, heating pad) after 48 to 72 hours of cold treatments if the swelling is gone. Some experts say to switch back and forth between heat and cold.

3. Compression (RICE)

◆ Wrap the injured area with an elastic (Ace) bandage or compression sleeve to reduce swelling. Do not wrap it too tightly. If the area below it feels numb, tingles, or feels cool, loosen the wrap.

◆ A tightly wrapped sprain may fool you into thinking you can keep using the joint. With or without a wrap, the joint needs total rest for 1 to 2 days.

4. Elevation (RICE)

◆ Prop up the injured area on pillows whenever you use ice and anytime you are sitting or lying down.

◆ Try to keep the injury at or above the level of your heart to help reduce swelling and bruising.

RICE: Rest, Ice, Compress (wrap), and Elevate

More

Other Tips

You may prevent further damage and feel better faster if you:

◆ Splint an arm, leg, finger, or toe that you think is broken until you can see your doctor. See Splinting on this page. You can also use a sling to protect an injured arm or shoulder until you see a doctor. Do not put an arm sling on a baby.

A homemade sling can protect an injured arm until you see a doctor.

◆ Remove all rings, watches, and bracelets from a hurt finger or hand right away. Swelling may make it hard to remove these items later.

◆ Take an over-the-counter medicine like acetaminophen (Tylenol) or ibuprofen (Advil, Motrin) for pain. Read and follow all instructions on the label.

◆ Start gentle exercise as soon as the initial pain and swelling have gone away. If you have a broken bone or a severe sprain, your doctor may put the limb in a cast.

Splinting

These splinting methods are for short-term first aid only. Your doctor will give you a splint or cast that is right for your injury.

If you think a bone is broken, you can splint it so that it doesn't move. This prevents further injury until you can see a doctor. Splinting may also help after a snakebite while you wait for help to arrive.

There are two ways to splint a limb:

Method 1: Tie the injured limb to a stiff object, such as rolled-up newspapers or magazines, a stick, or a cane. You can use a rope, a belt, or anything else that will work as a tie. Do not tie too tightly. Place the splint so the hurt limb cannot bend. Try to splint from a joint above the suspected break to a joint below it. For example, splint a broken forearm from above the elbow to below the wrist.

Method 2: Tape a broken finger or toe to the next finger or toe, with padding between them. Tie a hurt arm across the chest to keep it from moving.

Stroke

A stroke occurs when a blood vessel to the brain bursts or is blocked by a blood clot. Within minutes, the nerve cells in that part of the brain die. As a result, the part of the body controlled by those cells cannot work properly.

The effects of a stroke may range from mild to severe. They may get better, or they may last the rest of your life. A stroke can affect vision, speech, behavior, thought processes, and your ability to move. Sometimes it can cause a coma or death.

Get help as soon as you notice stroke symptoms. Quick treatment may reduce the damage in your brain so that you have fewer problems after the stroke.

What's a TIA?

TIAs—transient ischemic attacks—are often called "mini-strokes" because their symptoms are like those of a stroke. The difference is that TIA symptoms usually go away within 10 to 20 minutes.

A TIA is a warning that you may soon have a stroke. It can also occur months before a stroke occurs. You may have one or more TIAs before a stroke. If you think you have had a TIA, see your doctor right away.

Suicide

When to Call a Doctor

Call 911 if you or someone you know is about to attempt or is attempting suicide.

Call a doctor, your local suicide hotline, or the national suicide hotline at 1-800-273-8255 (1-800-273-TALK) if:

◆ You are thinking about suicide.

◆ You think or know that someone has made suicide plans.

If you are very depressed or feel hopeless, you may sometimes think of taking your own life. Occasional, fleeting thoughts of death are normal. But if thoughts of suicide continue, or if you have made suicide plans, you need help today.

People who are thinking about suicide are often unsure whether they want to live or die. With help and compassion, they may choose to live.

Home Treatment
For yourself

◆ Do not use alcohol or illegal drugs. They may make you more likely to do things you would not do when sober.

◆ Talk about your thoughts with someone you trust—a friend or family member, a clergy member, or a doctor. Or call a suicide hotline.

◆ If you think you are in a moment of crisis, ask someone you trust to stay with you until the crisis has passed or until you can get help.

Warning Signs of Suicide

◆ Saying that you are going to kill yourself. Most people who commit suicide tell someone about it.

◆ Past suicide attempt. Failed attempts are often followed by a completed attempt.

◆ Giving away your favorite things.

◆ Being preoccupied or obsessed with death. A suicidal person may talk, read, draw, or write about death.

◆ Feeling depressed and socially isolated. A suicidal person may stop seeing or calling friends and stop doing his or her normal activities.

If you are worried about someone else

◆ Do not ignore warning signs, thinking that the person will "snap out of it."

◆ Talk about the problem as openly as you can. Show understanding and compassion. Do not argue with or challenge the person.

◆ Encourage the person to get professional help today. Do what you can to make it happen. Help the person set up the appointment, and make sure the person has a way to get there. Follow up to find out how the treatment is going.

◆ Use common sense and a direct approach to find out if the suicide risk is high. Ask the person:

  ❖ Do you feel there is no other way?

  ❖ Do you have a suicide plan?

  ❖ How and when do you plan to do it?

◆ If you think the risk is high, do not leave. Stay with the person until the crisis has passed or until you can get help.

Sunburn

When to Call a Doctor

Call 911 if you are sunburned and have signs of heatstroke, such as confusion, fainting, or skin that is red, hot, and dry. See page 39.

Call a doctor if:

◆ You have symptoms of heat exhaustion (dizziness, nausea, headache) even though you have cooled off.

◆ Symptoms of mild dehydration (dry mouth, dark urine, not much urine) get worse even with home treatment.

◆ You have severe blistering (more than one-fourth of the affected body part).

◆ You have severe pain with fever, or you feel very sick.

◆ Your temperature is 102°F or higher.

A sunburn is usually a minor (first-degree) burn to the skin's outer surface. Unless a sunburn is severe, it's usually something you can treat at home. Bad sunburns can be serious in babies, small children, and older adults.

Home Treatment

◆ Drink plenty of water, and watch for signs of dehydration (especially in babies or children). See page 31. Also watch for signs of heat sickness. See page 39.

◆ Take a cool bath or use a cool, wet cloth to soothe the skin. Take an over-the-counter medicine like acetaminophen (Tylenol) or ibuprofen (Advil, Motrin) for pain or mild fever. Read and follow all instructions on the label.

◆ Use a moisturizing lotion to help with itching. There is nothing you can do to prevent peeling. It's part of the healing process.

More ▶

Don't Get Sunburned

Anytime you are going to be outdoors for more than 15 minutes:

◆ Wear light-colored, loose-fitting, long-sleeved clothes, and a broad-brimmed hat to shade your face. Wear sunglasses that have UV protection. Look for clothing with UV protection.

◆ Use a sunscreen with SPF 15 or higher. Use one labeled "broad spectrum."

❖ Apply sunscreen at least 30 minutes before you will be in the sun.

❖ Put sunscreen on all skin that will be exposed, including the nose, ears, neck, scalp, and lips.

❖ Reapply sunscreen at least every 2 to 3 hours, and more often if you are swimming or sweating a lot.

◆ Avoid the sun between 10 a.m. and 4 p.m., when the burning rays are strongest. Seek shade whenever you can.

For Your Kids

The sun can be very hard on a child's tender skin. And repeated sunburns increase the risk for skin cancer later in life (see page 235).

◆ Teach your children safe sun habits early. Have them wear hats and sunscreen.

◆ Use a sunscreen with SPF 15 or higher on babies and children.

◆ Keep babies younger than 6 months out of the sun. If you cannot avoid the sun, use a hat and clothing to protect your baby's skin. Use a small amount of sunscreen on any bare skin.

Tooth Injury

When to Call a Dentist

◆ You knock out a permanent tooth. The dentist may be able to reimplant it. This works best within 30 minutes of the injury. (After 2 hours, it probably won't work.) Pick up the tooth at its top, not by the root. Place the tooth in a small container of milk to take to your dentist. Use tap water if you don't have milk.

◆ You chip a permanent tooth. A blow that was hard enough to chip a tooth may have moved several teeth out of place or broken the bone that holds the tooth in place. Also, a chipped tooth can be repaired.

◆ A baby tooth gets knocked out. Make an appointment within 2 weeks. Baby teeth need to come out anyway, but your child may need a spacer until the permanent tooth comes in.

Unconsciousness and Fainting

When to Call a Doctor

Call 911 if a person is unconscious for more than a few seconds.

Call a doctor if:

◆ A person faints for a second or two and is now awake.

◆ A person with diabetes faints, even if he or she is now awake. This could be a low or high blood sugar emergency.

◆ Fainting has occurred more than once.

If the person has a head injury, see page 37.

A person who is unconscious is completely unaware of what's going on and cannot make purposeful movements.

When you faint, you lose consciousness briefly—usually only for a few seconds. This is most often caused by a brief drop in blood flow to the brain. When you fall or lie down, blood flow improves and you "wake up." Stress or injury can also make you faint.

Fainting is usually not a cause for concern. But if it happens often, there may be a problem.

Staying unconscious for more than a few seconds usually is a sign of a serious problem. There are many reasons why this might happen. These include stroke, epilepsy, very low or very high blood sugar, head injury, not being able to breathe, alcohol or drug overdose, shock, bleeding, heartbeat problems, and heart attack.

Home Treatment

◆ Make sure the person is breathing. If the person is not breathing, start CPR. See page 19.

◆ Lay the person on his or her side.

◆ Look for a medical alert bracelet, necklace, or card that says the person has a problem like epilepsy, diabetes, or a drug allergy.

◆ Treat any injuries.

◆ Do not give the person anything to eat or drink.

Common Health Problems

More

Symptom Guides

Look on the left side of the chart to find the symptoms that most closely match yours. Then look on the right to see examples of what can cause those symptoms and where to go to learn more. The charts do not include all possible causes for each symptom.

Skin Problems	
Symptoms	**Possible Causes**
Raised, red, itchy welts or fluid-filled bumps after an insect bite or taking a drug	Allergies, p. 76 Hives, p. 194 Insect or spider bite, p. 14
Red, painful, swollen bump under the skin	Boils, p. 102
Red, flaky, itchy skin	Dry skin, p. 142 Atopic dermatitis, p. 83 Fungal infections, p. 169 Psoriasis, p. 224 Also see Rashes, p. 225.
Crusty, honey-colored rash, most often between the nose and upper lip	Impetigo, p. 195
Rash that develops after wearing new jewelry or clothing, being exposed to poisonous plants, eating a new food, or taking a new drug	Allergies, p. 76 Also see Rashes, p. 225.
Red, itchy, blistered rash	Poison ivy, oak, or sumac, p. 226 Chickenpox, p. 121
Painful blisters in a band around one side of the body	Shingles, p. 122
Change in the shape, size, or color of a mole, or a persistently irritated mole; a sore that does not heal	Skin cancer, p. 235
Cracked, blistered, itchy, peeling skin between the toes	Athlete's foot (see Fungal Infections, p. 170)
Red, itchy, weeping rash on the groin or thighs	Jock itch (see Fungal Infections, p. 170)
Scaly, itchy, bald spots or sores on the scalp	Ringworm (see Fungal Infections, p. 170) Also see Hair Loss, p. 174.
Flaky, silvery patches of skin, especially on the knees, elbows, or scalp	Psoriasis, p. 224
Sandpapery skin rash with sore throat and a "raspberry" tongue	Scarlet fever (see Sore Throat, p. 239)
Sores on the lip or in the mouth	Canker sores, p. 115 Cold sores, p. 123

Headaches

If Headache Occurs:	Possible Causes
Suddenly (like an explosion) and is very severe	Bleeding in the brain. **This may be an emergency.**
Right when you wake up	Tension headache, p. 176
	Allergies, p. 76
	Sinusitis, p. 232
	Neck pain, p. 211
	TM disorder, p. 199
In jaw area or in both temples	TM disorder, p. 199
	Tension headache, p. 176
Each afternoon or evening; after hours of desk work; with sore neck and shoulders	Tension headache, p. 176
	Neck pain, p. 211
On one side of the head, with vision problems or runny nose	Migraine headache, p. 176
	Cluster headache, p. 178
After a blow to the head	Head injury, p. 37
After exposure to chemicals (paint, varnish, insect spray, smoke)	Chemical headache. Get into fresh air. Drink water. Call a doctor if headache does not get better.
With fever, runny nose, or sore throat	Flu, p. 165
	Sore throat, p. 239
	Colds, p. 124
	Sinusitis, p. 232
With fever, stiff neck, nausea, and vomiting	Encephalitis or meningitis, p. 161. **This may be an emergency.**
With runny nose, watery eyes, and sneezing	Allergies, p. 76
With fever and pain in the cheekbones or over the eyes	Sinusitis, p. 232
When you drink less caffeine than usual	Caffeine withdrawal. Cut back slowly. See p. 177.
After a stressful event	Tension headache, p. 176
At the same time during the menstrual cycle	Premenstrual syndrome, p. 219
	Migraine headache, p. 176
With new medicine	Drug allergy. Call your doctor.
With severe eye pain	Acute closed-angle glaucoma, p. 172. **This may be an emergency.**
With dizziness and vomiting, and everyone in the household feels the same	Carbon monoxide poisoning. **This may be an emergency.** Get everyone out of the house.

Eye and Vision Problems

Symptoms	Possible Causes
Sudden vision loss that does not clear	Stroke, p. 53 Closed-angle glaucoma, p. 172 **You may need urgent care.**
Sudden onset of severe eye pain, blurred vision, reddened eyeball, or halos around lights	Object in the eye, p. 35 Chemical burn, p. 27 Closed-angle glaucoma, p. 172 **You may need urgent care.**
Sudden increase in floaters (dark spots, specks, or lines); new flashes of light that do not go away; shadow or "curtain" across your field of vision; new or sudden vision loss	Retinal detachment. **You may need urgent care.** (If you have had a few floaters or flashes for a while, mention it at your next eye exam.)
Red, itchy, watery eyes	Allergies, p. 76. Think about allergy to eye care products, makeup, or smoke. Contact lens problem, p. 154
Discharge or crust from eye; red, swollen eyelids; sandy feeling	Pinkeye, p. 151 Contact lens problem, p. 154 Blepharitis (eyelid inflammation). Try home treatment for styes. See p. 244.
Pimple or swelling on eyelid	Styes, p. 244
Pain in the eye	Object in the eye, p. 35 Contact lens problem, p. 154 Pinkeye, p. 151 Chemicals or fumes, p. 27 Migraine or cluster headache, p. 176 Sinusitis, p. 232 Closed-angle glaucoma, p. 172
Red spot or blood on white of eye	Blood in the eye, p. 154
Dry, scratchy eyes	Dry eyes, p. 153 Allergies, p. 76
Eye twitches	Stress or fatigue. Call a doctor if twitching affects other face muscles or lasts longer than a week.
Black eye	Bruises, p. 24
Gradual loss of side vision; tunnel vision	Glaucoma, p. 172
Gradual onset of cloudy, filmy, or fuzzy vision, or halos around lights	Cataracts, p. 118

Ear and Hearing Problems

Symptoms	Possible Causes
Earache and fever; pulling at ears by babies and small children, especially with constant crying	Ear infections, p. 143 Object in the ear, p. 33
Pain when you chew; headache	TM disorder, p. 199
Pain when you wiggle your ear or chew; itching or burning in ear	Swimmer's ear, p. 143
Discharge from ear	Swimmer's ear, p. 143 Eardrum rupture, p. 144
Feeling of fullness in ear, with runny or stuffy nose, cough, fever	Colds, p. 124 Ear infections, p. 143
Feeling of something moving or "bumping around" in ear	Object in the ear, p. 33
Hearing loss; not paying attention	Hearing loss, p. 180 Earwax, p. 147 Fluid in the ear, p. 145
Ringing or noise in the ears	Tinnitus, p. 181

Nose and Throat Problems

Symptoms	Possible Causes
Stuffy or runny nose with watery eyes, sneezing	Allergies, p. 76 Colds, p. 124
Cold symptoms with fever, headache, severe body aches, fatigue	Flu, p. 165
Thick green, yellow, or gray nasal discharge with fever and facial pain	Sinusitis, p. 232
Bloody nose	Nosebleeds, p. 43
Foul odor from nose; swollen, painful nasal tissue	Object in the nose, p. 42 Sinusitis, p. 232
Sore throat	Sore throat, p. 239
Sore throat with white spots on tonsils, swollen lymph nodes, fever of 101°F or higher	Strep throat, p. 240
Swollen tonsils, sore throat, fever	Tonsillitis, p. 239
Swollen lymph nodes in the neck	Swollen lymph nodes, p. 245 Tonsillitis, p. 239
Hoarseness, loss of voice	Laryngitis, p. 203

Chest, Heart, and Lung Problems

Symptoms	Possible Causes
Wheezing or fast, shallow, or troubled breathing	Allergies, p. 76 Asthma, p. 266 Bronchitis, p. 108 COPD, p. 271 Heart failure, p. 291 Also see Breathing Problems, p. 107.
Cough, fever, yellow-green or rust-colored mucus (sputum), and trouble breathing	Bronchitis, p. 108 Pneumonia, p. 216
Chest pain or pressure with sweating or quick pulse	**Call 911**. Possible heart attack. See p. 38. Also see Chest Pain, p. 119.
Shortness of breath and coughing	Asthma, p. 266 Bronchitis, p. 108 COPD, p. 271 Heart failure, p. 291 Also see Breathing Problems, p. 107.
Burning, pain, or discomfort behind or below the breastbone	Angina, p. 276 Heartburn, p. 183 Also see Chest Pain, p. 119.
Coughing	See Cough, p. 132.
Pounding or racing heartbeat; heart skipping or missing a beat	Heart palpitations, p. 181 Anxiety, p. 80
Chest pain when you cough or breathe deeply	Pneumonia, p. 216 Pleurisy, p. 120 Also see Chest Pain, p. 119.
Pain when you press on the chest	Chest-wall pain, p. 121 Costochondritis, p. 121 Also see Chest Pain, p. 119.

Digestive Problems

Symptoms	Possible Causes
Belly pain (may be in a certain spot or all over)	See Abdominal Pain, p. 68.
Increasing pain in the lower right belly, with fever, nausea, and vomiting	Appendicitis, p. 69 Also see Abdominal Pain, p. 68. **You may need urgent care.**
Feeling sick to your stomach; vomiting (throwing up)	Vomiting and nausea, pp. 258 and 260 Drug reaction, p. 77 Food poisoning, p. 167
Frequent, watery stools	Diarrhea, pp. 136 and 138 Food poisoning, p. 167 Irritable bowel syndrome, p. 197
Stools are dry and hard to pass	Constipation, p. 130 Irritable bowel syndrome, p. 197
Bloody or black, tarry stools	Ulcers, p. 249 Diarrhea, pp. 136 and 138 Rectal problem, p. 187 **Also see Bleeding Emergencies, p. 17.**
Pain during bowel movements; bright red blood on surface of stool or on toilet paper	Hemorrhoids or other rectal problem, p. 187 Constipation, p. 130
Painless lump or swelling in groin that comes and goes	Hernia, p. 189
Burning or discomfort behind or below breastbone or in upper belly	Heartburn, p. 183 Ulcers, p. 249 Also see Chest Pain, p. 119.
Bloating and gas with diarrhea, constipation, or both	Irritable bowel syndrome, p. 197
Women only: Lower belly cramps, bloating, diarrhea, or constipation just before or during menstrual period	Menstrual cramps, p. 209 Also see Abdominal Pain, p. 68.

Urinary Problems

Symptoms	Possible Causes
Pain or burning when you urinate	Urinary tract infections, p. 251 Prostatitis, p. 223 Sexually transmitted infection, p. 229 Kidney stones, p. 200
Trouble urinating or weak urine stream (males)	Prostate enlargement, p. 222 Prostatitis, p. 223
Leaking urine or loss of bladder control	Bladder control problem, p. 100 Prostate enlargement, p. 222 Prostatitis, p. 223
Blood in urine (Eating beets, blackberries, or foods with red food coloring can briefly turn your urine pink or red. Some medicines can also change the urine's color.)	Urinary tract infections, p. 251 Kidney stones, p. 200 Groin injury Very hard exercise (such as running a marathon) Call your doctor if you think you have blood in your urine.

Abdominal Pain

When to Call a Doctor

Bellyaches are very common and not often serious. Use the guide below to help you decide when you need to spend your time and money on a doctor visit and when you can take care of the problem yourself.

Call 911 if:

◆ You have belly pain and you faint.

◆ You have pain in your upper belly with chest pain or pressure, especially if it occurs with any other symptoms of a heart attack. See page 38.

◆ You have severe pain after a blow or injury to the belly. See page 12.

◆ You vomit a lot of blood or what looks like coffee grounds.

◆ You have severe rectal bleeding. Severe means you are passing a lot of stool that is maroon or mostly blood.

Call your doctor if:

◆ You have new, severe belly pain for several hours or more.

◆ You have steady or increasing pain in just one area of your belly for more than 4 hours.

◆ You have pain throughout the belly or cramping pain that has lasted longer than 24 hours and is not getting better.

◆ You are dehydrated and cannot keep down fluids. See page 31.

◆ Pain gets worse when you move or cough and does not feel like a pulled muscle.

◆ Any new belly pain lasts longer than 3 days.

If you did not find your symptoms here, check the index or the Digestive Problems chart on page 66.

Abdominal pain—pain in the belly—is very common. You can get clues about the cause of pain and how serious the problem may be by asking:

◆ **How bad is the pain?** People usually need to see a doctor when severe belly pain comes on suddenly and continues, or when new or different pain gets worse over several hours or days.

◆ **Does it hurt all over or just in one spot?**

  ❖ When your belly hurts all over and you cannot point to a specific spot that hurts, there is usually no reason to worry. This type of pain is very common and will usually go away on its own. Heartburn, stomach flu, food poisoning, and other common illnesses can cause this type of bellyache.

  ❖ When your belly hurts in just one spot, it can be a sign of a more serious problem. This is especially true if the pain is bad, starts suddenly and does not go away, or gets worse when you move or cough. It may be a sign of a problem such as appendicitis, pancreatitis, diverticulitis, an ovarian cyst, or gallbladder disease.

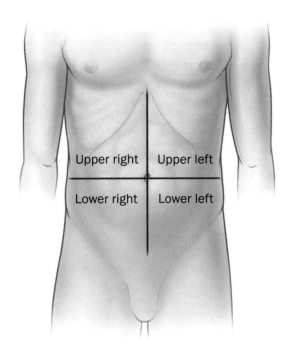

Upper right | Upper left
Lower right | Lower left

If you have belly pain, your doctor may ask you where it hurts. Lower right? Upper left? All over?

Home Treatment

Most of the time, belly pain goes away on its own. The best home treatment may depend on what other symptoms you have, such as diarrhea or vomiting. Be sure to review the home treatment for any other symptoms you have. Use the index to find what you need, or check the Digestive Problems chart on page 66.

If you have mild belly pain without other symptoms, these tips might help:

◆ Rest until you feel better.

◆ Drink plenty of fluids to avoid dehydration (see page 31). Taking small, frequent sips may be easier on your stomach than drinking a lot at once.

◆ Do not eat solid foods until the pain starts to go away. Then try several small meals instead of two or three large ones. Eat mild foods, such as rice, dry toast, crackers, bananas, and applesauce. Avoid spicy foods, alcohol, caffeine, and fruits other than bananas until 48 hours after all symptoms have gone away.

Appendicitis

The appendix is a small sac attached to the large intestine. (See the picture on page 171.) If the appendix gets blocked, it can swell and get infected. This is called appendicitis.

Symptoms may include:

◆ Pain that begins around the belly button or a little higher and then gets worse and moves to the lower right part of your belly. (See the picture on this page.) The pain is steady and gets worse when you walk or cough.

◆ Loss of appetite, nausea, vomiting, or constipation.

◆ Fever.

◆ A hard, swollen belly.

Call your doctor if you have these symptoms. You may need to have your appendix taken out right away. If not, it could burst and spread infection all through your belly.

Abuse and Violence

When to Call a Doctor

Call 911 if:

◆ You or someone you know is in danger right now.

◆ You or someone you know has just been physically or sexually abused or has been the victim of violence. Abuse is a crime no matter who does it.

Call a counselor or doctor if:

◆ You are worried about violence or abuse in your own relationship or that of a family member or friend.

◆ You need help controlling your anger, or someone in your family needs help. Also see Anger and Hostility on page 79.

◆ You suspect abuse, neglect, or maltreatment of a child, or a child reports this kind of treatment to you. You may also call local child protective services or the police.

Anger and disagreement are normal parts of healthy relationships. Threats and violence are not normal or healthy.

Abuse is an all-too-common problem. It often starts with threats, name-calling, and slamming doors or breaking dishes. It then gets worse with pushing, hitting, and other violent acts. Every year thousands of people are hurt or killed by their partners, spouses, or other family members.

Signs of Abuse

If you are not sure whether your relationship is abusive, there are signs to look for. This can be the first step in solving the problem. Ask yourself:

◆ Does my partner limit where I can go, what I can do, and whom I can talk to?

◆ Does my partner call me names or tell me that I'm crazy?

◆ Does my partner criticize what I do and say or criticize how I look?

◆ Does my partner "check up on me" at work, home, or school?

◆ Does my partner hit, shove, slap, kick, punch, or choke me?

◆ Does my partner blame me for the abuse he or she commits?

◆ Does my partner force me to have sex?

◆ Does my partner hurt my pets or destroy things that are special to me?

◆ Does my partner threaten to hurt or kill me?

If you answered yes to any of these questions, or if your partner could answer yes, you may be in an abusive relationship.

What You Can Do

Physical, verbal, or sexual abuse is never acceptable. There is no excuse for it. No one deserves to be abused.

◆ Know that there are people who can help you—friends, family, neighbors, police, health professionals, social workers, clergy. Talk to someone you trust. Do not feel that you have to hide what's going on. Everyone has the right to be in a safe relationship.

- Be alert to warning signs, such as threats or heavy drinking. This may help you avoid danger.

- If you can, make sure there are no guns or weapons in the house.

- Have a plan for how to leave your house and where to stay in case of an emergency. Put some money aside if you can, or at least make sure you will be able to get to your money after you leave. Do not tell the person who has been abusing you about your plan. Your local YMCA, YWCA, police, hospital, or clinic can tell you about shelters and safe homes near you. Or call the National Domestic Violence Hotline toll-free at 1-800-799-7233.

Preventing Violence Starts at Home

Violence is a learned behavior. It's important to teach your children that violence is not a healthy solution to conflict. Disagreeing is fine. Verbal or physical abuse is not.

Help your children learn that it's not okay to hurt people or to let other people hurt them. And model that behavior yourself. Try discipline techniques such as the "time-out" method that don't involve spanking or hitting your child. If you need help with discipline, take a course or read books on parenting skills, or talk to a counselor.

Acne

When to Call a Doctor

- Acne has not improved after 6 to 8 weeks of home treatment.

- Your skin is very red or purple, or you have hard bumps under your skin.

- Your pimples are large and hard or filled with fluid.

- Scars or marks form as acne heals.

- You get acne after starting a new medicine.

- Acne occurs with other symptoms, such as facial hair growth in women, or bone and muscle pain.

Acne is a skin problem that occurs when oil and dead skin cells clog your pores. This causes pimples, blackheads, and whiteheads, most often on the face, neck, and upper body. Acne usually starts during the teen years and often lasts into adulthood. Many adult women get a few pimples just before their menstrual periods.

Stress and some birth control pills may make acne worse. (However, some birth control pills may help treat acne.)

You can control most mild acne by gently cleansing your skin each day. Nonprescription acne products can also help. If home treatment does not work, or if your acne is severe, your doctor may pre-scribe stronger creams or lotions, antibiotics that you take by mouth, or other drugs such as isotretinoin (Accutane).

More

Treatment for acne often works very well, but you may not see progress for up to 8 weeks. Sometimes acne gets worse before it gets better, even with treatment. Try to be patient.

Home Treatment

◆ Keep your skin clean. Once or twice a day, gently wash your face, shoulders, chest, and back with warm (not hot) water and a gentle soap, such as Aveeno, Cetaphil, Neutrogena, or Basis. Do not scrub too hard. Do not use soaps that dry out your skin, such as deodorant soaps. Always rinse well.

◆ Wash your hair each day, and keep it off your face and shoulders.

◆ Try not to touch any areas that have acne.

◆ Do not squeeze or pick at pimples. This can cause infection and scars.

◆ Use an acne cream, lotion, or gel that contains benzoyl peroxide. After cleansing your skin, apply a thin layer of the medicine on all the places you get pimples, not just where you have them now. Start with the lowest strength, and increase the strength of the medicine if your skin can tolerate it. Keep in mind that it may take up to 2 months to work. Mild redness and dryness is normal, but if your skin gets too dry and scaly or red and sore, reduce the amount. Do not use more than 5% benzoyl peroxide unless your doctor tells you to.

◆ Use only water-based, oil-free lotions, makeup, and sunscreens that don't clog skin pores. These products may be labeled noncomedogenic. Don't use any product that seems to make your acne worse.

Alcohol and Drugs

When to Call a Doctor

Call 911 if:

◆ A person is unconscious or has trouble breathing after drinking alcohol or taking drugs.

◆ A person who has been drinking alcohol or using drugs threatens to hurt himself or herself or someone else.

◆ A person who suddenly stops using alcohol has trembling, hallucinations, seizures, or other severe withdrawal symptoms.

Call a counselor or doctor if:

◆ You are worried about an alcohol or drug problem in someone close to you.

◆ You think you have an alcohol or drug problem and are ready to get help. (See Are You a Problem User? on page 74.) Treatment can help you quit.

The overuse or abuse of alcohol or other drugs is called substance abuse. It is common, costly, and can lead to many problems.

Alcohol Problems

You have an alcohol use problem if you keep drinking even though it's interfering with your health or daily life.

People abuse alcohol in different ways. Some people get drunk every day. Some drink large amounts of alcohol at once. Others may be sober for a long time and then go on drinking binges for weeks or months. All of these are problems.

Long-term heavy drinking causes liver, nerve, heart, and brain damage; high blood pressure; depression; stomach problems; sexual problems; and cancer. Alcohol abuse can also lead to violence, accidents, and trouble at work, at home, or with the law.

Signs of an alcohol problem:

◆ Not remembering what happened while you were drinking (blackouts).

◆ Drinking more and more for the same high.

◆ Being uncomfortable when you can't drink alcohol.

◆ Gulping or sneaking drinks.

◆ Drinking alone or early in the morning.

◆ Getting "the shakes."

If your body is dependent on alcohol and you suddenly stop drinking, you may have severe withdrawal symptoms (such as trembling, delusions, hallucinations, sweating, and seizures). It's very hard to stop drinking without help if you are dependent on alcohol. You may need to go through "detox" under medical care.

Drug Problems

Drug abuse includes the use of marijuana, cocaine, meth, heroin, and other illegal drugs. It also includes the abuse of legal prescription drugs. People most often misuse tranquilizers, sedatives, pain medicines, and amphetamines, but it's not always on purpose. Some people turn to drugs as a way to get a high or deal with stress.

Signs of a drug problem:

◆ Constant red eyes, sore throat, dry cough, and fatigue. This can also just be allergies.

◆ Major changes in sleeping or eating habits.

◆ Being moody, hostile, or abusive.

◆ Work or school problems, especially being absent a lot.

◆ Losing interest in favorite activities.

◆ Withdrawing from friends, or finding a new group of friends.

◆ Stealing, lying, and having poor family relationships.

More ➤

Drug dependence or addiction occurs when you develop a physical or psychological need for a drug. You may not know you are dependent on a drug until you try to stop taking it suddenly. Withdrawing from the drug can cause muscle aches, diarrhea, depression, seizures, and other symptoms.

The usual treatment for drug dependence is to reduce the dose of the drug slowly until it can be stopped. This often needs to be done under a doctor's care.

Are You a Problem User?

Answer the questions below honestly. They ask about your use of alcohol and drugs, including prescribed and illegal drugs.

◆ Have you ever felt that you ought to cut down on your drinking or drug use?

◆ Have you ever been annoyed when others criticized your drinking or drug use?

◆ Have you ever felt guilty about your drinking or drug use?

◆ Have you ever taken an early-morning drink or used drugs first thing in the morning to steady your nerves or get the day started?

If you answer yes to two or more of these questions, you may have a problem with alcohol or drugs. Talk about it with your doctor or a counselor.

Home Treatment

◆ Pay attention to early signs that alcohol or drug use is becoming a problem. See Are You a Problem User? on this page.

◆ Go to an Alcoholics Anonymous (AA) or Narcotics Anonymous (NA) meeting. These support groups help members get sober and stay sober.

◆ If you are worried about a friend's or family member's alcohol or drug use:

❖ Don't ignore it. Discuss it as a health problem.

❖ Build up the person's self-esteem. Help the person see that he or she can succeed without alcohol or drugs. Offer your support.

❖ Ask if the person will accept help. If the person agrees, **act that very day** to get help. Call a doctor, AA, or NA for an immediate appointment. Make it easy for the person to get help. If the person says no to help, keep trying.

❖ Go to a few meetings of Al-Anon, a support group for family and friends of alcoholics. Read some 12-step program information. Many programs use the 12-step approach for dealing with addiction.

Alcohol, Drugs, and Your Children

You can have a strong influence on whether your children will use alcohol or drugs. Here are some ideas to help you deal with this issue.

1. Talk with your children before any substance use has occurred. Help them understand the risks:

   ◆ Remind them that it's against the law.

   ◆ Talk about how alcohol and drug use can lead to poor decisions about school and sex and can hurt their chances of going to college or getting a job.

   ◆ Stay focused on what matters to people their age. Children and teens live in the moment. Lecturing them about long-term health risks may not have much effect.

2. Tell your children what you expect from them and what the punishment will be if they don't follow the rules. If they break the rules, enforce the punishment you agreed on. Be clear, be fair, and be consistent.

3. Talk about what to do if their peers pressure them to drink or use drugs.

4. Be a good role model. If you drink, drink responsibly. If you have a substance abuse problem, get help. Never drink and drive.

5. If you suspect that your child is using alcohol or drugs, check it out now. Do not take a wait-and-see approach.

 For help with what to do if your child may have a drinking or drug problem, go to the Web site on the back cover and enter **k511** in the search box.

Allergies

Most allergies are caused by pollen, dust, and other things in the air. You can often find the cause of an allergy by noting when symptoms occur.

◆ Symptoms that happen at the same time each year are often caused by mold spores or tree, grass, or weed pollen. You are most likely to have problems during spring, early summer, or early fall.

◆ Allergies that last all year may be caused by dust, dust mites, cockroaches, different kinds of mold, or animal dander.

◆ An animal allergy is often easy to spot: Your symptoms clear up when you stay away from the pet or its bedding.

Allergies to pollen often cause **hay fever**. If you have hay fever, you already know the symptoms: itchy, watery eyes; sneezing; runny, stuffy, or itchy nose; and fatigue. You may also get dark circles under your eyes.

Allergies seem to run in families. Parents with hay fever often have children with allergies.

Home Treatment

Decongestants and antihistamines may help with some allergies. Talk to your doctor about the best choice for you, and use caution when you take these drugs. Some antihistamines (Alavert, Claritin, Zyrtec) are less likely to make you sleepy. Before you use these medicines, check the label. They may not be safe for young children or for people with certain health problems.

If you know what you are allergic to, the best treatment is to avoid it whenever you can. Keep a record of your symptoms and the plants, animals, foods, medicines, or chemicals that seem to trigger them.

In general:

◆ Avoid yard work, which stirs up both pollen and mold. If you must do yard work, wear a mask, and take an antihistamine before you start. Before you use an antihistamine, check the label. It may not be safe for young children or for people with certain health problems.

◆ If you smoke, quit. See page 316 for help.

◆ Do not use aerosol sprays, perfumes, room deodorizers, or cleaning products that trigger allergy symptoms.

For seasonal symptoms caused by pollen or mold spores:

◆ Keep your house and car windows closed. Do not open your windows at night.

◆ Limit the time you spend outside when pollen counts are high.

◆ Wash dogs and other pets often, or leave them outside. They can bring lots of pollen into your house.

For year-round symptoms caused by dust or dust mites:

◆ Keep your bedroom and other places where you spend a lot of time as dust-free as you can. Remove "dust collectors," such as stuffed toys, wall hangings, books, knickknacks, and artificial flowers.

◆ Dust and vacuum 1 or 2 times a week. This stirs up dust and makes the air worse until the dust settles, so wear a mask if you do the cleaning yourself. Damp mop tile, wood, or stone floors.

◆ Try not to use carpets, upholstered furniture, and heavy drapes that collect dust. Vacuum cleaners pick up dust but not dust mites. Use leather, vinyl, or plastic furniture that you can wipe clean and small rugs that you can wash.

◆ Cover your mattress, pillows, and box spring with dustproof cases, and wipe them clean weekly. Wash all bedding in hot water once a week.

◆ Use an air conditioner so you can keep the windows closed.

◆ Use an air purifier with a HEPA filter. Rent one before you buy it to see if it helps.

◆ Change or clean heating and cooling system filters often. Keep the humidity below 50 percent. Do not use a humidifier.

Life-Threatening Allergic Reactions

A few people have severe allergies to insect stings, nuts or other foods, or drugs, especially antibiotics such as penicillin. The reaction is sudden and severe and may cause dangerous swelling in the throat and mouth, trouble breathing, and a drop in blood pressure. This is called anaphylaxis. It needs emergency care.

If you have ever had a severe allergic reaction, your doctor may suggest that you carry an allergy kit (such as an EpiPen). These kits include pills and a shot that you can give yourself in case you are exposed to the same thing that caused your severe reaction before. The shot can help prevent a bad reaction and give you time to get help. To learn how to give an epinephrine shot, go to the Web site on the back cover and enter **u410** in the search box.

If you have ever had an allergic reaction to a drug, wear medical alert jewelry that lists your allergies.

More ▶

For year-round symptoms caused by mold or mildew:

◆ Keep your home aired out and dry. Keep the humidity below 50 percent. Use a dehumidifier when the weather is humid.

◆ Use an air conditioner, which keeps humidity lower.

◆ Change or clean heating and cooling system filters often.

◆ Clean bathroom and kitchen surfaces often with bleach.

◆ Use exhaust fans in the bathrooms and kitchen.

If you are allergic to a pet:

◆ Keep the animal outside, or at least out of your bedroom.

◆ If your symptoms are severe and your efforts to reduce dander exposure do not help, the best answer may be to find a new home for the pet.

What About Allergy Shots?

For many people who have allergies to insect stings, pollen, dust and dust mites, mold, animal dander, or cockroaches, allergy shots can reduce or prevent symptoms.

◆ Shots may take 3 to 5 years to complete.

◆ You may need to get them once a week at first and then once a month.

◆ It may take up to a full year of shots before you see any change in your symptoms.

You will also need skin and blood tests to find out what you are allergic to.

Getting allergy shots takes time and money. But they work for many people and may be worth it for you if:

◆ Your allergies bother you a lot, and medicines do not help well enough.

◆ You can't avoid the things you are allergic to, and your efforts to control them don't solve the problem.

◆ You have had a severe reaction to an insect sting, or your reactions have gotten worse over time.

◆ Allergy shots work for what you are allergic to. For example, they help with allergies to insect stings, but they do not help with many food allergies.

 Go to Web

For help deciding whether to try allergy shots, go to the Web site on the back cover and enter **d751** in the search box.

Food Allergies in Children

Food allergies are not common. Many parents think that their child has a food allergy when the child really has a food intolerance. Unlike a food allergy, a food intolerance does not cause severe symptoms and usually does not come on quickly. A good example is lactose intolerance (see page 139).

By slowly adding simple foods to your child's diet, you may be able to spot an allergy quickly. Eggs, milk, peanuts, wheat, soy, and fish cause most allergic reactions in children.

◆ Most children outgrow allergies to milk, wheat, eggs, and soy between ages 3 and 5.

◆ Allergies to peanuts, fish, or shellfish often last a lifetime.

If your child was allergic to a food when younger, talk to your doctor before you have your child try the food again. A child with a severe food allergy may have a dangerous reaction to even a tiny bit of that food.

If your child has a severe food allergy:

◆ Make sure that school or day care knows about it.

◆ Keep an allergy kit nearby at all times.

◆ Have your child wear medical alert jewelry.

Anger and Hostility

When to Call a Doctor

Call 911 if you or someone you know is in immediate danger.

Call a counselor if:

◆ Anger has led or could lead to violence or harm to you or someone else.

◆ Anger or hostility upsets your work, family life, or friendships.

Anger tells your body to prepare for a fight. It can be a normal response to daily events. And it is a healthy response to any situation that's a real threat. You can sometimes use anger as a positive, driving force behind your actions.

Hostility is being ready for a fight all the time. Hostile people are often stubborn, impatient, hotheaded, or have an "attitude."

Feeling angry and hostile all or much of the time is not good for you. It keeps your blood pressure high and may make you more likely to have a heart attack, stroke, or other health problem. Constant anger also cuts you off from the people in your life. It may lead to abuse and violence (see page 70).

More

Home Treatment

◆ Try to understand why you are angry. Is it the current situation that's making you angry or something that happened earlier?

◆ Notice when you start to get angry, and take steps to deal with your anger in a healthy way. Do not ignore your anger until you "blow up."

❖ Think before you act. Count to 10 or use some other form of mental relaxation. When you have calmed down, you'll be better able to deal with the problem.

❖ Give yourself a "time-out." Go someplace quiet so you can calm down.

❖ Go for a short walk or jog.

❖ Talk with a friend about your anger.

❖ Draw or paint to release the anger, or write about it in a journal.

◆ If you are angry with someone, listen to what the other person has to say. Try to understand his or her point of view. Use "I" statements, not "you" statements, to discuss your anger. Say "I feel angry when my needs are not being met" instead of "You make me mad when you are so inconsiderate."

◆ Forgive and forget. Forgiving lowers your blood pressure and eases muscle tension so you can feel more relaxed.

◆ Focus on the things in your life that make you happy.

◆ Read books about anger and how to handle it, or explore other resources through your job or community.

Anxiety and Panic

When to Call a Doctor

Call a counselor or your doctor if:

◆ Anxiety or fear upsets your daily life.

◆ Sudden, severe attacks of fear or anxiety seem to occur for no reason.

◆ Symptoms of anxiety are still severe after 1 week of home treatment.

◆ You have nightmares or flashbacks to traumatic events.

◆ You cannot feel certain about things (for example, whether you unplugged the iron) no matter how many times you check, especially if it interferes with your daily life.

Feeling worried, anxious, and nervous is a normal part of life. Everyone frets or feels anxious from time to time.

Your body tells you when you are anxious:

◆ You may tremble, twitch, or shake.

◆ You may feel lightheaded or dizzy.

◆ You may feel "butterflies" in your stomach.

◆ Your breathing and heartbeat may speed up.

◆ Your throat or chest may feel full.

◆ You may sweat, and your muscles may get tense.

◆ You may have sleep problems.

Anxiety also affects your emotions:

◆ You may feel hyper, annoyed, or edgy.

◆ You may worry a lot or fear that something bad is going to happen.

◆ You may not be able to concentrate.

◆ You may feel sad all the time.

A specific situation or fear can cause these symptoms for a short time. When the situation passes, the symptoms go away.

When you have an **anxiety disorder**, you get these symptoms for reasons that are not clear or do not make sense. This type of anxiety is not normal and can be overwhelming. People with an anxiety disorder may have fears, called **phobias**, of common places, objects, or situations.

Panic disorder is a problem related to anxiety. People with panic disorder have periods of sudden, intense fear and anxiety when there is no clear cause or danger. These panic attacks can cause scary (but not dangerous) symptoms, such as a pounding heart, shortness of breath, and a sense that you are about to lose control or die.

People who have had panic attacks may try hard to avoid anything that might trigger another attack. This often causes an even higher level of anxiety.

Many people manage anxiety and panic with counseling and medicines. The right medicines—especially when used with counseling—can even help prevent anxiety or panic attacks. They usually start to work within a few weeks, but you may need to take medicines for a year or more to get long-lasting results.

 For help deciding if medicines are right for you, go to the Web site on the back cover and enter **q880** in the search box.

Home Treatment

Try these tips to relieve anxiety. They can also help if you are getting treatment for anxiety or panic disorder.

◆ Accept your anxiety. When a situation makes you feel anxious, say to yourself, "This is not an emergency. I feel uneasy, but I'm not in danger. I can keep going even if I feel anxious."

◆ Be kind to your body:

  ❖ Relieve stress and tension with exercise, massage, warm baths, walks, or whatever works for you.

  ❖ Learn and use a relaxation technique. See page 320.

  ❖ Get enough rest. If you have trouble sleeping, see Sleep Problems on page 236.

  ❖ Avoid alcohol, caffeine, and nicotine. They can increase anxiety, cause sleep problems, or trigger a panic attack.

◆ Use your mind. Do things you enjoy, like going to a funny movie or taking a walk or a hike.

◆ Plan your day. Having too much or too little to do can make you more anxious.

◆ Keep a daily record of your symptoms. Discuss your fears with a good friend or family member, or join a support group. Talking to others about the problem sometimes relieves stress.

◆ Join a social group, or volunteer to help others. Being alone may make things seem worse than they are.

Arthritis

When to Call a Doctor

Call 911 if sudden back pain occurs with weakness in the legs or loss of bowel or bladder control.

Call a doctor if:

◆ You have fever or a skin rash along with severe joint pain.

◆ You have sudden, unexplained swelling, redness, warmth, or pain in one or more joints.

◆ A joint hurts so much that you cannot use it.

◆ Joint pain lasts for more than 6 weeks, and home treatment is not helping.

◆ You have side effects (stomach pain, nausea, heartburn, or stools that look black or tarry) from aspirin or other arthritis medicines.

Joint problems that cause pain, swelling, and stiffness are called arthritis. Arthritis can occur at any age but affects older people most often.

There are many types of arthritis. The chart on page 83 describes three common ones.

Home Treatment

The tips here will help with many types of arthritis and joint pain. The goal is to ease your pain, protect your joints, and help you stay active.

◆ Take a warm shower or bath to help relieve morning stiffness. Keep moving so your joints don't stiffen up.

◆ If a joint is stiff or sore, put moist heat on it for 20 to 30 minutes, 2 or 3 times a day. You may also try cold packs for 10 to 20 minutes once an hour. Do what works for you.

◆ When joints are sore, avoid activities that put weight or strain on them for a few days. Give your joints short rest breaks all through the day.

◆ Put each of your joints gently through all of its possible movements 2 or 3 times a day.

◆ Exercise regularly to help your muscles and joints stay strong and flexible. Swimming, doing water aerobics, biking, and walking are great ways to be active. They do not stress your joints as much as other exercises. Do some stretching every day. To learn how to exercise safely with arthritis and see examples of good exercises, go to the Web site on the back cover and enter **d288** in the search box.

◆ Stay at a healthy weight. Being overweight puts extra strain on your joints. If you need to lose weight, see page 300 for help.

◆ Take an over-the-counter medicine like acetaminophen (Tylenol) or ibuprofen (Advil, Motrin) for pain. Talk to your doctor about whether these medicines are safe for you and how much to take.

Common Types of Arthritis

Type	Symptoms	Comments
Osteoarthritis (breakdown of joint cartilage)	Pain and stiffness; common in knees, fingers, hips, and back; morning stiffness that lasts for less than 1 hour	Most common after age 50; most common type of arthritis
Rheumatoid arthritis (inflammation of tissue lining the joint)	Pain, stiffness, warmth, and swelling in joints on both sides of the body; common in hands, wrists, elbows, feet, knees, and neck; morning stiffness that lasts for more than 1 hour	Often starts around age 40; more common in women
Gout (buildup of uric acid crystals in joint fluid)	Sudden burning pain, stiffness, and swelling; usually in the big toe or in the midfoot, ankle, knee, wrist, or elbow	Most common in men 30 to 50; alcohol, illness, or surgery may make gout worse

◆ Use helpful devices such as special doorknobs, kitchen tools with padded handles, and a higher toilet seat. Braces, splints, canes, or walkers can give your joints a rest and can help you get around.

◆ Join a support group, or take a course on how to manage your arthritis. People in these programs often have less pain and fewer limits on what they can do.

Looking for the Asthma topic? See page 266.

Atopic Dermatitis

When to Call a Doctor

◆ You have new blisters or bruises and do not know why.

◆ The rash spreads and looks like a sunburn.

◆ There are crusting or oozing sores or serious scratch marks.

◆ Fever occurs with the rash.

◆ Joint aches or body aches occur with the rash.

◆ Itching is severe, and home treatment does not help.

◆ You cannot control atopic dermatitis with home treatment.

More

Atopic dermatitis (also called atopic eczema) causes intense itching and a red, raised, scaly, or rough rash. When the rash is severe, it may have fluid-filled blisters. The blisters can get infected, especially if you scratch them too much.

Where the rash is depends partly on age:

◆ In babies, the rash is usually on the face, scalp, arms, thighs, and torso.

◆ In older children, it tends to occur in areas that bend, like elbows and knees.

◆ In adults, it may affect the hands, neck, face, genitals, or legs. The rash is usually smaller than in children.

Atopic dermatitis often occurs in young children who have asthma, hay fever, and other allergies, though it can occur at any age. Most children outgrow it by their early teens.

Home Treatment

◆ Take short baths or showers with warm (not hot) water. For areas that need soap (armpits, feet, groin), use a nondrying cleanser, such as Aveeno, Dove, Basis, or Neutrogena.

◆ Right after bathing, apply a moisturizer while your skin is still damp. Use a cream such as Lubriderm, Moisturel, or Cetaphil that doesn't irritate the skin.

◆ Keep cool, and stay out of the sun.

◆ Use a humidifier in your bedroom if the air is dry.

◆ Avoid things that make the rash worse, like cleaning products, chemicals, or certain fabrics. Wear gloves when you have to work with an irritating product.

If Your Child Has Atopic Dermatitis

Atopic dermatitis can be very hard on children. Both the child and the parents may avoid touching, which is a vital part of their bonding. The child avoids it because the skin hurts, and the parents avoid it because the skin feels rough and looks bad.

The child may also feel set apart from other children because of restrictions (on diet or sports, for instance). He or she may feel unattractive because of the rash. And the child may be fussy and hard to deal with because he or she is so itchy.

Here's how you can help:

◆ Talk to your child, and offer support. Spend time with your child every day.

◆ Try to be sure your child takes part in activities with other kids.

◆ Help your child find things to do that keep his or her hands busy and distracted from the itching. (This may take a lot of effort on your part, but it can help.)

◆ Help your child with proper skin care. Provide soft clothes and bedding. Keep your child cool. Watch for things that make the problem worse, and remove them if you can.

- When you wash clothes and bedding, use mild detergent and rinse at least twice. Don't use fabric softener if it irritates your skin. Avoid scratchy fabrics.

- Keep fingernails trimmed and filed smooth so you don't hurt your skin if you scratch. Put mittens or cotton socks on your baby's hands.

- Use cold, wet cloths to reduce itching. An oral antihistamine (such as Benadryl) may also help. Some types (Alavert, Claritin, Zyrtec) are less likely to make you sleepy. Before you use these medicines, check the label. They may not be safe for young children or for people with certain health problems. Do not use antiseptic and antihistamine creams and sprays. Also see Relief From Itching on page 142.

Back Pain

When to Call a Doctor

Call 911 if:

- Back pain occurs with chest pain or other symptoms of a heart attack (see page 38).

- You have severe back pain after an injury or fall (see page 49).

- You suddenly lose bowel or bladder control, even if you were not injured.

- You cannot walk or stand at all because of weakness and not just because it hurts too much.

Call a doctor if:

- You have new numbness in the buttocks, genital or rectal area, or legs.

- You have leg weakness that is not solely due to pain. Many people with low back pain say their legs feel weak. If leg weakness is so bad that you cannot bend your foot upward, get up out of a chair, or climb stairs, see your doctor.

- You have new or increased back pain with fever, painful urination, or other signs of a urinary tract infection. See page 251.

- You have a dramatic increase in your chronic back pain, especially if it's not related to physical activity.

- You have a history of cancer or HIV infection, and you have new or increased back pain.

- You have severe pain that does not improve after a few days of home treatment.

- Pain wakes you from sleep.

- You have a new, severe pain in your lower back that does not change when you move and is not related to stress, muscle tension, or a known injury.

- Pain does not improve after 2 weeks of home treatment.

More

Your back is the whole area from your neck to your tailbone. It includes the bones (vertebrae) and joints of the spine, the spinal discs that separate the bones and absorb shock as you move, and the muscles and ligaments that hold them all together. You can stress or hurt any of these parts of your back.

What causes most back pain?

◆ Repeating movements or staying too long in positions that strain the back

◆ Moving suddenly or awkwardly in ways that twist the back

These kinds of movements or postures can strain or sprain the ligaments, muscles, or the joints between the spine and the pelvic bones (sacroiliac joints).

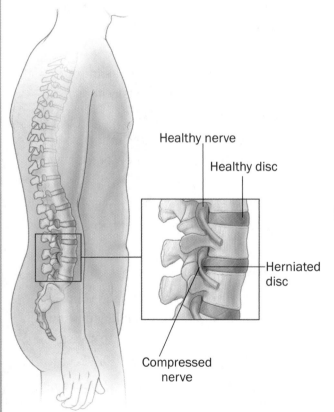

A bulging (herniated) disc can press on a nerve, causing pain.

You can hurt a disc in your back the same way, causing it to bulge or tear (rupture). This is called a **herniated disc**. If the tear is large enough, the gel inside the disc may leak out and press against a nerve.

A sprain or strain can cause 2 to 3 days of pain and swelling, followed by slow healing and a gradual decrease in pain. Pain from a herniated disc may last much longer. You may feel the pain in your low back, in your buttock, or down one leg.

With good self-care, most of these back injuries will heal in 6 to 12 weeks. Home treatment can help relieve pain, promote healing, and prevent reinjury.

Back pain can also be caused by problems that affect the bones and joints of the spine.

◆ **Arthritis** pain may be a steady ache, unlike the sharp, sudden pain of back strain and disc injuries. If you think arthritis may be causing your back pain, combine the home treatment for back pain with the treatment for arthritis on page 82.

◆ **Osteoporosis** can weaken the bones of the spine and cause them to break or collapse. See page 214.

Home Treatment

◆ Follow the First Aid for Back Pain guidelines on page 87. These include relaxation, medicines (if needed), heat or ice, and short walks.

◆ Sit or lie in positions that feel good and reduce your pain, especially any leg pain.

◆ Avoid sitting for long periods of time. Do not sit up in bed, and avoid soft couches and twisted positions. Follow the tips for good body mechanics on page 89.

- When you lie down or rest, try one of the following positions (see pictures on page 90):

  ❖ Lie on your back with your knees bent and supported by large pillows. Or lie on the floor with your legs on the seat of a sofa or chair.

  ❖ Lie on your side with your knees and hips bent and a pillow between your legs.

- Take an over-the-counter medicine like acetaminophen (Tylenol) or ibuprofen (Advil, Motrin) for pain. Read and follow all instructions on the label.

- Relax your muscles. See page 320.

Two to three days after the injury, you can try the following:

- Keep using ice, heat, or both if it seems to help. Do what works for you.

- Keep taking walks (10 to 20 minutes) 3 or 4 times a day.

- Try swimming. It may hurt right after a back injury, but lap swimming or kicking with swim fins often helps prevent pain from coming back.

- When your pain has improved, try easy exercises that don't increase your pain. One or two of the exercises described on pages 91 to 94 may be a good place to start. Start with 8 repetitions, 3 to 4 times a day, and increase to 12 repetitions if it does not cause pain.

First Aid for Back Pain

When you first feel a strain in your back, try these steps to avoid or reduce pain. These are the most important home treatments for the first few days of back pain.

1. **Relax:** Lie down in a comfortable position. This will let your back muscles relax. See ways to lie down on page 90.

2. **Walk:** Take a walk (10 to 20 minutes) on a flat, level surface every 2 to 3 hours. Walk only as far as you can without pain. If your back or legs hurt, stop.

3. **Pain medicine:** If you need it, take an over-the-counter medicine like acetaminophen (Tylenol) or ibuprofen (Advil, Motrin). It's best to take them on a regular schedule instead of waiting until the pain is severe. Read and follow all instructions on the label.

4. **Ice or heat:** Put an ice pack or heating pad on your back every 2 to 3 hours (use ice for 10 to 15 minutes; use heat for 15 to 20 minutes). Use whichever works best for you. Or try switching back and forth between ice and heat. Always put a thin cloth between the ice and your skin.

More ▶

Who to See for Back Pain

Medical doctors

A doctor (MD or DO) can:

◆ Diagnose the cause of back pain and assess injuries.

◆ Help you develop an exercise and home care plan or a modified work plan if you need it.

◆ Prescribe muscle relaxants, anti-inflammatory drugs, and pain medicines.

◆ Prescribe physical therapy.

◆ Help you decide if you need back surgery.

Physical therapists

After basic first aid, a physical therapist can:

◆ Identify specific muscle or disc problems.

◆ Use hands-on treatment (such as massage or spinal manipulation) to help relax muscles, loosen tight tissues, or align joints.

◆ Develop an exercise program to help you recover and teach you how to prevent future problems.

Chiropractors, osteopaths, and physiatrists

A chiropractor, an osteopath, or a physiatrist can relieve some types of back pain through spinal manipulation. Spinal manipulation usually works best if you have had symptoms for less than 4 weeks. If your symptoms do not improve after 1 month of treatment, stop the treatment and talk to your doctor about other treatments.

For help deciding whether to see a chiropractor, go to the Web site on the back cover and enter **i018** in the search box.

Other health professionals

Acupuncturists, massage therapists, and others can also provide treatments that may give short-term relief.

Sciatica

Sciatica is an irritation of the sciatic nerve, which is formed by the nerve roots that come out of the spinal cord into the lower back. The nerve extends down through the buttock to the foot. Sciatica can occur when a damaged disc presses against a spinal nerve root.

The main symptom is pain, numbness, or weakness that extends from your back down into your leg. The pain is usually worse in the leg.

For relief, see Home Treatment on page 86, and follow these tips:

◆ Do not sit unless you have to (unless it's more comfortable to sit than to stand).

◆ Switch between lying down and taking short walks. You can slowly increase how far you walk as long as it does not cause pain.

◆ Put ice or heat on the middle of your lower back every 2 to 3 hours (use ice for 10 to 15 minutes; use heat for 15 to 20 minutes). Or switch back and forth between ice and heat. Always put a thin cloth between the ice and your skin.

How to Have a Healthy Back

The keys to preventing back pain are to:

◆ Use good body mechanics.

◆ Stretch and strengthen your back.

◆ Practice good health habits, such as getting regular exercise, staying at a healthy weight, and not smoking (nicotine weakens the discs in your back).

Some of the tips presented here are things you'll want to do every day, not only because they're good for your back, but because they're good for your overall health. The rest will come in handy if you ever have back pain. They include:

◆ Good body mechanics.

◆ Exercises to make your back stronger and more flexible.

◆ Exercises to avoid.

Good Body Mechanics

The goal of good body mechanics is to sit, stand, sleep, and move in ways that reduce the stress on your back. Use good body mechanics all the time, not just when you have back pain.

Sitting

◆ Try not to sit in the same position for more than an hour at a time. Get up or change positions every 20 to 30 minutes.

◆ If you must sit a lot, the extension exercises starting on page 91 are particularly important.

◆ If you work at a desk or computer, set up your workstation to reduce stress on your back and neck.

❖ Use a chair that you can adjust and that does not upset the normal curve of your back.

❖ Keep your feet flat on the floor or on a footrest.

❖ Keep your screen at or just below eye level so you do not have to tilt your head or look sideways.

◆ If your chair does not give enough support, use a small pillow or rolled-up towel to support your lower back.

Adjust your chair, keyboard, and screen to reduce back and neck stress.

◆ When you drive, pull your seat forward so that you can easily reach the pedals and steering wheel. Stop often to stretch and walk around. A small pillow or rolled-up towel behind your lower back might help too.

More ➡

Lifting

◆ Keep your upper back straight. Do not bend forward at the waist.

◆ Bend your knees, and let your arms and legs do the work. Tighten your buttocks and belly to support your back.

◆ Keep the load as close to your body as you can, even if the load is light.

◆ While holding a heavy object, use your feet to turn, not your back. Try not to turn or twist your body.

◆ Do not lift heavy objects above shoulder level.

◆ For heavy or awkward items, use a hand truck or ask someone to help you.

When you lift heavy objects, keep your upper back straight, bend your knees, and keep the load close to your body.

Lying down

◆ If you have back pain at night, your mattress may be the problem. Try a firmer mattress. Or if you think your mattress is too firm, try a softer one.

◆ If you sleep on your back, you may want to use a rolled-up towel to support your lower back or put a pillow under your knees.

◆ If you sleep on your side, try placing a pillow between your knees.

◆ Sleeping on your stomach is fine if it does not cause back or neck pain.

Try placing pillows between or under your knees to relieve back pain while lying in bed.

Exercise

Regular exercise helps you stay fit and flexible and strengthens the muscles that support your back. It also helps you stay at a healthy weight, which reduces the strain on your lower back.

Although there is no clear evidence that specific exercises can help prevent back pain, the exercises described here are a common, practical approach to helping you stay strong and flexible. You may want to make them a part of your regular fitness routine.

Do not do these exercises if you have just hurt your back. Instead, see First Aid for Back Pain on page 87.

It helps to do both extension exercises and flexion exercises. Extension exercises strengthen your lower back muscles and stretch the stomach muscles. Flexion exercises stretch the lower back muscles and strengthen the stomach muscles—the reverse of extension.

◆ You do not need to do every exercise. Do the ones that help you the most.

◆ If any exercise makes your back pain worse, stop it and try something else. Stop any exercise that makes the pain spread into your buttocks or legs, either during or after the exercise.

◆ Start with 8 repetitions, 3 to 4 times a day, and gradually increase to 12 repetitions. Do all exercises slowly.

Extension exercises

Press-ups

This is a good exercise to start and end with.

◆ Lie on your stomach, supporting your body with your forearms.

◆ Press your elbows down into the floor to raise your upper back. As you do this, relax your stomach muscles and allow your back to arch without using your back muscles. As you press up, do not let your hips or pelvis come off the floor.

Press-up (shading shows where you should feel the stretch)

More

Backward bends

These help a lot if you work in a bent-forward position.

◆ Stand with your feet slightly apart. Back up to a countertop if you want extra support.

◆ Place your hands in the small of your back, and gently bend backward. Keep your knees straight (not locked), and bend only at the waist. Hold the backward stretch for about 6 seconds.

Backward bend
(keep neck straight
and chin down)

Flexion exercises

Curl-ups

These strengthen your stomach muscles, which help support your spine.

◆ Lie on your back with knees bent, feet flat on the floor, and arms crossed on your chest. Do not hook your feet under anything.

◆ Slowly curl up using your abdominal (belly) muscles until your shoulder blades barely rise from the floor. Keep your lower back pressed to the floor. To avoid neck problems, remember to lift your shoulders, and do not force your head up or forward. Hold for 1 to 2 seconds (don't hold your breath), and then curl down very slowly.

Curl-up (keep neck straight and chin tucked in)

Knee-to-chest stretch

This stretches the lower back and butt muscles and relieves pressure on the joints in your spine.

◆ Lie on your back with knees bent and feet close to your buttocks.

◆ Bring one knee to your chest, keeping the other foot flat on the floor (or the other leg straight, if that is more comfortable for your lower back). Keep your lower back pressed to the floor. Hold for 15 to 30 seconds.

◆ Relax and lower your knee to the starting position. Repeat with the other leg.

Knee-to-chest stretch (shading shows where you should feel the stretch)

Hamstring stretch

This stretches the muscles in the back of your thigh, which will let you bend your legs without stressing your back.

◆ Lie on your back in a doorway. Keep one leg resting on the floor of the doorway, and extend the leg you want to stretch straight up, resting the heel on the wall next to the doorway.

◆ Keep the leg straight, and slowly move your heel up the wall until you feel a gentle pull in the back of your thigh. Stretch as far as you can without pain.

◆ Relax in this position for at least 1 minute to begin. Then try to lengthen the time you hold the stretch to as long as 6 minutes. Then bend the knee to relieve the stretch. Repeat with the other leg.

Hamstring stretch (shading shows where you should feel the stretch)

More

Other strengthening and stretching exercises

Prone buttocks squeeze

This strengthens the butt muscles, which support the back and help you lift with your legs. You may need to place a small pillow under your stomach for comfort.

- Lie flat on your stomach with your arms at your sides.

- Slowly tighten your buttocks muscles and hold for about 6 seconds. Do not hold your breath. Relax slowly.

Hip flexor stretch

This stretches the muscles in the front of your hip.

- Kneel on one knee with your other leg bent in front of you.

- Slowly sink your hips so your weight shifts onto your front foot. The knee of your forward leg should be in a straight line with your ankle. Hold for 15 to 30 seconds. You should feel a stretch in the groin of the leg you are kneeling on. Repeat with the other leg.

Pelvic tilts

This exercise gently moves the spine and stretches the lower back.

- Lie on your back with knees bent and feet flat on the floor.

- Slowly tighten your stomach muscles and press your lower back against the floor. Hold for about 6 seconds while breathing smoothly. Slowly relax.

Pelvic tilts

Exercises to Avoid

These common exercises actually increase the risk of low back pain.

- Sit-ups with your legs straight out in front of you.

- Bent-leg sit-ups when you have back pain.

- Lifting both legs while lying on your back.

- Lifting heavy weights above the waist (military press, biceps curls while standing).

- Toe touches while standing.

Hip flexor stretch (shading shows where you should feel the stretch)

Back Surgery

Rest, pain medicines, and exercise can relieve almost all back problems. And back pain usually gets better within 6 to 12 weeks.

Most back surgeries are done to treat problems that have not improved with time. You may need surgery if you have a broken bone in your spine, a spinal infection, or another serious problem. Or you may think about surgery if you have a disc problem that has not improved with time and other treatment.

If you are thinking about having surgery to treat your back pain, get all the facts. Find out:

◆ How likely it is to help your problem. For some kinds of surgery, there is no clear evidence about whether it will help.

◆ What risks it has.

◆ How much it will cost.

 For help deciding whether surgery is right for you, go to the Web site on the back cover and enter **f952** in the search box.

If you do plan to have surgery, using good body mechanics and doing exercises for your back are very important. Having a strong, flexible back will help you recover more quickly after surgery.

Bed-Wetting

When to Call a Doctor

Your doctor can rule out or treat any physical causes of bed-wetting and help you and your child manage the problem.

Call your doctor if:

◆ Bed-wetting occurs with pain or burning during urination or other signs of a urinary infection. See page 251.

◆ Bed-wetting occurs in a child older than 6 years, and home treatment has not worked after 4 to 5 weeks.

◆ Your child starts wetting the bed more often, even with home treatment.

◆ Bed-wetting occurs in a child who had been dry for several months.

◆ A child age 4 or older is wetting the bed and leaking stool.

◆ A child over age 3 who has been toilet-trained has bladder control problems during the day.

More

Bed-wetting in children who have never been dry is common. Most children will outgrow it by age 5 or 6.

In some cases, a child who has not wet the bed for several months may start to wet the bed again. This can happen without a clear cause, or it may be caused by a urinary tract infection or emotional problems.

Home Treatment

There are a lot of ways to deal with bed-wetting if there is not an infection or other physical cause behind it. Ask your doctor for advice.

◆ Do not punish, embarrass, or blame your child. Praise and reward your child for dry nights.

◆ Limit how much your child drinks before bedtime.

◆ Have your child empty his or her bladder before bed.

◆ Remind your child to get up during the night to urinate. A night-light may help.

◆ Let your child choose whether to wear diapers, Pull-Ups, or absorbent under-wear at night. Use a thick pad or a vinyl mattress cover to protect the mattress.

◆ If your child is old enough, let him or her help with changing clothes, putting a dry towel down on the bed, and changing the sheets after wetting the bed.

◆ Add ½ cup vinegar to the wash water to get rid of odor in clothes and bedding.

Birth Control

Birth control helps prevent pregnancy. But no birth control method works every time and is risk-free. The only way to be sure you will not get pregnant is to not have sex.

This topic briefly describes the most common types of birth control. Be sure to think about their pros and cons, including cost and how well one type works compared to another, if you are trying to choose a method.

For more help with your options, go to the Web site on the back cover and enter **j225** in the search box. Talk to your doctor about it as well.

Use birth control exactly as your doctor or the package instructions say. Birth control works best when you use it right every time.

Hormonal Birth Control

This includes birth control pills, shots (Depo-Provera), implants under the skin (Implanon), the patch (Ortho Evra), and the vaginal ring (NuvaRing). These types of birth control either stop the release of an egg each month (ovulation) or thicken the mucus at the opening of the uterus so sperm cannot get through to the egg.

These types of birth control work very well if you use them right. All of them require a doctor's prescription. They do not protect you from sexually transmitted infections (STIs), also called sexually transmitted diseases.

IUD (Intrauterine Device)

The IUD is a piece of plastic or metal that your doctor can place in your uterus. There are two types.

◆ The copper IUD can stay in place for at least 10 years.

◆ The hormonal IUD (Mirena) works for at least 5 years, and it reduces menstrual bleeding and cramping.

Both types of IUDs damage or kill sperm. IUDs also change the lining of the uterus so that the fertilized egg does not attach there.

IUDs work better than most other types of birth control (IUDs work about as well as surgery). They may not be the best choice for all women, such as those who have an STI or have never been pregnant. Rarely, an IUD can come out without your noticing it. Some women have problems with IUDs during the first few months of use and decide to have them removed. IUDs don't protect you from STIs.

Condoms

The male condom is a thin, stretchy tube of latex, polyurethane, or animal skin that is placed over the erect penis before sex. The female condom fits inside the vagina.

Latex condoms are the best protection against STIs, including HIV. If you are allergic to latex, polyurethane condoms are the next best choice. See page 323. Lambskin condoms do not protect against HIV or other STIs.

Condoms are cheap, and you can get them without a prescription. But many people don't use them the right way, and they can break or slip off. For best protection against STIs and pregnancy, use condoms with another birth control method. For tips on how to use condoms right, see page 322.

Emergency Birth Control

Emergency birth control can help prevent pregnancy if you use it soon after you have sex. Sometimes called the morning-after pill, it is usually a high-dose form of birth control pills (Plan B or Next Choice). Inserting a copper IUD (intrauterine device) also works, but a doctor has to do this.

You can take Plan B or Next Choice up to 5 days after having sex. But the sooner you take it, the better your chance of not getting pregnant. The IUD can be used up to 7 days after sex.

Use emergency birth control right away if you want to avoid pregnancy and:

◆ You just had sex without birth control.

◆ You just had sex and your birth control failed. (For instance, a condom slipped or broke, or you skipped a pill.)

Anyone 17 or older with proof of age can buy Plan B or Next Choice without a prescription in most states. If you are younger than 17, you will need to get a prescription. Call your doctor or local clinic.

For next time

Accidents can happen. It's a good idea to keep a set of the pills on hand in case you ever need it. But don't rely on emergency birth control. Ask your doctor to help you find a good method of birth control you can use every time you have sex.

More ➤

Diaphragm and Cervical Cap

These are small rubber caps that you fill with spermicide and put in the vagina to cover the opening of the uterus (cervix) before you have sex. You have to leave them in place for 6 hours or longer after sex. And you have to see a doctor to have the diaphragm or cervical cap fitted.

The diaphragm or cervical cap prevents pregnancy better if you use it with another method, such as condoms. The diaphragm offers a little protection from STIs, but condoms are by far the best choice for this.

Spermicide

Spermicides are foams, jellies, films, and suppositories that kill sperm. You can buy them without a prescription.

Used by itself, spermicide is not a very good birth control method. For better protection, use it with another form of birth control, like a condom, diaphragm, or cervical cap. Spermicide does not protect you from STIs at all and may increase your risk for HIV. It can also irritate the vagina.

Surgery

◆ For men: In a vasectomy, the tubes (vas deferens) that carry sperm from the testicles are clamped or cut off. (See the picture on page 224.) This means there are no sperm in the semen when you ejaculate. After this surgery, you need to use birth control until a test shows that you are not releasing sperm.

◆ For women: Tubal ligation ties off the tubes that carry eggs from the ovaries to the uterus. (See the picture on page 329.) This keeps eggs from being fertilized or implanting in the uterus.

Surgery is the most effective form of birth control. Both types of surgery are permanent, though you can sometimes reverse them with a second surgery. Surgery does not protect you from STIs.

Tubal Implants

Implants are coils placed in the tubes that carry eggs from the ovaries to the uterus. Scar tissue forms around the coils and blocks the tubes. This keeps eggs from being fertilized. Putting the coils in takes about an hour and can be done while you are awake. Implants often cost less than tubal ligation.

Implants are permanent. You need to use another form of birth control for 3 months, until an X-ray shows that your tubes are blocked.

Natural Family Planning

Natural family planning helps a couple know when the woman is most likely to get pregnant (just before or during ovulation). This is sometimes called fertility awareness.

The woman records her temperature, checks her vaginal discharge, and tracks her periods. You can also buy urine test strips that help tell when ovulation occurs.

People may use natural family planning methods to know:

◆ When *not* to have sex if they don't want to get pregnant.

◆ When to have sex if they want to get pregnant.

Like other birth control, these methods work best when you use them correctly. If you don't want to get pregnant, make sure you don't have sex on fertile days. Or you'll need to use another type of birth control on those days. Natural family planning does not protect you from STIs.

How Well Does Birth Control Work?

Method	Pregnancies per 100 Women*

Surgery:
  Tubal ligation (women)
  Vasectomy (men)
	Fewer than 1

Intrauterine device (IUD):
  Hormonal (Mirena)
  Copper T (ParaGard)
	Fewer than 1

Tubal implants (women)	Fewer than 1
Implants under the skin (Implanon)	Fewer than 1
Shot every 3 months (Depo-Provera)	3
Birth control pills	8
Patch (Ortho Evra)	8
Vaginal ring (NuvaRing)	8
Male condom (latex or polyurethane) **Female condom**	15 21
Diaphragm (with spermicide)	16
Cervical cap (with spermicide)	16 to 32
Natural family planning (basal body temperature, mucus, or rhythm/calendar method)	25
Withdrawal (pulling out)	27
Spermicide by itself (jelly, cream, foam, suppositories)	29
No birth control	85

*Typical number of accidental pregnancies per 100 women in 1 year. If you use birth control exactly as directed every time, pregnancy rates are lower.

Abramowicz M (2007). Choice of Contraceptives. Treatment Guidelines from The Medical Letter, 5(64): 101–108.

Adapted from: Trussell J (2007). Choosing a Contraceptive: Efficacy, safety, and personal considerations. In RA Hatcher et al., eds., *Contraceptive Technology*, 19th ed., pp. 19–47. New York: Ardent Media.

Bladder Control

When to Call a Doctor

Call 911 if you suddenly lose bladder control.

Call a doctor if:

◆ You have to urinate frequently but cannot pass much urine.

◆ Your bladder does not feel empty after you urinate.

◆ You have trouble urinating even when your bladder feels full.

◆ It burns or hurts when you urinate. See Urinary Tract Infections on page 251.

◆ Your urine has blood in it.

◆ Your urine smells strange.

◆ You want help with your bladder control problem.

If you sometimes cannot control your bladder—a problem called **urinary incontinence**—you are not alone. It happens to many people.

The two most common bladder control problems are stress incontinence and urge incontinence.

If you have **stress incontinence**:

◆ Small amounts of urine leak out when you exercise, cough, laugh, or sneeze. This is more common in women.

◆ Kegel exercises may help. See page 101.

If you have **urge incontinence**:

◆ The need to urinate comes on so fast that you don't have time to get to the toilet.

◆ There may be an illness or disease causing the problem. This can include bladder infection, prostate enlargement, tumors that press on the bladder, and nerve problems such as those caused by Parkinson's disease, multiple sclerosis, and stroke.

Bladder control problems often can be controlled or cured if you can find and correct the cause. Water pills (diuretics) and other common medicines can cause short-term problems. Constipation, urinary tract infections, kidney stones, pregnancy, and being overweight are other causes.

Try not to let a bladder control problem embarrass you. Work with your doctor to treat it.

Home Treatment

◆ Avoid caffeine. It can make symptoms worse.

◆ Do not cut down on fluids. You need them to stay healthy. If having to get up at night bothers you, cut down on fluids before bed.

◆ If you smoke, quit (see page 316). This may reduce your coughing, which may help with bladder control.

◆ Lose weight if you need to.

◆ Practice "double voiding." Empty your bladder as much as you can, relax for a minute, and then try to empty it again.

◆ If you have trouble controlling your bladder when you laugh, sneeze, cough, or exercise, try doing Kegel exercises every day. See page 101.

- Urinate on a schedule, perhaps every 3 to 4 hours during the day, whether you have the urge or not. This may help you restore control.

- Wear clothing that you can take off quickly, such as pants with an elastic waist.

- Clear a path from your bed to the bathroom, or place a portable toilet by your bed.

- Use absorbent pads or briefs, such as Attends or Depend. No one will know you're wearing an absorbent pad.

- Keep skin in the genital area dry to prevent rashes. Use Vaseline or Desitin ointment to help protect the skin from irritation caused by urine.

- Ask your doctor or pharmacist whether any medicines you take, including non-prescription drugs, can affect bladder control. Do not stop taking your medicine without first talking to your doctor.

Kegel Exercises

Kegel exercises strengthen the pelvic muscles that control the flow of urine. This can help cure or improve some bladder control problems.

- To locate the muscles, repeatedly stop your urine in midstream and start again.

- Practice squeezing these muscles while you are not urinating. If your belly or buttocks move, you are not using the right muscles.

- Hold the squeeze for 3 seconds; then relax for 3 seconds.

- Repeat the exercise 10 to 15 times a session.

Do at least 3 sessions of Kegel exercises each day. You can do them anywhere, anytime. No one else will know you're doing them.

Blisters

When to Call a Doctor

- You have signs of infection. These may include increased pain, swelling, redness, or warmth; red streaks leading from the blister; pus; and fever.

- You get blisters often and do not know why.

- You have a band of painful blisters on one side of your body or face. See Shingles on page 122.

- You have diabetes or peripheral artery disease, and you get blisters on your hands, feet, or legs.

Home Treatment

- If a blister is small and closed, leave it alone. Use a loose bandage to protect it. Avoid the activity or shoes that caused the blister. (Blisters are usually caused by something rubbing against the skin.)

- If a small blister is in a weight-bearing area like the bottom of the foot, protect it with a doughnut-shaped moleskin pad. (Moleskin has soft felt on one side and a sticky backing on the other.) Leave the area over the blister open.

Blister

Use a doughnut-shaped pad to protect the blister.

Use a needle to puncture a large blister.

◆ If a blister is large and painful, it is usually best to drain it. Here is a safe method:

❖ Wash your hands.

❖ Wipe a needle or straight pin with rubbing alcohol.

❖ Gently poke a hole in the edge of the blister.

❖ Press the fluid in the blister toward the hole so it can drain out.

After you have opened a blister, or if it has torn open:

◆ Wash the area with soap and water. Do not use alcohol, iodine, or any other cleanser.

◆ Do not remove the flap of skin over a blister unless it's very dirty or torn or there is pus under it. Gently smooth the flap flat over the tender skin.

◆ Apply an antibiotic ointment and a clean bandage.

◆ Change the bandage once a day or anytime it gets wet or dirty. Remove it at night to let the area dry.

Boils

When to Call a Doctor

If needed, your doctor can drain the boil and treat the infection. **Call your doctor if:**

◆ The boil is on your face, near your spine, or in the anal area.

◆ You have any other lumps near the boil, especially if they hurt.

◆ You are in a lot of pain or have a fever.

◆ The area around the boil is red or has red streaks leading from it.

◆ You have diabetes or peripheral artery disease and you get a boil.

◆ The boil is the size of a Ping-Pong ball or larger.

◆ The boil has not improved after 5 to 7 days of home treatment.

◆ You get many boils over several months.

A boil is a red, swollen, painful bump under the skin. It may look like an overgrown pimple. Boils are often caused by infected hair follicles. A boil can become large and cause severe pain.

Boils occur most often where there is hair and rubbing. The face, neck, armpits, breasts, groin, and buttocks are common sites.

Home Treatment

◆ Do not squeeze, scratch, drain, or open the boil. Squeezing can push the infection deeper into the skin. Scratching can spread the infection.

◆ Wash with an antibacterial soap. Dry the area well.

◆ Put hot, wet cloths on the boil for 20 to 30 minutes, 3 or 4 times a day. Do this as soon as you notice a boil. The heat and moisture can help bring the boil to a head, but it may take 5 to 7 days. A hot pack or a waterproof heating pad placed over a damp towel may also help.

◆ Keep using heat for 3 days after the boil opens. Apply a bandage so the draining fluid does not spread. Change the bandage every day.

◆ Do not wear tight clothing over the area.

Breast Problems

When to Call a Doctor

◆ You find a lump in your breast, armpit, or chest area that concerns you, especially if it is hard and not like the rest of your breast tissue.

◆ You find a breast lump after menopause.

◆ You have a bloody or greenish discharge from a nipple, or you have a watery or milky discharge that occurs without pressing on the nipple or breast.

◆ You have a change in a nipple, such as crusty or scaly skin or a nipple that turns in rather than points out.

◆ One of your breasts changes shape or seems to pucker or pull when you raise your arms.

◆ The skin looks dimpled like an orange peel.

◆ You have a change in the color or feel of the skin of a breast or the darker area around a nipple.

◆ You have new pain in one breast that lasts longer than 1 or 2 weeks and was not caused by an injury.

◆ You have any signs of infection in a breast, such as pain, redness, warmth, or swelling.

◆ You are a man and you find a lump in your chest area.

More

Breast Pain

Many women's breasts get achy, heavy, or sore a week or so before their periods. This is caused by normal hormone changes. The symptoms usually go away at the end of a woman's period.

It may help to:

◆ Avoid salty foods just before your period starts.

◆ Take 400 mg of magnesium each day.

◆ Take evening primrose oil.

◆ Take an over-the-counter medicine like acetaminophen (Tylenol) or ibuprofen (Advil, Motrin) for pain. Read and follow all instructions on the label.

◆ Wear a more supportive bra, especially when you exercise.

You will probably stop having this type of breast pain after you complete menopause.

Stress, estrogen therapy, and the use of certain medicines can make breast pain worse. Sore breasts can also be a sign of pregnancy.

Breast pain that is not related to your periods or an injury is usually sharp or burning. This pain tends to be on one side only and may reach up to the armpit. It may come and go. Pain in one spot that does not go away should be checked by a doctor.

Breast Lumps

Breast lumps are common, especially in women between ages 30 and 50. Many women's breasts feel lumpy right before their periods. Women also may have lumps when they are breast-feeding. Breast lumps usually go away after menopause, but they may occur in women who take hormones after menopause.

Most breast lumps are not cancer. A lumpy texture in both breasts is very common, but still have a doctor check any lump or thickness that is not like the rest of your breast tissue. (It may be bigger or harder or feel different.)

How dense or lumpy a woman's breasts are tends to run in the family. If your mother had lumpy breasts, you are likely to as well. It is also common for one breast to be denser than the other. The important thing is to watch for a change in the breast tissue.

Breast Cancer

Here are a few things you should know:

◆ Breast cancer can often be cured if you find it early.

◆ Regular mammograms can help find breast cancer early and save lives.

◆ Self-exams can help you learn what is normal for your breasts and may make you aware of changes sooner. See page 330.

◆ Your risk for breast cancer goes up after age 50. In general, women younger than 50 are at lower risk for breast cancer.

◆ If your mother or a sister had breast cancer before menopause, you are at increased risk for breast cancer. Talk with your doctor about when to start mammograms and other tests.

What You Can Do to Prevent Breast Cancer

◆ Do not have more than 1 alcoholic drink a day. Moderate to heavy drinking increases your risk for breast cancer.

◆ Get regular exercise. See page 311.

- Eat a low-fat diet (see page 305). It is not proven that a diet low in fat will prevent cancer, yet women in cultures that eat a high-fat diet are more likely to die of breast cancer than women in cultures that eat a low-fat diet.

- Talk to your doctor about starting mammograms at age 40.

- Have a mammogram every 1 to 2 years starting at age 50. See page 330.

- If you have a strong family history of breast cancer, you may need to have mammograms earlier.

 For help deciding when to start having mammograms, go to the Web site on the back cover and enter **a000** in the search box.

Are you at high risk for breast cancer? To learn about some risks, go to the Web site on the back cover and enter **a888** in the search box. You'll learn options to lower risk, such as taking medicine like tamoxifen or having other treatments.

Breast-Feeding

When to Call a Doctor

Call your doctor if you are nursing and:

- You have signs of a breast infection, such as breast pain, swelling, redness, warmth, or a fever.

- You gain or lose more than 1 pound a week for several weeks in a row.

- You need to take a medicine and have not talked to your doctor about whether it is safe.

- You have trouble breast-feeding and want help.

- You think that your milk supply is not enough for your baby.

Home Treatment for Sore Breasts

- Use ice or cold packs on the sore breast for 10 to 15 minutes at a time. Put a thin cloth between the ice and your skin.

- Wear a supportive nursing bra.

- Take an over-the-counter medicine like acetaminophen (Tylenol) or ibuprofen (Advil, Motrin). Read and follow all instructions on the label. These will not affect your breast milk.

- To soften your breasts before feedings, put a warm, wet cloth on them, massage gently, and use your hands to squeeze a little milk from both breasts.

- Although painful for you, breast-feeding from your sore breast is safe for your baby. If starting with the sore breast hurts too much, start feeding on the other side, then switch sides after your milk lets down. If your nipple hurts too much to breast-feed from that breast, use a breast pump to empty the breast of milk each time that you cannot breast-feed.

More

Health Tips for Breast-Feeding Mothers

◆ Eat 500 extra calories a day, and drink extra fluids. Although you do not need to drink milk to make milk, extra calcium and protein are important. Your doctor may have you keep taking your prenatal vitamins.

◆ Do not smoke.

◆ Do not drink alcohol.

◆ Limit caffeine to 1 or 2 drinks a day.

◆ Talk to your doctor before you take any medicine. Some medicines may pass through the breast milk to your baby.

Football hold

Cradle hold

Breast-feeding in the right position will help your baby latch on and breast-feed correctly. Above are two positions you can try.

Thinking About Breast-Feeding?

Breast milk is the perfect food for babies and the only food they need for the first 6 months.

◆ Breast milk helps your baby resist infections and other diseases. Breast-fed babies have fewer colds and ear infections.

◆ Breast milk is easier for your baby to digest than formula. Breast-fed babies have less diarrhea and vomiting.

◆ Breast-fed babies have a lower risk of problems like obesity and high blood pressure later in life.

For these reasons, the American Academy of Pediatrics recommends that babies be breast-fed for at least the first year.

Breast-feeding also helps your body recover from pregnancy. And it may lower your risk of breast and uterine cancer and diabetes later in life. But whether you breast-feed and for how long also depends on you, your child, and your situation. Babies can get great nutrition from formula too.

If this is your first baby, you may want to take a breast-feeding class before your child is born. Many hospitals offer them. The La Leche League and the Nursing Mothers Counsel are other good sources of breast-feeding advice and support.

To learn how to breast-feed and how to deal with problems that might come up, go to the Web site on the back cover and enter **g021** in the search box.

Breathing Problems

When to Call a Doctor

Call 911 if:

◆ You cannot breathe, or you have severe trouble breathing. For signs of severe trouble breathing, see page 19.

◆ You have shortness of breath with chest pain or pressure or other symptoms of a heart attack. See page 38.

◆ Your tongue or throat swells quickly and makes it very hard to breathe. This can be caused by an allergic reaction. See page 77.

Call your doctor if:

◆ You wheeze when you breathe. Wheezing is a high-pitched sound you may make if you have a problem in your airways.

◆ You tire quickly when you talk or eat, or you often have to stop to catch your breath.

◆ You wake up in the night short of breath.

◆ You have trouble breathing or cough a lot when you exercise.

◆ You have any trouble breathing that lasts longer than an hour and is not related to a cold, flu, or other illness.

Be sure to check the Chest, Heart, and Lung Problems chart on page 65 if you do not find your symptoms here.

Breathing problems have many possible causes, from asthma to anxiety to heart problems. A breathing problem can be a sign of something serious, though this is not always the case. See When to Call a Doctor to find out whether you need medical care and how soon you need it.

If you have already been diagnosed with allergies, asthma, COPD (chronic obstructive pulmonary disease), or heart failure, one of these topics may help:

◆ Allergies, page 76

◆ Living Better With Asthma, page 266

◆ Living Better With Heart Failure, page 291

◆ Living Better With COPD, page 271

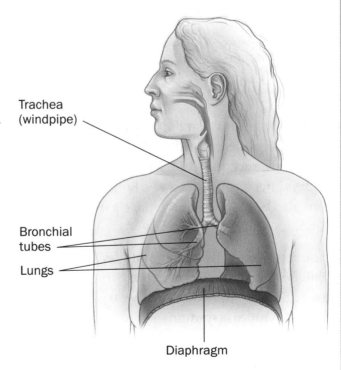

Trachea (windpipe)

Bronchial tubes

Lungs

Diaphragm

The respiratory tract

Bronchitis

When to Call a Doctor

Any of these symptoms may mean that your bronchitis is getting worse or that you have a bacterial infection that needs treatment.

Call your doctor if:

◆ A cough occurs with new wheezing or new trouble breathing.

◆ You cough up blood.

◆ You cough up yellow, green, or rust-colored mucus from your lungs (not from your nose or the back of your throat) for more than 2 days, and you have a fever.

◆ You have a fever of 104°F or higher.

◆ You have a fever higher than 101°F with shaking chills and a cough that brings up mucus.

◆ You still have a fever after using home treatment. Bronchitis may cause fevers of 102°F or higher for up to a day. But call a doctor if the fever stays high. See the fever guidelines on pages 158 and 160.

◆ Your breathing is fast or shallow, and you are short of breath.

◆ You have pain in the muscles of your chest (chest-wall pain) when you cough or breathe.

◆ You are more tired than you would be with a typical cold.

Also call if:

◆ You cannot drink enough fluids and are dehydrated, or you cannot eat at all.

◆ The sick person is a baby, an older adult, or someone who has lung problems or another long-term disease.

◆ Any cough lasts longer than 2 weeks.

Bronchitis means that the airways leading to the lungs are irritated. It is usually caused by a virus, such as a cold, and may start 3 to 4 days after a cold goes away. But bronchitis can also be caused by bacteria, cigarette smoke, or air pollution.

You may have a dry cough, mild fever, fatigue, pain or tightness in the chest, and wheezing. As your cough gets worse, it may bring up mucus (sputum).

If you get bronchitis often—especially if you smoke—you may reach a point where your airways are inflamed and irritated all the time. This is called chronic bronchitis. If you smoke, you are also at high risk for emphysema. Chronic bronchitis, emphysema, and other lung diseases are known as **COPD (chronic obstructive pulmonary disease)**. If you have COPD, see page 271.

Home Treatment

◆ If your doctor prescribes medicine, take it as directed. But don't be surprised if your doctor does not prescribe medicine. Bronchitis often goes away without it.

◆ Drink plenty of water to stay hydrated.

◆ Get some extra rest.

◆ Take an over-the-counter medicine like acetaminophen (Tylenol) or ibuprofen (Advil, Motrin) for fever and body aches. Read and follow all instructions on the label. Do not give aspirin to anyone younger than 20.

◆ Use a nonprescription cough suppressant with dextromethorphan. This may help quiet a dry, hacking cough so you can sleep. Read the label on the bottle, and find a cough medicine that treats only coughs.

◆ Before you use cough or cold medicines, check the label. They may not be safe for young children or for people with certain health problems.

◆ Breathe moist air from a humidifier, a hot shower, or a sink filled with hot water. The heat and moisture can help thin mucus so you can cough it out.

◆ Do not smoke. If you need help quitting, see page 316.

◆ If you have classic flu symptoms, try home treatment for flu, and see how you're doing after another day or two. See Flu on page 165.

Bunions and Hammer Toes

When to Call a Doctor

◆ You have sudden, severe pain in your big toe.

◆ Your big toe starts to partly cover your second toe.

◆ You have diabetes, poor blood flow, peripheral artery disease, or a weak immune system, and you develop any kind of foot problem. Irritated skin over a bunion or hammer toe can easily get infected.

◆ You have a sore over a bunion or hammer toe.

◆ Pain does not get better after 2 to 3 weeks of home treatment.

A **bunion** is a bump on the outside of the joint at the bottom of your big toe. You get a bunion when the big toe bends toward and sometimes partly covers the second toe.

Bunion

A **hammer toe** is a toe that bends up at the middle joint.

These foot problems sometimes run in families. Tight or high-heeled shoes increase the risk of both. If you already have a foot problem, wearing tight shoes or high heels may make it worse.

Hammer toe

Home Treatment

When you have a bunion or a hammer toe, there is usually no way to get rid of it unless you have surgery. Home treatment will help relieve pain and keep the problem from getting worse.

◆ Wear roomy, low-heeled shoes that have wide, deep toe areas and good arch support. To find the best footwear for your problem, go to the Web site on the back cover and enter **v561** in the search box.

◆ Cushion the joint with moleskin or a doughnut-shaped pad to prevent rubbing and pressure. (Moleskin has soft felt on one side and a sticky backing on the other.)

What About Foot Surgery?

If you have tried home treatment but you have severe pain or an oddly shaped joint that affects your walking, you may want to think about surgery.

◆ Surgery can help reduce pain and help you walk better, but it may not cure the problem.

◆ If you want surgery to improve how your foot looks rather than to relieve pain, you may not be happy with the result.

◆ Surgery can sometimes cause other problems.

◆ Surgery costs a lot.

 For help deciding whether surgery is worth the cost and risks, go to the Web site on the back cover and enter **b064** in the search box.

◆ Take an old pair of shoes, and cut out the area over the toe. Wear these shoes around the house. Or wear comfortable sandals that do not press on the area.

◆ Take an over-the-counter medicine like acetaminophen (Tylenol) or ibuprofen (Advil, Motrin) for pain. Read and follow all instructions on the label. Ice or cold packs may also help. See page 243.

◆ Ask your doctor about bunion pads, arch supports, or custom-made supports called orthotics. Orthotics can hold your foot in a healthy position and help take pressure off your big toe.

Bursitis and Tendon Injury

Bursitis and tendon injuries are common reasons for pain and swelling in the ankles, knees, hips, wrists, elbows, and shoulders.

A bursa is a small sac of fluid that helps the tissues around a joint slide over one another easily. Injury, overuse, or constant direct pressure on a joint can cause pain, redness, heat, and swelling of the bursa. This is called **bursitis**. Bursitis often develops quickly, over just a few days.

Tendons are tough, ropelike fibers that connect muscles to bones. A **tendon injury** develops when wear and tear or overuse of a tendon causes tiny tears in the tissue. This leads to pain, inflammation, and breakdown in the tendons or the tissues surrounding them.

Both bursitis and tendon injuries can be caused by jobs, sports, or things you do around the house that require a lot of twisting or fast moving of the joints or constant pressure on a joint (kneeling, for example).

The same home treatment is good for both problems.

Home Treatment

Bursitis or a tendon injury will usually get better in a few days or weeks if you avoid the activity that caused it. But the mistake many people make is thinking that the problem is gone when the pain is gone.

To keep the problem from coming back, you will need to strengthen and stretch the muscles around the joint and change the way you do some activities.

Pelvis

Bursa

Thighbone (femur)

The fluid-filled bursa helps cushion a joint like the hip.

More

111

◆ Rest the area. Change the way you do the activity that causes pain so that you can do it without pain. See the joint-specific guidelines later in this topic. To stay fit, try activities that do not stress the area.

◆ As soon as you notice pain, use ice or cold packs for 10 to 15 minutes at a time, several times a day. Put a thin cloth between the ice and your skin. See Ice and Cold Packs on page 243. Keep using ice as long as it relieves pain.

◆ You can also use a warm, moist cloth or take hot baths if they make you feel better. Or switch back and forth between heat and cold.

◆ Take an over-the-counter medicine like acetaminophen (Tylenol) or ibuprofen (Advil, Motrin) for pain. But do not use the medicine to control the pain while you keep overusing the joint. Read and follow all instructions on the label.

◆ To prevent stiffness, gently move the joint through all of its possible movements as much as you can without pain. As the pain gets better, add exercises that strengthen the muscles around the joint.

◆ When you are ready to try the activity that caused the pain, start slowly and do it for short periods only or at a slower speed. Increase the intensity slowly and only if the pain does not come back.

◆ Warm up before and stretch after the activity. Use ice after exercise to prevent pain and swelling.

Along with the home treatment information for bursitis and tendon injuries above, the following tips will help for problems with a specific joint.

Wrists

Wrist pain may be caused by a tendon injury. Although this is not the same as carpal tunnel syndrome, the same home care may help. See page 116.

Elbows

Elbow pain is often caused by a tendon injury in the forearm or bursitis in the elbow.

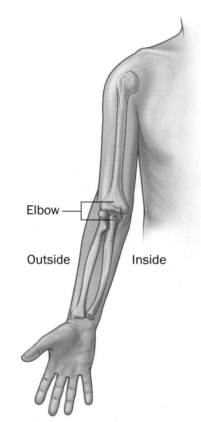

Elbow — Outside — Inside

Tennis elbow causes pain on the outside of the elbow. Golfer's elbow hurts on the inside.

To relieve elbow pain and prevent further injury:

◆ Rest the elbow and give it time to heal.

◆ Wear a brace or elbow sleeve.

◆ Support a sore elbow with a sling for 1 to 2 days (see page 52). Do exercises that help you move your elbow through all of its possible movements daily.

◆ Strengthen the wrist, arm, shoulder, and back muscles.

◆ Avoid activities that make you repeat a wrist motion many times.

◆ Make changes in your activities so you don't irritate the tendon:

  ❖ Use tools with larger handles.

  ❖ Avoid leaning on the point of your elbow for long periods.

  ❖ Switch hands during activities such as raking, sweeping, or gardening.

Shoulders

Shoulder pain that occurs on the outside of the upper arm is often caused by bursitis or a tendon injury around the shoulder joint. Pain on the top of the shoulder or in the neck may be caused by tension in the trapezius muscles, which run from the back of the head across the back of the shoulders. See Neck Pain on page 211.

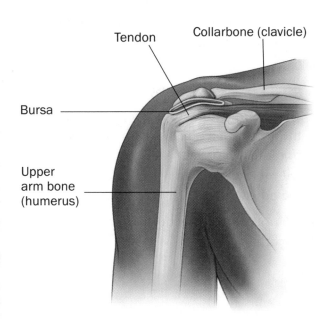

Bursitis, a tendon injury, and muscle tension are common causes of shoulder pain.

Common symptoms of shoulder bursitis or a tendon injury are pain, pinching, and stiffness when you raise your arm. The symptoms are often brought on by doing repeated overhead movements. Pain and swelling can occur when you keep using your shoulder without giving it time to rest.

To relieve shoulder pain and stiffness:

◆ Avoid activities that involve overhead reaching, but keep using your shoulder.

◆ Try the "pendulum" exercise: Bend forward and hold the back of a chair with the hand of your healthy arm. Let the other arm hang straight down from the shoulder. Move the hanging arm in circles; start with small circles and slowly make them bigger. Then switch directions. Again, go from small circles to large ones. Next, swing the arm forward and backward, then from side to side. Do this exercise 10 times a day.

◆ Use proper throwing techniques for baseball and football.

◆ Use a different swim stroke. Try breaststroke or sidestroke instead of the crawl or butterfly.

◆ Gently move your shoulder through all of its possible movements every day.

Hips

Hip pain may be caused by a tendon injury or bursitis. You may feel it at the side of your hip when you rise from a chair and take the first few steps, while you climb stairs, or while you drive. If pain is severe, sleeping on your side may also hurt.

Pain in the front of the hip may also be caused by arthritis (see page 82).

More

Hip pain can also cause knee or thigh pain. This is called referred pain.

To relieve hip pain and avoid further problems:

◆ Wear well-cushioned shoes. Do not wear high heels.

◆ Avoid activities that force one side of your pelvis higher than the other, such as running in only one direction on a track or working sideways on a slope.

◆ Sleep on your "good" side with a pillow between your knees, or on your back with pillows under your knees.

◆ See the hip flexor stretch on page 94. Stretch after activity, when your muscles are warm.

Knees

Knee pain may be caused by bursitis or a tendon injury. Also see Knee Problems on page 201.

Legs and Feet

Heel or foot pain may be caused by plantar fasciitis or an Achilles tendon injury. See page 185. Pain in the front of the lower leg may be due to shin splints. See page 205.

Calluses and Corns

When to Call a Doctor

◆ A callus or corn breaks open and starts to hurt.

◆ A callus or corn bleeds, looks red or black, or drains pus.

◆ You have diabetes or peripheral artery disease and get a callus or corn.

Calluses and corns are areas of skin that have gotten thick and hard because of rubbing and pressure. Calluses are common on the soles of the feet, the heels, and the hands. Corns are often on the toes.

Home Treatment

◆ If you have diabetes or peripheral artery disease, talk to your doctor before you try to remove a callus or corn on your own.

◆ If a callus or corn hurts, soak your foot in warm water for 5 to 10 minutes. Then rub the callus or corn with a towel or pumice stone. You may need to repeat this a few times over several days until the thickened skin is gone.

◆ You can also use a nonprescription product for removing calluses and corns.

◆ To prevent pain and rubbing, cushion the area with a doughnut-shaped pad or moleskin patch. (Moleskin has soft felt on one side and a sticky backing on the other.)

◆ Do not try to cut or burn off a callus or corn.

Canker Sores

When to Call a Doctor

- You have canker sores and a fever.

- You get canker sores after you start a new medicine or after you go to the dentist.

- A canker sore does not heal in 2 weeks, or you get several sores.

- A canker sore hurts a lot, or it goes away and then comes back.

- You have white spots in your mouth that are not canker sores and that have not gone away after 1 to 2 weeks.

Canker sores are painful, open sores on the inside of the mouth. The sores usually heal in 7 to 14 days. You can get them because of stress, a mouth injury, an infection, certain foods, poor nutrition, hormone changes, and other reasons.

Home Treatment

- Avoid coffee, spicy and salty foods, nuts, chocolate, and citrus fruits when you have open sores in your mouth.

- Use a nonprescription canker sore medicine (such as Anbesol, Orabase, or Zilactin) to protect the sore, ease pain, and speed healing. Or put a thin paste of baking soda and water on the sore to relieve pain.

- Rinse your mouth with an antacid (such as Maalox or Mylanta) or with a mixture of 1 tablespoon of hydrogen peroxide in 8 ounces of water.

- Do not smoke or chew tobacco. If you need help quitting, see page 316.

- Use a soft-bristled toothbrush to brush your teeth and gums.

Carpal Tunnel Syndrome

When to Call a Doctor

- You have tingling, numbness, weakness, or pain in your fingers and hand even after 2 weeks of home treatment.

- You often have little or no feeling in your fingers or hand.

- You cannot do simple hand movements, or you drop things a lot because you can't hold on to them.

- You cannot pinch your thumb and first finger together, or you have no thumb strength.

- You have problems at work because of pain in your fingers or hand.

- Your hand muscles, especially the muscles of the thumb, look smaller.

More

Carpal Tunnel Syndrome

The carpal tunnel is a narrow space in your wrist. The nerve that controls feeling in some of your fingers and controls some of the hand muscles passes through this space.

Carpal tunnel syndrome develops when there is pressure on the nerve where it goes through the carpal tunnel.

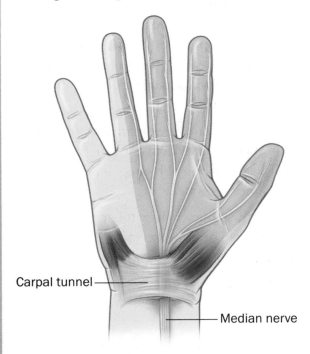

Carpal tunnel —

— Median nerve

Carpal tunnel syndrome causes pain and tingling in the shaded area.

You may have:

◆ Numbness or pain in your hand or wrist that wakes you up at night.

◆ Numbness or tingling in your fingers, except for the little finger and half of the ring finger.

◆ Numbness or pain that gets worse when you use your hand or wrist, especially when you grip an object or flex your wrist.

◆ Aching pain in your arm between your hand and your elbow. The pain may come and go.

◆ A weak grip.

◆ Loss of muscle mass in your hand, especially of your thumb.

Activities that make you use the same wrist or hand movements over and over can cause carpal tunnel syndrome or make it worse. You may do things at work, at home, or during sports or hobbies that cause this problem.

Home Treatment

◆ Stop any activity that you think may be causing numbness or pain. If the problem improves when you stop, return to that activity slowly. Try to keep your wrist straight or only slightly bent.

When you type, keep your fingers lower than your wrists. Try to keep your wrist straight or only slightly bent.

◆ Watch your posture. When you type, keep your fingers lower than your wrists. A keyboard wrist support and arm supports on your chair may help. When your arms are at your sides, relax your shoulders.

◆ Use your whole hand (not just your fingers and thumb) to hold objects.

◆ Reduce the speed and force of repeated hand movements. For instance, type a little slower, and don't hit the keys too hard.

◆ Switch hands and change positions often when you have to repeat the same motions a lot.

◆ Rest your hands frequently.

◆ Take an over-the-counter medicine like acetaminophen (Tylenol) or ibuprofen (Advil, Motrin) for pain. Read and follow all instructions on the label.

◆ Use ice or a cold pack on the palm side of your wrist. Put a thin cloth between the ice and your skin. See Ice and Cold Packs on page 243.

◆ Don't sleep on your hands.

◆ Ask your doctor about a wrist splint. This can relieve pressure and keep your wrist in a good position when you sleep.

Losing weight, quitting smoking, reducing alcohol and salt, and controlling diabetes may help reduce swelling in your wrist. Use the index in the back of the book to find information that can help.

What About Surgery?

Most cases of carpal tunnel syndrome can get better without surgery. If you are thinking about surgery, learn as much as you can about its pros and cons, including the cost of the surgery.

To help you decide whether surgery is right for you, go to the Web site on the back cover and enter **b941** in the search box.

Preventing Carpal Tunnel Syndrome

You are more likely to get carpal tunnel syndrome if:

◆ You spend a lot of time doing activities that make you repeat the same wrist and hand movements.

◆ You work with tools or machines that vibrate in your hand, like sanders or drills.

◆ You do a lot of activities with your wrist bent downward.

But there are ways you can reduce your risk, as well as any pain or weakness you already have. To learn how to keep your wrist healthy, go to the Web site on the back cover and enter **v714** in the search box.

Cataracts

When to Call a Doctor

- You have eye pain.
- You have a change in your vision, such as vision loss, double vision, or blurred vision. A sudden change could be a sign of a serious problem.
- You need to change your eyeglasses prescription often.
- Daytime glare is a problem.
- You have trouble driving at night because of glare from headlights.
- Vision problems are affecting your daily life.

A cataract is a painless, cloudy area in the lens of the eye (see the picture on page 172). By blocking some of the light that comes into the eye, a cataract may cause cloudy, foggy, filmy, or double vision. Glare is also a common problem.

Cataracts can be caused by:

- Normal changes in your eyes as you get older.
- Eye injury.
- Certain medicines.
- Eye disease and other health problems, especially diabetes.

Some children are born with cataracts.

Home Treatment

Home treatment may help you avoid or delay cataract surgery. There are many things you can do to make the changes in your vision easier to live with.

- Move room lights and use window shades to prevent glare.
- Use more lighting or higher-watt bulbs in your home.

Do You Need Surgery?

For most adults, the need for cataract surgery depends on how much the cataract affects their quality of life. Most cataracts grow slowly. At first, you may just need stronger glasses. Many people get along very well with the help of glasses, contact lenses, and other vision aids.

Later, if the cataract grows and starts to seriously affect your vision, you can have surgery to remove it. Some cataracts, such as those caused by injury, need to be removed right away.

Go to Web For most people with cataracts, whether and when to have surgery is up to them. For help with your decision, go to the Web site on the back cover and enter **p502** in the search box.

118

- Use contrasts in color and brightness to make things easier to find. For example, use dark switch plates on light-colored walls. Use bright labels to "color code" medicines, spices, and stove dials.

- Use a magnifying glass to help you read. Look for large-print books and other reading material. You sometimes can get bank checks, medicine labels, and other items in large print.

- Have your eyes checked regularly. Update your glasses when needed.

- Wear sunglasses to reduce glare and block out harmful sunlight. Buy sunglasses that screen out UVA and UVB rays.

- If you smoke, quit. Smoking can make cataracts worse. If you need help quitting, see page 316.

Chest Pain

Are You Having a Heart Attack?

You may be having a heart attack if:

❏ You have chest pain or pressure, or a strange feeling in your chest. You may feel tightness, squeezing, crushing, intense burning, or aching in your chest.

❏ The pain or pressure lasts longer than 5 minutes and does not go away with rest or nitroglycerin.

Other signs include:

❏ Sweating.

❏ Shortness of breath.

❏ Nausea or vomiting.

❏ Pain, pressure, or a strange feeling in your back, neck, jaw, upper belly, or one or both shoulders or arms.

❏ Lightheadedness or sudden weakness.

❏ A fast or irregular heartbeat.

The more boxes you check, the more likely it is that you are having a heart attack. Some people, especially women, may not have chest pain but may have some of the other symptoms.

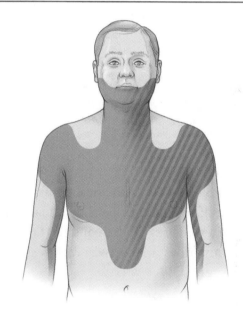

A heart attack may cause discomfort in any of the shaded areas as well as the upper back.

Angina

Angina is chest pain or pressure, or a strange feeling in your chest. It occurs when your heart does not get enough oxygen. You may feel pain or pressure in your chest, back, neck, jaw, upper belly, shoulders, or arms. This can happen during activity or moments of stress, or when you do anything that works your heart too hard. The pain stops when you stop and rest or take a medicine called nitroglycerin.

More ➤

When to Call a Doctor

Call 911 if:

◆ You think you may be having a heart attack. Do not wait to see if you feel better. See Are You Having a Heart Attack? on page 119.

◆ You have been diagnosed with angina, and your angina does not go away with rest or is not getting better within 5 minutes after taking a dose of nitroglycerin.

After you call 911, the operator may tell you to chew 1 adult-strength aspirin or 2 to 4 low-dose aspirin (unless you are allergic to it).

If you can't get an ambulance, have someone drive you to the hospital. Do not drive yourself.

Call a doctor if:

◆ You think you have angina, and you have not seen a doctor about it.

◆ You have been diagnosed with angina and it's getting worse or lasting longer than usual, or you start getting it more often.

◆ You have any chest pain and have a history of heart disease or blood clots in the lungs.

◆ You have mild but constant chest pain that does not go away with rest.

◆ You have chest pain with other symptoms of pneumonia. See page 216.

◆ Mild chest pain lasts longer than 2 days without getting better.

Unlike angina, a heart attack is caused by blocked blood flow to the heart muscle, not just lack of oxygen. The pain of a heart attack is usually more severe than angina, lasts longer, and does not go away with rest or nitroglycerin.

Angina is a sign of **coronary artery disease**. Having coronary artery disease means you are at high risk for a heart attack. To learn how to reduce your risk, see page 276.

Are You At Risk for a Heart Attack?

To find out your chance of having a heart attack in the next 10 years, go to the Web site on the back cover and enter **u149** in the search box.

Other Causes of Chest Pain

◆ Heartburn (see page 183) or gas can cause chest pain.

◆ Hyperventilation (see page 23) can also cause chest pain.

◆ Chest pain that gets worse when you take a deep breath or cough may be a sign of pneumonia (see page 216) or an illness called **pleurisy**.

◆ An ulcer (see page 249) can cause chest pain, usually below the breastbone. The pain may be worse when your stomach is empty.

◆ Gallstones (see page 170) may cause pain in the right side of the chest or around the shoulder blade. The pain may get worse after a meal or in the middle of the night.

◆ Shingles (see page 122) may cause a sharp, burning, or tingling pain that feels like a tight band around one side of the chest.

A shooting pain that lasts a few seconds or a quick pain at the end of a deep breath is usually not a cause for concern.

Chest-Wall Pain

If you can point to the exact spot in your chest that hurts and it hurts more when you press on it, you probably have chest-wall pain.

If you have chest-wall pain, you may have strained a muscle in your chest or hurt a rib. Or the cartilage in your chest wall could be inflamed for no clear reason. This is called **costochondritis**. It usually goes away in a few days.

Home Treatment

If you have angina caused by coronary artery disease, there are many things you can do to control it. See page 276.

For chest-wall pain caused by injury

◆ Take an over-the-counter medicine like acetaminophen (Tylenol) or ibuprofen (Advil, Motrin) for pain. Read and follow all instructions on the label.

◆ Use an ice pack to help relieve pain after an injury. See page 243.

◆ You can also use heat for the pain. Use a heating pad set on low or heat that is no warmer than bathwater. Don't go to sleep while using a heating pad.

◆ Use products such as Bengay or Icy Hot to help soothe sore muscles.

◆ Avoid any activity that strains the chest. As your pain gets better, slowly return to your normal activities.

Chickenpox

When to Call a Doctor

◆ A child who takes steroid medicines, is being treated for cancer, or has a weak immune system gets chickenpox or is exposed to it.

◆ You are pregnant and have never had chickenpox, and someone in your household gets chickenpox.

◆ A baby younger than 3 months has a fever of 100.4°F or higher.

◆ A child with chickenpox has a fever of 102°F or higher for 2 days. Also see pages 158 and 160.

◆ Bruising appears for no clear reason.

◆ Your child has sores in his or her eyes.

◆ Your child has signs of a serious illness called **encephalitis** (see page 161). These include:

❖ Fever, severe headache, and stiff neck.

❖ Unusual sleepiness or lack of awareness.

❖ Vomiting.

◆ A teenager or adult gets chickenpox.

◆ You cannot control severe itching.

Chickenpox is a common viral infection. In most children, it is a minor illness.

◆ For the first few days, your child will feel ill with a fever and headache. He or she may not want to eat and will feel very tired.

◆ Red spots will appear. There may be as few as 30 spots, or the rash may cover the whole body, including the throat, mouth, ears, groin, and scalp. The rash itches a lot.

◆ The spots turn into blisters that break open and crust over.

◆ More spots will appear for 1 to 5 days and then go away over 1 to 2 weeks.

Chickenpox spreads easily. Symptoms usually start 14 to 16 days after you come in contact with the virus. You can spread chickenpox 2 to 3 days before the rash appears (when there is a fever) and until all the spots have crusted over.

Most of the time, children can go back to school or day care after the spots have crusted over and the fever is gone. The same rule applies to adults going back to work.

Preventing Chickenpox

◆ **Children 12 months and older:** Make sure they get the chickenpox vaccine. See page 325.

◆ **Teens and adults who have not had the vaccine or the illness:** Get the vaccine. Until then, avoid anyone who has chickenpox or shingles (see this page). Chickenpox can be serious if you get it as an adult.

◆ **Pregnant women who have not had the vaccine or the illness:** Avoid anyone who has chickenpox or shingles. The virus can harm your unborn baby, and the vaccine is not given to pregnant women.

Shingles

If you have ever had chickenpox, you still have the virus in your body. If the virus becomes active again, years after the first illness, it is called **shingles**.

Shingles often affects one or two of the large nerves that spread outward from the spine. This causes pain and a rash, often in a band or small area on one side of the chest, belly, or face. The rash will blister and scab, then clear up over a few weeks.

If you think you have shingles, call your doctor right away. There is medicine that can limit the pain and rash. It works best if you start it as soon as symptoms appear. If you are 50 or older, ask your doctor about the shingles vaccine.

Avoid close contact with people until your blisters have healed. A person who has not had chickenpox can get it from exposure to your rash. Avoid contact with pregnant women, babies, and anyone who has a hard time fighting infections (such as someone with HIV, diabetes, or cancer).

Home Treatment

◆ Use an over-the-counter medicine like acetaminophen (Tylenol) or ibuprofen (Advil, Motrin) to relieve fever if your child feels bad or has a high or fast-rising temperature. Read and follow all instructions on the label. Do not give aspirin to anyone younger than 20.

◆ Reduce itching with an oral antihistamine (such as Benadryl or a non-drowsy kind, like Claritin). Before you use these medicines, check the label. They may not be safe for young children or for people with certain health problems. Warm baths with baking soda or Aveeno colloidal oatmeal added to the water also help. Do not use antihistamine creams, because they make it hard to control how much medicine you are using.

◆ Cut your child's nails short to prevent scratching. If he or she scratches off the scabs too early, the sores may get infected and leave scars.

Looking for the Chronic Obstructive Pulmonary Disease (COPD) topic? See page 271.

Cold Sores

When to Call a Doctor

◆ You have cold sores and a fever.

◆ A sore lasts longer than 2 weeks.

◆ You often have outbreaks of cold sores. Your doctor can prescribe a medicine that may help.

Cold sores (fever blisters) are small, red blisters on the lips and outer edge of the mouth. They often weep a clear fluid and scab over after a few days.

Sometimes people confuse cold sores with impetigo (see page 195), which is usually between the nose and upper lip. The fluid from impetigo is cloudy and honey-colored, not clear like the fluid from a cold sore.

The herpes simplex virus causes cold sores. Herpes viruses (chickenpox is another kind) stay in the body after the first infection. Later, something triggers the virus to become active again. You can get a cold sore after a cold, a fever, or stress. A woman's menstrual period can be another trigger.

Sometimes you get cold sores for no clear reason.

Sunlight triggers cold sores in some people. Wear lip balm with sunscreen in it when you are going to be outdoors.

Home Treatment

◆ Do not kiss or have oral sex with anyone while you have a cold sore. This can spread the virus.

◆ Put ice or a cool, wet cloth on the area 3 times a day. This may help reduce redness and swelling.

◆ Use petroleum jelly to ease cracking and dryness.

◆ Apply a nonprescription ointment, such as Abreva, Zilactin, or Ziladent. These products may speed healing.

◆ Use a lip protector such as Blistex or Campho-Phenique to ease the pain. Do not share the product with anyone else.

◆ Be patient. Cold sores usually go away in 7 to 10 days.

Colds

When to Call a Doctor

◆ You have trouble breathing.

◆ You have a high fever. See pages 158 and 160.

◆ You have new shortness of breath, or it gets worse.

◆ You cough up yellow, green, or bloody mucus (sputum) from your lungs and have a fever.

◆ Mucus from your nose is thick (like pus) or bloody.

◆ You have redness in your face or around your eyes, or you have pain in your face, eyes, or teeth that does not get better with home treatment.

◆ Your symptoms are worse than what you would expect with a cold, and you don't think you have the flu. See Flu on page 165.

Everyone gets a cold from time to time. The average child has six colds a year; adults have fewer.

Lots of different viruses cause colds, but the symptoms are usually the same:

◆ Runny nose and sneezing

◆ Red eyes

◆ Sore throat and cough

◆ Headaches and body aches

You will probably feel a cold come on over the course of a couple of days. As the cold gets worse, your nose may get stuffy with thicker mucus. Most colds last a week or two.

There is no cure for the common cold. Antibiotics will not help. If you catch a cold, treat the symptoms.

If you feel like you have a cold all the time, or if cold symptoms last more than 2 weeks, you may have allergies (see page 76) or sinusitis (see page 232).

Home Treatment

Sometimes a cold will lead to a worse infection like bronchitis or pneumonia. Good home treatment of a cold will help you feel better.

◆ Get extra rest. Slow down just a little from your usual routine. You don't need to stay home in bed, but try not to expose others to your cold.

◆ Drink plenty of fluids to stay hydrated. Hot water, herbal tea, or chicken soup will help relieve a stuffy nose and head.

◆ Take an over-the-counter medicine like acetaminophen (Tylenol) or ibuprofen (Advil, Motrin) to relieve aches. Read and follow all instructions on the label. Do not give aspirin to anyone younger than 20.

◆ Use a humidifier in your bedroom and take hot showers to relieve a stuffy nose and head.

◆ If you have streaks of mucus in the back of your throat (postnasal drip), gargle with warm water.

- Use throwaway tissues, not handkerchiefs. This will reduce the chance of spreading the cold to others.

- If your nose is red and raw from rubbing it with tissues, put a dab of petroleum jelly on the sore area.

- Before you use cough or cold medicines or decongestants, check the label. They may not be safe for young children or for people with certain health problems.

- Do not take cold remedies that use several drugs to treat different symptoms. Treat each symptom on its own. Take a decongestant for a stuffy nose and a cough medicine for a cough. See Home Treatment for coughs on page 132.

- Do not use nasal decongestant sprays (such as Afrin) for more than 3 days in a row. Doing so may lead to a "rebound" effect, which makes the mucous membranes in your nose swell up even more.

- Do not take antihistamines for a cold. They don't help.

How to Avoid Colds

- Wash your hands often! Be extra careful during the winter and when you are around people with colds.

- Keep your hands away from your nose, eyes, and mouth. These are the most likely places for a cold virus to enter your body.

- Eat well, and get plenty of sleep and exercise. This keeps your body's immune system strong.

- Do not smoke. If you need help quitting, see page 316.

Colic

When to Call a Doctor

Colic does not need medical care unless it occurs with vomiting, diarrhea, or other signs of a more serious illness. If your baby looks healthy and acts normally when he or she is not crying, and if your emotions can stand the noise for the first 3 to 4 months, you do not need to worry.

But if colic lasts more than 4 hours a day, or if you feel like you need help, call your doctor for advice.

In rare cases, colic may be so severe that you and your doctor may consider a medicine for the baby. Ask about side effects.

Does Your Baby Have Colic?

All babies cry, but colic usually follows the "rule of three": Crying starts in the first 3 to 6 weeks after birth and goes on for more than 3 hours a day, on more than 3 days a week, for more than 3 weeks. The crying tends to be worse at night.

There is no way to prevent colic. It is equally common among boys and girls and among breast-fed and bottle-fed babies.

The good news is that colic goes away as the baby gets older, almost always by the end of the fourth month. It ends sooner for many babies.

More ▶

Home Treatment

A colicky baby may cry no matter what you do, but there are several things you can try. What works one time may not work the next. Be creative, and don't give up.

- Most important: Stay calm. If you start to lose control, take a minute to calm down. Never shake a baby. It can cause brain damage and even death. If you have the option, let family members or friends take a turn trying to comfort the baby.

- Make sure your baby is getting enough to eat, but not too much. The problem may be hunger, not colic.

- Make sure your baby does not swallow too much air while eating.

  - Feed the baby slowly, holding him or her almost upright. Burp your baby regularly. Prop up your baby for 15 to 30 minutes after feeding.

  - If your baby is bottle-fed, use nipples with holes large enough to drip at least 1 drop of cold formula per second. Babies will swallow more air from around the nipple if the hole is too small.

- Heat formula to body temperature. Don't make it too hot.

- Babies may need to suck on something for up to 2 hours a day to be satisfied. If feedings are not enough, use a pacifier.

- Set a schedule for meals, naps, and play. Keep feedings calm and quiet.

- Make sure that your baby does not have a dirty diaper, is not too hot, and is not bored.

- Try to keep the environment around your baby calm. Some babies cry because there is too much light, noise, or activity, or there are too many people around them.

- Try rocking or walking your baby. Putting him or her stomach-down over your knee or arm may help.

- Calm your baby with a car ride or a walk outside. The hum of a clothes dryer, dishwasher, or bubbling fish tank may soothe your baby.

- Don't worry about spoiling a baby during the first few months of life. Comforting a baby makes both of you feel better.

- Do not leave your baby alone for more than 5 to 10 minutes while he or she is crying. After 10 minutes, try the suggestions here again.

Colorectal Cancer

When to Call a Doctor

- Your bowel habits have changed for no clear reason.

- You have bleeding from your rectum or blood in your stools.

- You have constant or frequent diarrhea, constipation, or a feeling that your bowel does not empty completely.

- Your stools have become very thin (they may be as thin as a pencil).

- You have frequent belly pain or new problems with gas or bloating.

- You are losing weight and don't know why.

- You have a family member with colon cancer and want to know how to prevent it in yourself.

- You want to talk about your test options.

Cancer of the colon and rectum is a leading cause of cancer deaths in the United States. Treatment works very well early in the disease and can cure the cancer. But because the cancer usually does not cause symptoms early on, it is often not found until later.

This is why screening tests are important. These tests can help find cancer early, when treatment can work the best. They can also find growths and changes in the colon before they lead to cancer.

Screening Tests

Your doctor may suggest one or more of these or other tests:

Colonoscopy. For this test, doctors use a flexible lighted tube to view the rectum and all of the colon. Doctors can remove any growths or polyps at the same time. Colonoscopy is one of the most thorough screening tests. It also costs more than most of the other tests and is probably the least convenient (you have to do some preparation at home). But if the first result is normal and you are not at high risk, you would only need to have the test every 10 years.

Flexible sigmoidoscopy. As in a colonoscopy, the doctor uses a lighted tube to look for growths and cancers. But the doctor can only view the rectum and the lower part of the colon. If the test finds any growths, you may need a colonoscopy. If the first result is normal and you are not at high risk, you would need to have a sigmoidoscopy every 5 years.

Fecal occult blood test. This test can find hidden blood in your stool. It does not cost much and is easy to do at home, but it's only a first step. If the test finds blood in your stool, you will need more tests. If this is your only screening test, you need it every year.

You may have the option to have other screening tests, such as a test that looks for gene markers in your stool or a test known as virtual colonoscopy.

More

Who Should Get Tested?

◆ All adults ages 50 to 75. If you are older than 75, talk to your doctor about whether testing is a good choice for you.

◆ Adults who are at high risk. You are at high risk if you have a family history of this cancer, are African American, or if you have had colon polyps, ulcerative colitis, or Crohn's disease.

Which test should you have? Some tests may cost less, but you need to have them more often. And in some cases, you may wind up having to have a more expensive test anyway.

 For help deciding which tests are right for you and how often you need them, go to the Web site on the back cover and enter **i924** in the search box. Then talk with your doctor.

Confusion and Memory Loss

When to Call a Doctor

Call 911 if:

◆ Confusion occurs with other signs of a stroke, such as sudden, severe headache; new trouble seeing or speaking; new weakness or numbness; and loss of balance. See page 53.

◆ Confusion and memory loss develop quickly, over a few hours or days. This is called **delirium**. It can be a sign of many serious problems, such as a medicine problem, an infection, an alcohol or drug problem, or a worsening of a long-term illness like heart disease or diabetes.

Call a doctor if:

◆ You are worried that confusion or memory loss is caused by medicine or a health problem.

◆ Confusion or memory loss occurs with changes in behavior or personality.

◆ You have new trouble with familiar things, like how to read or how to tell time, or you get lost in places you know well.

◆ Confusion or memory loss starts to upset your daily life.

It's normal to forget a person's name or lose a set of keys from time to time. But more serious confusion or memory loss needs to be checked out by a doctor. If it comes on quickly, it may be caused by something that needs urgent care.

We all forget things as we get older. It also may take a little longer to remember things as you age. This is normal. But if your memory keeps getting worse—especially if you start to have problems with thinking or emotions too—see your doctor.

Home Treatment

The best way to keep your mind sharp and avoid the problems that can cause confusion is to stay healthy and fit.

◆ Eat a healthy diet, and drink plenty of water (unless your doctor has told you to limit fluids).

◆ Get enough sleep. If you have trouble sleeping, see Sleep Problems on page 236.

◆ Try to reduce stress. Slow down and focus on what you're doing. People often forget things because they have too much on their minds. See Dealing With Stress on page 318.

◆ Keep your body active. Try to get some exercise throughout the week.

◆ Keep your brain active. This is the "use it or lose it" approach.

  ❖ Learn new things. Read. Take a class.

  ❖ Play "brain" games like cards and Scrabble. Do crossword puzzles or other word or number games.

  ❖ Spend time with other people.

◆ Do not drink alcohol.

◆ Do not use illegal drugs.

◆ If you feel depressed (see Are You Depressed? on page 156), tell your doctor. Treatment can help.

Some people take an herb called ginkgo biloba to help with memory. Talk to your doctor before you use this or any other treatment to make sure it works or is safe.

Alzheimer's Disease

Alzheimer's disease damages the part of the brain involved in memory, problem solving, judgment, language, and behavior. It is the most common type of dementia in older adults.

Alzheimer's usually starts with mild memory loss and gets worse over a few years. Medicines may improve some of the thinking and memory problems for a short time, but they do not cure the disease. Over time, Alzheimer's robs people of the ability to take care of themselves. They may become confused and frightened and may strike out at others.

You may wonder how to tell whether memory loss is normal or related to Alzheimer's. Early on, it's not always clear.

But there are some signs you can look for. For example, a person may:

◆ Have trouble making decisions.

◆ Be confused about what time and day it is.

◆ Get lost in places he or she knows well.

◆ Have trouble learning and remembering new information.

◆ Have trouble finding the right words to say what he or she wants to say.

◆ Have more trouble doing daily tasks like cooking a meal or paying bills.

◆ Lose things in strange places, like putting an iron in the freezer or a wristwatch in the sugar bowl.

More

Be Careful With Medicines

Misuse of medicines is a common cause of confusion. This is especially true in older adults, but it can happen at any age. You can help prevent problems by using medicines safely. This includes over-the-counter medicines and supplements.

◆ Take as few medicines as possible. Do not take medicines that you don't need. If you have a medicine and are not sure what it's for, take it to your pharmacist or doctor and ask.

◆ Keep a list of the medicines, vitamins, and herbal products you use. Review the list with your doctor, and bring a copy to anyone who treats you or any pharmacist who fills a prescription for you. Some medicines do not work well together and can cause a bad reaction.

◆ Always take your medicines exactly as your doctor says. Take them at the right time and in the right amount. If you are supposed to take a medicine with food, then do so.

◆ For people who have to take several medicines, it can be hard to keep track of them all. Use a calendar or notepad to list each medicine and what time of day you should take it. Post it on your refrigerator or bathroom cabinet—anyplace where you will see it several times a day. Your pharmacist may be able to suggest products, such as medicine organizers, to help you stay on schedule.

◆ Never take someone else's prescription medicine.

Constipation

When to Call a Doctor

◆ Constipation gets worse or does not improve with home treatment.

◆ Rectal bleeding is heavy (more than a few bright red streaks) or your stools look like black tar.

◆ Rectal bleeding lasts longer than 2 to 3 days after constipation has improved, or any bleeding occurs more than once.

◆ You have sharp or severe belly pain.

◆ You still have rectal pain after you pass a stool, or pain keeps you from passing stools at all.

◆ You have any leaking of stool.

◆ Stools have become consistently thinner (they may be as thin as a pencil).

◆ You cannot pass stools unless you take laxatives.

Constipation means you have trouble passing stools. Some people pass stools 3 times a day. Others do it 3 times a week. No matter what your normal schedule is, if your stools are soft and pass easily, you are not constipated.

Constipation causes cramping and pain in the rectum that gets worse when you try to pass hard, dry stools. If a stool gets stuck in the rectum, mucus and fluid may leak out around it. This may cause you to go back and forth between constipation and diarrhea.

Lack of fiber and too little water in the diet are common reasons for constipation. Other causes include not getting enough exercise, delaying bowel movements, taking certain medicines, and using laxatives too often. Irritable bowel syndrome (see page 197) may also cause constipation.

Toilet training may lead to constipation in young children. Kids who are playing or busy and ignore the urge to pass stools may get constipated. Children and adults who do not like to use toilets away from home may get constipated.

Home Treatment

- Eat more fiber (see page 308).
  - Eat plenty of fruits, vegetables, and whole grains.
  - Eat bran cereal that has at least 10 grams of bran in a serving.
  - Add 2 tablespoons of wheat bran to cereal or soup.
  - Try a product that contains a bulk-forming agent, such as Citrucel, FiberCon, or Metamucil. Start with a dose or less (check the label), and drink extra water to avoid bloating.

- Avoid foods that are high in fat and sugar.
- Drink plenty of water and other fluids.
- Get some exercise every day. A walking program is a good start.
- Set aside a relaxed time for each bowel movement. Urges usually occur sometime after meals. A daily routine (after breakfast, for example) may help.
- Go when you feel the urge, and teach your children to do the same. The bowel sends signals when a stool needs to pass. If you ignore it, the urge will go away and the stool will become dry and hard.
- If you need more help, use a stool softener or a very mild laxative such as Milk of Magnesia. Do not give laxatives or enemas to a child without talking to your child's doctor first. And don't use mineral oil or any other laxative for more than 2 weeks unless your doctor tells you to.

If your child is constipated and has pain, try this:

- Put the child in a warm bath, and add about ½ teaspoon of baking soda to the tub. This may help relax the muscles that keep stool inside the rectum.
- If your child is 6 months old or older and the warm bath doesn't work, use 1 or 2 glycerin suppositories to make the stool easier to pass. Use these suppositories only once or twice. If they don't help, talk to your doctor.

Looking for the Coronary Artery Disease topic? See page 275.

Cough

When to Call a Doctor

◆ You have a fever and a cough that brings up yellow, green, or bloody mucus from the lungs.

◆ You are in poor health, and coughing makes you feel weak or very tired.

◆ Any cough lasts longer than 2 weeks.

◆ You are short of breath.

Coughing is the body's way of keeping the lungs clear.

◆ **Productive coughs** bring up mucus (sputum) from the lungs. If you have this kind of cough, you should not try to stop it with cough medicine.

◆ **Nonproductive coughs** are dry coughs that do not bring up mucus. You may get a dry, hacking cough after a cold or after being exposed to dust or smoke. A dry cough that follows a viral illness like a cold may last up to 2 weeks and get worse at night.

Longtime smokers often have a frequent dry cough. If you have a "smoker's cough," it means your lungs are always irritated.

A common type of blood pressure medicine can cause a dry cough. If your cough began after you started taking an ACE inhibitor for high blood pressure, tell your doctor. You may need to switch to another medicine.

Chronic coughs are often caused by the backflow (reflux) of stomach acid into the lungs and throat. If you think problems with stomach acid reflux may be causing your cough, see Heartburn on page 183.

Home Treatment

◆ Drink plenty of water to stay hydrated. Water helps soothe the throat. Or try hot tea or hot water with honey or lemon juice in it. Do not give honey to a child younger than 1 year.

◆ Suck on cough drops or hard candy if your throat hurts. Expensive, medicine-flavored cough drops do not work any better than cheap, candy-flavored ones or hard candy.

◆ To ease a dry cough at night, use extra pillows to raise your head.

◆ Do not take cold remedies that use several drugs to treat different symptoms. Treat each symptom on its own.

◆ Use cough medicines wisely. Coughing can be good, because it brings up mucus from the lungs and helps prevent infection. People with asthma and other lung diseases need to cough. But if you have a dry, hacking cough that doesn't bring anything up, ask your doctor to suggest a good cough suppressant.

◆ Before you use cough or cold medicines or decongestants, check the label. They may not be safe for young children or for people with certain health problems.

◆ Do not take anyone else's prescription cough medicine.

◆ Avoid dust and smoke, or wear a mask to protect yourself.

◆ If you smoke, quit. See page 316 for help.

Type of Cough	Possible Causes and Treatment
Baby's loud cough like a seal's bark	Croup (see below)
Dry cough in the morning that gets better as the day goes on	Dry air; smoking. Drink more fluids. Humidify the bedroom. Stop smoking. Also see Cough, p. 132.
Hacking, dry cough; may be worse at night. Common for several weeks after a cold.	Postnasal drip, smoking, or mild asthma. Drink more fluids. Try a decongestant. Stop smoking. Also see Cough, p. 132, and Asthma, p. 266.
Cough that brings up mucus. Common after a cold or flu.	Bronchitis, p. 108; pneumonia, p. 216; sinusitis, p. 232
Dry cough that starts suddenly after a choking episode, most often in a baby or young child	Object in the throat. See Choking, p. 28.

Croup

When to Call a Doctor

Call 911 if:

◆ Your child stops breathing or starts to turn blue.

◆ Your child has serious trouble breathing. It can be hard to know for sure, but a child who is having trouble breathing may:

❖ Breathe very fast.

❖ Drool or grunt with each breath.

❖ Not be able to speak, cry, or make sounds.

❖ Use the neck, chest, and belly muscles to breathe. The skin may "suck in" between the ribs with each breath, and the child may need to sit up and lean forward to tilt the nose up.

❖ Flare the nostrils with each breath.

❖ Have a gray, blotchy, or blue color to the skin. Look for color changes in the nail beds, lips, and earlobes.

Call a doctor if:

◆ Your child has a bad cough and some trouble breathing and does not get any better after 30 minutes of home treatment.

◆ Your child's cough has not started getting better after 2 days.

Croup can be scary but is not usually serious. The main symptom of croup is a harsh cough that sounds like a seal's bark. A fever up to 101°F is also common.

Croup may last 2 to 5 days. It usually gets worse at night, but it tends to get better with each passing night.

More ➤

Croup occurs most often in children from 6 months to 4 years of age. It usually happens when a child has a viral infection, like a cold.

Home Treatment

◆ Do whatever you can to calm your child. Crying can make it harder to breathe.

◆ Get moisture into the air to make it easier for your child to breathe. Use water in a cool humidifier. Set your child in your lap, and let the cool vapor blow into your child's face. Do not use a hot vaporizer to blow moisture directly into your child's face.

◆ If your child does not improve after several minutes, take him or her into the bathroom and turn on all the hot-water faucets to create steam. Close the door, and sit with your child while he or she breathes the moist air for several minutes.

◆ If your child's breathing still does not improve, bundle him or her up and go outside into the cool night air for a few minutes.

◆ Before you give cough or cold medicines to a child, check the label. They may not be safe for young children.

◆ Give your child an over-the-counter medicine like acetaminophen (Tylenol) or ibuprofen (Advil, Motrin). Read and follow all instructions on the label. Do not give aspirin to anyone younger than 20.

Dandruff

When to Call a Doctor

Call if daily shampooing or shampooing with a dandruff shampoo does not control dandruff.

You get dandruff when the skin cells of the scalp flake off. This flaking is natural and occurs all over your body. On the scalp, though, flakes can mix with oil and dust to form dandruff. Some people are more likely to get it than others.

Cradle Cap

Cradle cap is an oily, yellow scaling or crusting on a baby's scalp. It is caused by a buildup of normal oils on the skin.

If your baby has cradle cap:

◆ Wash your baby's head with baby shampoo once a day. Wet your baby's head, then gently scrub the scalp with a soft-bristled brush for a few minutes to remove the scales. A soft toothbrush works well. Shampoo and rinse well.

◆ It may help to rub mineral oil on your baby's scalp an hour before you shampoo it. This will loosen the scales.

◆ If baby shampoo doesn't work, try a dandruff shampoo, such as Selsun Blue, Head & Shoulders, or Sebulex. Be careful to keep these shampoos out of your baby's eyes.

◆ If the rash looks irritated and red, a mild hydrocortisone cream (such as Cortaid) may help.

Home Treatment

◆ Wash your hair every day with any shampoo you choose. This is often enough to control dandruff.

◆ If you have a lot of dandruff or itching, try a dandruff shampoo such as Head & Shoulders, Sebulex, T/Gel, or Tegrin. Work the shampoo into your scalp, and leave it on for several minutes. Then rinse well.

◆ You can treat eyebrows, ears, and beards with a gentle shampoo.

Looking for the Depression topic? See page 280.

Looking for the Diabetes topic? See page 284.

Diaper Rash

When to Call a Doctor

◆ The diaper rash is very red or raw, looks very sore, or has blisters, pus, peeling areas, or crusty patches.

◆ The rash is mainly in the skin creases. This may mean that your baby has a yeast infection.

◆ A rash does not get better after 3 days.

Diaper rash is a skin reaction, usually to the moisture and bacteria in a baby's urine and stools, to the soap used to wash diapers, or to the diapers. The rash is uncomfortable but usually not serious.

Symptoms of the rash are a red bottom and thighs. It will be easy to recognize diaper rash after you have seen it the first time.

Home Treatment

If your baby gets diaper rash often, these are good tips to follow all the time.

◆ Change wet or dirty diapers as soon as you can. Check the diaper at least every 2 hours. Use a washcloth and water to rinse the skin in the diaper area at every diaper change. Let the diaper area air-dry for 5 to 10 minutes when you can. Wash the area with a mild soap once a day.

◆ Do not use plastic pants. They trap moisture against the skin.

◆ Protect healthy skin near the rash with Desitin, Diaparene, A & D Ointment, or zinc oxide cream. Put the cream only on dry, unbroken skin. Stop using the cream if a rash develops or if it seems to slow down the healing.

◆ Try another brand of diapers. Some babies react to one kind better than another. Unscented, white diapers may not irritate the skin as much as scented or colored ones.

◆ Do not use bulky diapers or ones with lots of layers.

◆ If you use cloth diapers, wash them with mild detergent, and rinse twice. Do not use bleach or fabric softeners.

◆ Try changing laundry soaps if a rash does not clear.

Diarrhea, Age 11 and Younger

When to Call a Doctor

Call 911 if:

◆ Your child faints, or you cannot wake him or her.

◆ Your child has signs of severe dehydration. These include fast breathing and heartbeat, not acting alert, or having trouble waking up.

Call a doctor if:

◆ Your child has signs of moderate dehydration. These include sunken eyes, no tears, and a dry mouth and tongue; a sunken soft spot on your baby's head; little or no urine for 8 hours; or skin that sags when you pinch it.

◆ The diarrhea is bloody.

◆ The urine is bloody or cola-colored.

◆ Your child refuses to drink or cannot take in enough liquid to replace lost fluids.

◆ Severe diarrhea (large, loose stools every 1 to 2 hours) lasts longer than:

 ❖ 4 hours in a baby younger than 3 months.

 ❖ 8 hours in a baby 3 to 6 months old.

 ❖ 24 hours in a child 7 months to 11 years old.

◆ Mild to moderate diarrhea continues without a clear cause or other symptoms for longer than:

 ❖ 24 hours in a baby younger than 3 months.

 ❖ 1 to 2 days in a baby 3 to 6 months old.

 ❖ 4 days in a child 7 months to 11 years old.

◆ Your child has a fever with diarrhea for more than 12 hours. Also see the fever guidelines on pages 158 and 160.

◆ Your child has severe belly pain.

◆ Your child has pain in just one part of the belly, especially the lower right belly. See the picture on page 69. It may be hard to tell where the pain is in a small child.

For diarrhea in people age 12 and older, see page 138.

Diarrhea in children is often caused by:

◆ Eating unusual kinds or amounts of food. A baby's digestive system sometimes cannot handle large amounts of juice, fruit, or even milk. Breast-fed babies are less likely to get diarrhea.

◆ Viral stomach flu or another illness. Stomach flu often starts with vomiting that is followed in a few hours (sometimes 8 to 12 hours or longer) by diarrhea. Sometimes there is no diarrhea.

Babies and young children need special care when they have diarrhea because they can quickly get dehydrated. This means the body has lost too much fluid. If your child has bad diarrhea, watch for signs that he or she is looking sicker, and make sure your child gets enough fluids.

Home Treatment

Diarrhea in babies up to 1 year

◆ If your baby is breast-fed, breast-feed more often than usual to replace lost fluids.

◆ If your baby is formula-fed, feed him or her more often than usual with small amounts at each feeding to make up for lost fluids.

◆ If there are signs of dehydration (see When to Call a Doctor), give your child a children's oral electrolyte solution (such as Pedialyte) along with the feedings. The amount your baby needs depends on his or her weight and how dehydrated he or she is. You can give the electrolyte solution a little at a time in a dropper, spoon, or bottle. For children over 6 months, add a pinch of an artificial sweetener (such as NutraSweet), sugar-free flavored drink mix (such as Kool-Aid), or sugar-free gelatin dessert powder to make it taste better.

◆ Do not use oral electrolyte solutions as the only source of fluid for more than 12 to 24 hours.

◆ Do not use sports drinks, fruit juice, or soda to treat dehydration. These drinks have too much sugar and not enough of the minerals your baby needs.

◆ Do not give your baby plain water.

◆ Offer your baby solid foods that are easy to digest (cereal, strained bananas, mashed potatoes) if he or she was eating them before.

◆ Protect the diaper area with Desitin, Diaparene, A+D Ointment, or zinc oxide cream. Babies often get diaper rash after diarrhea.

Diarrhea in children 1 through 11 years

◆ Give ½ cup to 1 cup of a children's oral electrolyte solution, fruit juice mixed to half strength with water, or plain water (if the child is eating food) each hour. Add an artificial sweetener (such as NutraSweet) if needed. Let your child drink as much as he or she wants.

◆ Do not use an electrolyte solution as the only source of fluids and nutrients for more than 24 hours.

◆ Do not give your child full-strength juice, chicken broth, sports drinks, soft drinks, or ginger ale. These drinks do not have the right mix of minerals and sugar to restore lost fluids, and they may make the diarrhea worse.

◆ Give your child frequent small meals with foods that are easy to digest. Cooked cereal, crackers, mashed potatoes, applesauce, and bananas are good choices. Avoid foods that have a lot of sugar.

As the child gets better, the stools will be smaller and less frequent. Some types of diarrhea may cause watery stools for 4 to 6 days. You can treat the illness at home as long as the child gets enough fluids and nutrients, is urinating normal amounts, and seems to be getting better.

Diarrhea, Age 12 and Older

Diarrhea has many causes—stomach flu, food poisoning, antibiotics and other medicines, certain foods, and food additives such as sorbitol and olestra. For some people, stress or anxiety can be a cause. Irritable bowel syndrome (see page 197) may cause frequent or long-term diarrhea.

Drinking untreated water that contains parasites, viruses, or bacteria is another cause. Just because water looks clean does not mean it is. You may get diarrhea a few days to a few weeks later.

Home Treatment

◆ Do not eat any food for several hours or until you feel better. Keep taking small, frequent sips of water or a rehydration drink (see page 33).

◆ Do not take diarrhea medicines like Pepto-Bismol or Imodium during the first 6 hours. After that, use them only if you do not have a fever, cramping, bloody stools, or other symptoms.

  ❖ Do not take more than the label tells you to.

  ❖ Stop the medicine as soon as stools thicken.

◆ After the first 24 hours (or sooner, if you feel better), try some mild foods. Bananas, rice, applesauce, dry toast, and crackers are all good choices. Avoid spicy foods, fruits other than bananas, alcohol, and caffeine until 48 hours after all symptoms have gone away.

◆ Avoid dairy products for 3 days after all symptoms have gone away.

◆ Be careful not to get dehydrated. This can happen when your body loses a lot of fluids. See page 31.

Lactose Intolerance

People whose bodies produce too little of the enzyme lactase have trouble digesting the lactose (sugar) in milk. If you are lactose-intolerant, you may get gas, bloating, cramps, and diarrhea after you drink milk or eat milk products.

To reduce your symptoms:

◆ Do not eat or drink large amounts of milk products all at once.

◆ Try cheese instead of milk. It may be easier on your stomach, because most of the lactose is removed during processing.

◆ Eat yogurt made with active cultures. These have enzymes that digest the lactose in milk.

◆ Drink pretreated milk (such as Lactaid), or try enzyme tablets (such as Lactaid or Dairy Ease).

◆ You may be able to tolerate milk if you drink it with snacks or meals.

If you have severe lactose intolerance:

◆ Read food labels to avoid all forms of lactose.

◆ Be sure to include nondairy sources of calcium in your diet. You can get good calcium from tofu, broccoli, certain greens, and calcium-fortified orange juice. Ask your doctor or dietitian if you need to take a calcium supplement.

◆ Plan your diet so it gives you the nutrients that milk products would normally provide.

Dizziness and Vertigo

When to Call a Doctor

Call 911 if:

◆ Vertigo occurs with severe headache, confusion, loss of speech or sight, weakness in the arms or legs, or numbness in any part of the body.

◆ Lightheadedness occurs with chest pain or pressure or any other symptoms of a heart attack. See page 38.

◆ Someone who is feeling dizzy faints, and you cannot wake the person.

◆ Vertigo or loss of balance occurs with severe headache, stiff neck, fever, seizure, or feeling grouchy or confused.

◆ Severe lightheadedness lasts a long time and occurs with a sudden change in heart rate.

Call a doctor if:

◆ You are lightheaded or have vertigo after an injury.

◆ You have severe vertigo, or vertigo with hearing loss.

◆ You think a medicine may be making you dizzy.

◆ You have vertigo often and have not seen your doctor about it.

◆ Vertigo lasts longer than 5 days.

◆ Your vertigo is a lot different than past attacks.

◆ You feel lightheaded several times during just a few days.

◆ You feel lightheaded, and your pulse is less than 50 or more than 150 beats per minute. See page 48 to learn how to take your pulse.

Dizziness is a word people use for two different feelings: lightheadedness and vertigo. Knowing what these mean may help you and your doctor narrow down the list of possible problems.

Lightheadedness is a feeling that you are about to faint.

◆ You may feel unsteady but do not feel like you are moving.

◆ You may feel sick to your stomach, vomit, or faint.

◆ It usually improves when you lie down.

Feeling lightheaded now and then is common. There are many reasons why you might feel lightheaded. Some of the most common ones are in the chart on page 141.

Lightheadedness is usually not a cause for concern unless it is severe, happens often, or occurs with symptoms like heartbeat changes or fainting.

Problem	Possible Causes
Lightheadedness	Drop in blood pressure from getting up too fast
	Flu, cold, or allergies
	Dehydration, see p. 31
	Medicines
	Stress or anxiety, see p. 80
	Blood loss (could either be visible or hidden inside the body; see Bleeding Emergencies on p. 17)
	Heart rhythm problem, see p. 181
	Heart attack, see p. 38
Vertigo	Inner ear problem (benign positional vertigo, labyrinthitis, Ménière's disease)
	Migraine headache, see p. 176
	Multiple sclerosis or other nerve problems
	Stroke, see p. 53
	Brain tumor (rare)

Vertigo is the feeling that you or your surroundings are spinning, whirling, or tilting when there is no actual movement. It may make you sick to your stomach. You may have trouble standing or walking and may lose your balance.

Vertigo is often related to an inner ear problem. The most common form is triggered by moving your head. This is called **benign positional vertigo**. Or vertigo can be caused by a cold (viral labyrinthitis).

Home Treatment

◆ If you feel lightheaded, lie down for a minute or two. This lets more blood flow to your brain. Then sit up slowly. Stay seated for a minute or two before you slowly stand up.

◆ If you are having vertigo, do not lie flat on your back. Propping yourself up slightly may help. Keep your eyes open.

◆ If you have a cold or the flu, rest and drink extra fluids.

◆ Do not drive, operate machinery, or do anything else that might be dangerous if you have vertigo or feel lightheaded. You might hurt yourself if you fall or faint.

 There are balance exercises that can help if you have problems with vertigo. To learn how to do them, go to the Web site on the back cover and enter **t822** in the search box.

Dry Skin

When to Call a Doctor

◆ You itch all over your body, but there is no clear cause or rash.

◆ Itching is so bad that you cannot sleep, and home treatment does not help.

◆ You have open sores from scratching, or your skin is red and swollen.

Dry, itchy, flaky skin is the most common skin problem, especially in winter. Dry indoor air is a common cause. Taking a lot of hot showers or baths can also dry your skin.

Home Treatment

◆ Take baths instead of showers. Showers strip the natural oil that helps hold moisture in the skin. Baths are much kinder to the skin. If you take showers, keep them short and not too hot.

◆ Use bath oils when you bathe. Be careful not to slip.

◆ Use mild soaps, such as Dove or Cetaphil. You may only need to use soap under your arms and in the groin area.

◆ Use a moisturizing lotion right after you bathe.

◆ For very dry hands or feet, try this for a night: Apply a thin layer of petroleum jelly, and wear thin cotton gloves or socks to bed.

◆ Try not to scratch. It can damage the skin.

Relief From Itching

◆ Keep the itchy area well moisturized. Dry skin may make itching worse.

◆ Take an oatmeal bath: Wrap 1 cup of oatmeal in a cotton cloth, and boil as you would to cook it. Use this as a sponge, and bathe in cool-to-warm water without soap. Or try an Aveeno colloidal oatmeal bath.

◆ Use calamine lotion on itchy insect bites or plant rashes.

◆ Try a nonprescription 1% hydrocortisone cream for small itchy areas. Do not use it on the face or genitals. If itching is severe, your doctor may prescribe a stronger steroid cream or ointment.

◆ Try a nonprescription oral antihistamine such as Benadryl or Chlor-Trimeton. Some types, such as Claritin, Alavert, and Zyrtec, are less likely to make you sleepy. Before you use these medicines, check the label. They may not be safe for young children or for people with certain health problems.

◆ Cut nails short or wear gloves at night to prevent scratching.

◆ Wear cotton or silk clothing. Do not wear wool and acrylic fabrics next to the skin.

Ear Infections

This topic covers the two most common kinds of ear infections:

- **Swimmer's ear**, which affects the ear canal.

- **Middle ear infections.** These are very common in children. Middle ear infections are worse than ear canal infections because they are deeper in the ear and can cause more problems.

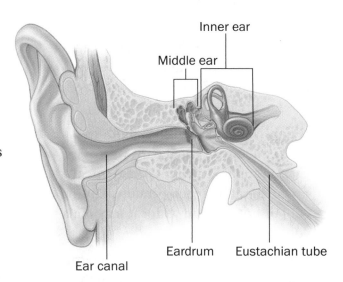

Infections can occur in the ear canal, middle ear, or inner ear.

Swimmer's Ear

When to Call a Doctor

- There is pus or blood draining from the ear.

- Both the ear canal and the outer ear are red.

- There is redness or swelling around or behind the ear.

- The ear canal is swollen, red, and very painful.

- Ear pain follows a cold.

- You have ear pain with fever.

- You feel dizzy or unsteady.

- Symptoms do not get better after 3 days of home treatment.

Swimmer's ear is an irritation or infection of the ear canal. It often develops after water, sand, or dirt gets in the ear canal.

Other causes include a cut inside the ear or an injury from a cotton swab or other object; too much earplug use; soap or shampoo buildup; and skin problems such as eczema and psoriasis.

If you have swimmer's ear, your ear will probably hurt, itch, and feel full. The ear canal may be swollen. A bad infection can cause discharge from the ear and possibly some hearing loss.

Unlike in a middle ear infection (see page 145), the pain of swimmer's ear is worse when you press on the "tag" in front of the ear, touch your earlobe, or chew.

More

Home Treatment

◆ Make sure there is not an object or insect in the ear. See page 33.

◆ If the eardrum may have ruptured or there is pus or blood draining from the ear, do not put eardrops or anything else into the ear unless a doctor has told you to.

◆ Gently rinse the ear using a bulb syringe and a mixture of equal parts white vinegar and rubbing alcohol. Make sure the mixture is at body temperature. Putting cool or hot fluids in your ear may make you dizzy.

◆ Keep water out of the ear until the irritation clears up. You can use cotton that is lightly coated with petroleum jelly as an earplug. Do not use plastic earplugs.

◆ If the ear itches, try nonprescription swimmer's eardrops before and after your ears get wet.

◆ To insert eardrops, have the person lie down with the ear facing up. Warm the drops by rolling the container between your hands. Place drops on the outer ear near the opening of the ear canal, and gently wiggle the ear until the drops flow in. Pulling the ear up and back will help.

Never stick a dropper into the ear canal.

◆ Put a warm, moist cloth on the ear to ease ear pain, or use a heating pad set on low. Do not use a heating pad on a baby or a child who cannot tell you if it's too hot. Do not send your child to bed with a heating pad.

◆ Take an over-the-counter medicine like acetaminophen (Tylenol) or ibuprofen (Advil, Motrin) for pain. Read and follow all instructions on the label. Do not give aspirin to anyone younger than 20.

Preventing Swimmer's Ear

◆ Keep ears dry. After you swim or shower, shake your head to get water out of the ear canals. (Never shake a baby's head.) Gently dry the ears with the corner of a tissue or towel. You can also use a hair dryer set on low.

◆ After you swim or shower, put a few drops of rubbing alcohol, or alcohol mixed with an equal amount of white vinegar, in the ear. Pull the ear up and back to let the liquid go deep into the ear canal. Then tilt your head and let it drain out. You can also use nonprescription drops (Star-Otic, Swim-Ear).

◆ Never use cotton swabs, hairpins, or other objects to clean wax out of the ears. This can damage the ear. See page 148 for tips on removing earwax safely.

◆ Avoid wearing earplugs for long periods of time.

◆ Try to keep soap and shampoo out of the ear canal. To remove dirt or sand that gets into the ear, spray a gentle stream of warm water from the shower or a bulb syringe into the ear; then tip your head to let the water drain out.

Middle Ear Infections

When to Call a Doctor

◆ Ear pain is severe or gets worse even with home treatment.

◆ Ear pain occurs with other signs of serious illness, such as headache with severe stiff neck, fever, or feeling grouchy or confused. See page 161.

◆ Your baby keeps pulling or rubbing an ear and seems to be in pain (crying, screaming).

◆ Your child has a fever over 102°F with other signs of an ear infection. Also see pages 158 and 160.

◆ A baby younger than 3 months has a fever of 100.4°F or higher.

◆ There is pus or blood draining from the ear.

◆ Your child is not getting better after 48 hours of treatment with an antibiotic.

◆ Your child has ear tubes and has an earache or ear drainage.

◆ There is redness or swelling around or behind the ear.

◆ Your child cannot move the muscles in his or her face normally.

◆ Mild ear pain lasts longer than 3 to 4 days.

A middle ear infection (otitis media) often develops during a cold. Colds can cause the eustachian tube, which connects the middle ear to the throat, to swell and close. Fluid then builds up in the middle ear. Bacteria or viruses can grow in the fluid, causing an infection.

Symptoms of a middle ear infection include:

◆ Ear pain. Children who can't talk yet may tug on their painful ears.

◆ Dizziness.

◆ Ringing or a feeling of fullness in the ear.

◆ Hearing loss.

◆ Fever, headache, and runny nose.

The trapped, infected fluid puts pressure on the eardrum. If there is pus or blood draining from the ear, the eardrum may have ruptured. Ear pain caused by an infection usually improves once an eardrum ruptures.

A single eardrum rupture usually is not serious. Repeated eardrum ruptures can lead to hearing loss.

Fluid buildup (effusion) in the middle ear may also occur after an infection has cleared. There may be no symptoms, or there may be minor hearing loss and mild discomfort. Fluid buildup that occurs after an infection usually does not need treatment unless it lasts longer than 3 or 4 months and causes hearing loss. See What About Ear Tubes? on page 147.

More ➡

Home Treatment

◆ Put a warm washcloth on the ear to relieve pain, or use a heating pad set on low. Do not use a heating pad on a baby or a child who cannot tell you if it's too hot. Do not send your child to bed with a heating pad.

◆ Give your child an over-the-counter medicine like acetaminophen (Tylenol) or ibuprofen (Advil, Motrin) for pain. Read and follow all instructions on the label. Do not give aspirin to anyone younger than 20.

◆ Have your child drink plenty of clear liquids.

◆ If the eardrum ruptures, avoid getting water in the ear for 3 to 4 weeks. Showers or baths are fine, but do not let your child soak his or her head in the tub.

Does Your Child Need Antibiotics?

Antibiotics can treat ear infections, but most children with ear infections get better without them. If the care you give at home relieves pain, and if your child is feeling better after a few days, your child may not need antibiotics.

There are exceptions to this. Your child may need antibiotics right away if:

◆ He or she is younger than 2. The risk of other problems is higher for very young children. Also, a loss of hearing for even a short time may affect how your child learns to talk.

◆ Your child is very ill, has a high fever, or is in severe pain.

◆ Your child has a serious long-term health problem (like heart disease or cystic fibrosis).

In most other cases, your doctor may suggest that you wait 48 hours before you give your child antibiotics. If after 48 hours your child has not improved and needs antibiotics, you will have to wait at least another 48 hours for the antibiotics to take effect.

There are good reasons not to use antibiotics unless you really need them:

◆ Antibiotics can cost a lot.

◆ You will probably have to see the doctor to get a prescription. This costs you time and money.

◆ Antibiotics can have harmful side effects, such as diarrhea, vomiting, and skin rashes.

◆ Your child could be allergic to the antibiotic.

◆ The most important reason of all: If you take antibiotics when you don't need them, they may not work when you do need them. Each time you take antibiotics, you are more likely to carry some bacteria that were not killed by the medicine. Over time, these bacteria get tougher and can cause worse infections. To treat them, you may need different, stronger, and more costly antibiotics.

 If you are not sure what's best for your child and need help deciding, go to the Web site on the back cover and enter **i279** in the search box.

Preventing Childhood Ear Infections

- If you can, breast-feed your baby. Breast-fed babies have fewer ear infections. If you bottle-feed your baby, hold the baby upright to drink. Never let a baby or young child lie down with or go to sleep with a bottle.

- Do not smoke in your home or around your children.

- Take your child to a smaller day care center. Being around fewer children means less contact with germs and illness.

- Wean your child from his or her pacifier by about 6 months of age. Babies who use their pacifiers after 12 months of age are more likely to get ear infections.

- Wash your hands and your child's hands often.

- Make sure your child's immunizations are up to date. See page 324.

What About Ear Tubes?

Some children seem to get ear infections all the time. These children often develop fluid behind the eardrum and hearing loss. The hearing loss is usually temporary, but it is more of a concern in children age 2 and younger. Normal hearing is important when young children are learning to talk.

If your baby or young child often has ear infections and fluid in the ear, you may want to talk to your child's doctor about ear tubes. Ear tubes are put in the eardrums to drain fluid and help restore good hearing.

The doctor may want to test your child's hearing first. If there is no hearing loss, you may choose to take a "wait and see" approach for a few months.

 To help you decide whether ear tubes are right for your child, go to the Web site on the back cover and enter **e339** in the search box.

Earwax

When to Call a Doctor

- Earwax is still hard, dry, and packed after 1 week of home treatment.

- Earwax causes ringing in your ears, a full feeling in your ears, or hearing loss.

- You have nausea or balance problems along with earwax.

- An earwax problem develops in a person who has a ruptured eardrum or ear tubes or who has had previous ear surgery.

Earwax helps keep the ears clean and keeps out dust and water. Normally, earwax drains freely from the ears and does not cause problems.

As a rule, it is best to leave earwax alone. You can avoid most earwax problems by not using cotton swabs in your ears.

More

Once in a while, earwax will build up, get hard, and cause some hearing loss or discomfort. Poking at the wax with cotton swabs, fingers, or other objects will only push the wax deeper into the ear canal and pack it against the eardrum.

You should be able to take care of most earwax problems with home treatment. But when wax is tightly packed, you may need professional help to remove it.

Home Treatment

Do not use home treatment if you think the eardrum is ruptured, if there is pus or blood draining from the ear, or if the person has ear tubes.

To remove earwax safely, try one of these methods:

◆ Place 2 drops of warm (body temperature) mineral oil in the ear twice a day for 1 or 2 days to soften and loosen the wax. Then use the spray from a warm, gentle shower or a bulb syringe to remove the wax. Spray the water into the ear, and then tip the head to let the wax drain out.

◆ Each night for 1 to 2 weeks, use a nonprescription wax softener (such as Debrox or Murine), then gently flush the ear with warm water from a bulb syringe. Make sure the water is warm but not hot. Putting cool or hot fluids in the ear may make you dizzy.

Eating Disorders

When to Call a Doctor

Call a counselor or your doctor if you notice any of these warning signs:

◆ Unrealistic body image or an intense fear of gaining weight

◆ Extreme weight loss in a short period of time

◆ Frequent vomiting

◆ Frequent use of laxatives or diuretics (water pills)

◆ Constant dieting or a constant focus on food

◆ Excessive, rigid exercise routines

◆ Loss of menstrual periods

◆ Withdrawal from family and friends

In a culture where "thin is in," many of us have skipped meals or dieted to try to lose weight. But unlike typical dieters, people who have eating disorders are affected by strong psychological issues that cause abnormal eating. The problem tends to run in families.

Anorexia, bulimia, and binge eating are the most common eating disorders.

Anorexia

People with anorexia force themselves to follow strict, severe diets even when they do not need to lose weight. The problem occurs most often in teenage girls and young women.

Signs of anorexia include:

◆ Refusing to eat but being focused on food.

◆ Exercising all the time.

◆ Extreme weight loss and loss of menstrual periods.

◆ Thinking you are fat when in fact you are very thin.

◆ Low self-esteem.

◆ Denying the problem.

Bulimia

People with bulimia eat large amounts of food at once and then vomit or use laxatives or diuretics to get rid of the food. This pattern is called binge eating and purging. Emotional stress, not hunger, usually triggers binges.

Signs of bulimia include:

◆ Dry skin and brittle hair.

◆ Depression and mood swings.

◆ Thinking you are fat when you are at a normal weight. Most people with bulimia look healthy.

◆ Secrecy. People with bulimia usually know they have a problem but will try to hide it.

Binge Eating

Binge eaters eat huge amounts of food at once. They will take in thousands of calories at a time, quickly and without pleasure. Because they do not purge the food (vomit), people with this problem often become obese.

What to Do

If you know or suspect that you or someone you know has an eating disorder, get help. Eating disorders need professional treatment. Without it, they can lead to major health problems or even death.

Treatment usually involves nutrition counseling, therapy for the person and the family, and medicine. In extreme cases, the person may need to stay in a hospital.

Teach Healthy Attitudes

You can help your children build healthy relationships with food and their bodies.

◆ Teach and model healthy eating and exercise habits at home and at school.

◆ Help young people build confidence and self-esteem. Accept them for who they are, not how they look.

◆ Be careful about urging a young person to lose weight. Let people know that you love them no matter how much they weigh.

◆ Set realistic expectations for your child. Trying to live up to unrealistic ones may lead to an eating disorder.

◆ Be alert to the stress in your child's life. Let your child know you are there to listen and help.

149

Erection Problems

When to Call a Doctor

◆ An erection lasts longer than 3 hours.

◆ You took an erection-producing medicine in the past 24 hours, and you are having chest pain. **Do not take nitroglycerin!** See Chest Pain on page 119.

◆ You cannot have an erection at all, or you think the cause may be physical.

◆ You have erection problems along with urinary problems, pain in your lower belly or lower back, or fever.

◆ Your erection problems started after a recent injury.

◆ You think your erection problems may be caused by a medicine.

Erection problems are common. At some time in their lives, most men have trouble getting an erection or having one that lasts long enough to have sex.

Having an erection problem from time to time is normal and is usually nothing to worry about. But if you often cannot get or maintain an erection, you may want to work with your doctor to find the cause.

Erection problems can be caused by:

◆ Problems with blood vessels, nerves, or hormones. These can be related to diabetes, heart disease, injuries, and other health problems.

◆ Medicines. Blood pressure medicines, water pills (diuretics), and mood-altering drugs can all have sexual side effects.

◆ Alcohol.

◆ Smoking.

◆ Depression, stress, grief, or relationship problems.

As you get older, it may take longer to get erections, and they may be less firm. But with the right approach, healthy men can have erections at any age.

Home Treatment

◆ Rule out medicines as a cause. Ask your doctor or pharmacist whether any that you take can have sexual side effects.

◆ Limit alcohol. Have no more than 2 drinks a day.

◆ If you smoke, quit. Smoking makes it harder for the blood vessels in the penis to relax and let blood flow in. If you need help quitting, see page 316.

◆ Try to reduce stress. See page 318. Regular exercise may help too.

◆ Take time for more foreplay.

◆ Talk to your partner about your concerns. If you and your partner have trouble talking about sex, see a therapist who can help you talk about it together. Reading books about sex with your partner may also help.

◆ Find out if you can have erections at other times. If you get erections when you masturbate or have them when you first wake up, the cause is more likely emotional than physical.

- Talk to your doctor about medicines that can help, such as Cialis, Levitra, or Viagra. These drugs can make heart problems worse in some people, so check with your doctor first. For help deciding whether these medicines are right for you, go to the Web site on the back cover and enter **j763** in the search box.

- There are also devices that can help with erections. Talk to your doctor if you want to learn more about them.

Eye Problems

This topic covers three common problems:

- Pinkeye
- Dry eyes
- Blood in the eye

If you have other symptoms, be sure to check the Eye and Vision Problems chart on page 63.

Pinkeye

When to Call a Doctor

- There is a new difference between the sizes of the pupils.
- The skin around the eye or eyelid is red.
- You have blurring or loss of vision that does not clear at all when you blink.
- You have pain in the eye, not just irritation.
- Light is very painful for your eye.
- You think you may have an object in the eye. See page 35.
- The eye is red, and there is a yellow, green, or bloody discharge that does not begin to go away in 24 hours. You may need antibiotics.
- Pinkeye lasts longer than 7 days.
- Your eye has not improved within 48 hours after you start using antibiotics.
- You wear contact lenses, and you have pinkeye.

More ➤

Pinkeye is inflammation of the conjunctiva, which lines the eyelid and the surface of the eye. Pinkeye is also called conjunctivitis.

Pinkeye may be caused by:

◆ Infection with a virus or bacteria. This kind of pinkeye spreads very easily from person to person.

◆ Dry air, allergies, smoke, and chemicals. This kind of pinkeye does not spread from person to person.

If you have pinkeye, you may have redness in the whites of your eyes, red and swollen eyelids, lots of tears, itching or burning, and a sandy feeling in your eyes. Light may hurt your eyes more than usual. And there may be fluid or pus in your eyes that crusts over and makes your eyelids stick together when you sleep.

Although pinkeye will often clear on its own in 7 to 10 days, pinkeye that is caused by a virus can last many weeks. Antibiotics will help if you have pinkeye that is caused by bacteria. If you have pinkeye because of allergies or chemicals, it will not go away unless you can avoid the cause. But home treatment can help your symptoms.

Home Treatment

Good home care will speed healing and help you avoid spreading pinkeye to others.

◆ Wash your hands often. Always wash them well before and after you treat pinkeye or touch your eyes or face.

◆ Put cold or warm wet cloths on your eye several times a day if your eye hurts.

◆ Use moist cotton or a clean, wet cloth to remove any crust. Wipe from the inside corner (next to the nose) to the outside. Use a clean part of the cloth for each wipe.

Wipe from the inside corner to the outside to remove any crust.

◆ Do not wear contact lenses or eye makeup until the pinkeye is gone. Throw away any eye makeup you were using when you got pinkeye. Clean your contacts and storage case. If you wear disposable contacts, use a new pair after it is safe to wear contacts again.

◆ If the doctor prescribes ointment or eye-drops, use them as directed.

❖ For older children and adults: Pull the lower lid down with two fingers to create a small pouch. Squeeze the drops or ointment into it. Close the eye for 30 to 60 seconds.

❖ For younger children: Ask the child to lie down with eyes closed. Put a drop in the inner corner of the eye. When the child opens the eye, the drop will run in.

❖ Be sure the bottle tip is clean and does not touch the eye, eyelid, or eyelashes. If the tip does touch the eye area, throw the bottle away and replace it.

Do not let the bottle tip touch the eye, eyelid, or eyelashes.

◆ Putting antibiotic ointment in the eye can be tricky, especially with children. If you can get it on the eyelashes, it will melt and get into the eye.

◆ Make sure any medicine you buy without a prescription is ophthalmic (for eyes), not otic (for ears).

◆ Do not share towels, pillows, eye makeup, or contact lens equipment while you have pinkeye.

Dry Eyes

When to Call a Doctor

Call a doctor if dry eyes are a problem and artificial tears do not help.

Eyes that do not have enough moisture in them may feel dry, hot, sandy, or gritty. Dry air, smoke, aging, and certain diseases can cause dry eyes. Some common medicines also can make your eyes dry. These include antihistamines, decongestants, drugs for depression, and birth control pills.

Home Treatment

◆ Rest your eyes. When you read, watch TV, or use a computer, take breaks often and close your eyes. As you work, try to blink your eyes more often.

◆ Try "artificial tears" eyedrops. Preservative-free eyedrops are the gentlest on your eye.

◆ Do not use eyedrops that reduce redness (such as Visine) to treat dry eyes. Your eyes may get even drier when you stop using the drops.

◆ Avoid smoke and fumes from chemicals.

More

Avoiding Problems With Your Contacts

If you wear contact lenses, these tips will help you avoid problems.

◆ Keep your lenses and anything that touches them (hands, storage cases, makeup) very clean. Wash your hands before you touch your contacts.

◆ Follow the cleaning instructions for your lenses, and use a store-bought contact lens solution. Generic brands are just as good as name brands, and they cost less. Do not make your own solution. It can get contaminated too easily.

◆ Never wet your lenses with saliva. It has bacteria that may infect the eye. Don't use tap water either.

◆ Put in your contacts before you put on eye makeup. Do not put makeup on the inner rim of the eyelid. Replace eye makeup every 3 to 6 months.

◆ If you use extended-wear contacts, follow the wearing and cleaning schedule your eye care professional recommends. When worn for long periods of time, these lenses are more likely to cause severe eye infections.

◆ Visit your eye doctor or optometrist as directed or at least once a year.

Symptoms of a possible problem with your contacts include redness, pain, or burning in the eye; discharge from the eye; blurred vision; or extreme sensitivity to light. Take out your lenses, clean them, and don't put them back in until your symptoms are gone. If symptoms last longer than 2 to 3 hours after you take out your contacts, call your eye doctor or optometrist.

Blood in the Eye

When to Call a Doctor

◆ Bleeding starts after a blow to the head or injury to the eye.

◆ There is blood in the colored part of the eye.

◆ Your eye is bloody and painful.

◆ You often get blood spots in your eyes.

◆ Bleeding occurs while you are taking blood thinners, such as warfarin (Coumadin) or large doses of aspirin.

Sometimes blood vessels in the whites of the eyes break and cause a red spot or speck. This is called a **subconjunctival hemorrhage**. The blood may look alarming, especially if the spot is large. But it usually is not a cause for concern, and the red spot will go away in 2 to 3 weeks.

If you have a black eye, see Bruises on page 24.

Fatigue and Weakness

When to Call a Doctor

◆ You have sudden muscle weakness, and you don't know why.

◆ You are so tired that you have to limit your usual activities for longer than 2 weeks.

◆ You have lost or gained weight for no clear reason.

◆ You do not feel better after 4 weeks of home treatment.

◆ Fatigue gets worse even with home treatment.

Fatigue is a feeling of being very tired or exhausted or not having any energy. Most fatigue is caused by lack of exercise, stress or overwork, lack of sleep, depression, worry, or boredom. You can usually treat fatigue with self-care.

Weakness is a lack of physical or muscle strength and the feeling that moving an arm, a leg, or any other part of your body takes a lot of extra effort. Unexplained muscle weakness is usually more serious than fatigue. It may be caused by diabetes (see page 284), thyroid problems, stroke (see page 53), or other problems related to the brain and spinal cord.

Colds, flu, and other short-term illnesses often cause fatigue and weakness while you are sick.

Low Thyroid

Not having enough thyroid hormone (hypothyroidism) is a common cause of fatigue, especially in middle-aged and older women. When your thyroid gland does not make enough thyroid hormone, your body slows down. This may make you feel tired and sluggish, have trouble concentrating or remembering things, and slowly gain weight.

A blood test can tell if your thyroid hormone is too low.

Low thyroid is an easy problem to treat with medicine. Most people with this problem need to take thyroid medicine for the rest of their lives.

Anemia

Anemia means that you do not have enough red blood cells, which carry oxygen to your body's tissues. This can make you pale, weak, and tired.

Lack of iron is the most common cause of anemia. You may not be getting enough iron in your diet, or your body may have trouble absorbing it. To boost your iron:

◆ Eat foods rich in iron, such as beef, shellfish, chicken, eggs, beans, raisins, whole-grain breads, and leafy green vegetables.

◆ Steam vegetables instead of boiling them (they lose iron if you boil them).

You can also get anemia from a gradual loss of blood, such as from heavy menstrual periods or from bleeding in your stomach or colon. If a health problem is causing your anemia, treating that problem may correct your anemia and help you feel better.

More

Home Treatment

These self-care tips help with most cases of fatigue. If you have low thyroid, anemia, or another health problem, talk to your doctor about what other home treatment you should do.

- Get some exercise every day. Daily exercise balanced with plenty of rest is often the best treatment for fatigue. If you feel too tired to exercise hard, try a short walk.

- Eat a healthy diet. This can help you stay at your best.

- Make sure you get enough sleep. See page 236.

- Do not ignore emotional problems like depression or anxiety. There are treatments that can help. See Living Better With Depression on page 280 and Anxiety on page 80.

- Take steps to control your stress and workload. See page 318.

- Ask your doctor or pharmacist whether any of your medicines can make you tired. Cold and allergy medicines are common causes of fatigue.

- Drink less caffeine and alcohol.

- If you smoke or chew tobacco, think about quitting. See page 316 for help.

- Watch less TV. Spend time with friends instead, or try new activities.

- Be patient. It may take a while before you feel energetic again.

Are You Depressed?

If you have been feeling very tired for no clear reason, you may want to think about whether you are depressed.

Depression is more than just the normal sadness and moodiness that come and go with the ups and downs of life. It's an illness. You may be depressed if:

- You feel sad, anxious, or hopeless much of the time, and these feelings do not go away.

- You have lost interest in many of the things you once enjoyed—hobbies, work, time with friends and family.

You may also have changes in your sleep or eating patterns, weight gain or loss, and trouble concentrating and making decisions. You may feel worthless or guilty for no reason and think about death a lot.

If you think you might be depressed and have felt this way for more than 2 weeks, talk to your doctor or a counselor. If you want to take a self-test for depression, go to the Web site on the back cover and enter **x453** in the search box. If you have already been diagnosed with depression, see Living Better With Depression on page 280.

Treatment can almost always help. If you are just mildly depressed, home treatment may be all you need. Or you may need to try counseling and antidepressant medicines. Without any treatment, your depression is likely to get worse.

Chronic Fatigue Syndrome

Chronic fatigue syndrome can make you so tired and weak that you can't do your normal activities. Even after you rest, you still may not have your usual energy. You may also have memory problems, headaches, a sore throat, painful lymph glands, muscle and joint pain, and sleep problems.

Chronic fatigue syndrome is hard to diagnose. Depression, thyroid problems, mono, and many other illnesses can cause the same symptoms. You may need tests to rule out some of these other causes. If fatigue and other symptoms go on for at least 6 months and there is no other explanation for them, your doctor may diagnose chronic fatigue syndrome.

Feeling tired and weak may make it hard to get through the day sometimes. But many people do get better over time. Your doctor may be able to help with specific symptoms.

To feel better overall:

◆ Look for ways to adjust your schedule so that it's easier on you. Schedule rest breaks. Resist the urge to do too much when you have energy. If you overdo it, you may get too tired. Then you may be even more tired the next day.

◆ If you have problems sleeping, try to improve your sleep habits. See page 236.

◆ Get light exercise every day. Gentle stretching, light aerobics, swimming, walking, and cycling can help relieve your symptoms.

◆ Eat a healthy diet. You may feel better if you avoid heavy meals and eat more fruits and vegetables.

◆ Join a support group with other people who have chronic fatigue syndrome. These groups can be a good source of information and tips for what to do to feel better.

Fever, Age 11 and Younger

When to Call a Doctor

The temperatures listed in this topic are rectal.

◆ Fever occurs with vomiting, severe headache, sleepiness, not acting alert, stiff neck, or a bulging soft spot on a baby's head. See page 161.

◆ Fever occurs with a seizure. See page 161.

◆ Fever occurs with:

  ❖ Fast, difficult breathing. See page 19.

  ❖ Drooling or inability to swallow. See page 19.

  ❖ A purple rash that does not lighten when you press on it. See page 161.

  ❖ Vomiting, diarrhea, and belly pain.

  ❖ Signs of dehydration. See page 31.

  ❖ Unexplained skin rash. See page 227 for common childhood illnesses that cause rashes.

  ❖ Ear pain. Babies often pull at painful ears. See Middle Ear Infections on page 145.

  ❖ Pain or crying when urinating.

❖ New swelling, pain, redness, or warmth in one or more joints.

❖ Any unusual or severe pain.

◆ A baby younger than 3 months of age has a fever of 100.4°F or higher.

◆ A child 3 months to 11 years old has a fever of:

  ❖ 104°F or higher.

  ❖ 102°F to 104°F for more than 12 hours.

  ❖ 100.4°F to 102°F for more than 24 to 48 hours.

◆ Your child has a fever and seems sicker than you would expect from a viral illness like a cold or the flu.

◆ Your child acts strangely, seems confused, or hallucinates.

◆ Your child's fever began after he or she took a new medicine.

For fever in people age 12 and older, see page 160.

Fever is usually defined as a rectal temperature of 100.4°F or higher. Rectal temperatures are the most accurate for checking for fever in a child. To learn how to take an accurate rectal temperature, see page 159.

In most but not all cases, fever means your child has an illness. (Sometimes it may mean your baby is dressed too warmly or the room is too warm.)

Common causes of fevers in children are:

◆ Colds, flu, chickenpox, and other infections caused by a virus. Flu can cause a high fever for 5 days or longer.

◆ Ear infections, strep throat, and other infections caused by bacteria.

Teething does not cause a fever. If a baby is teething and has a fever, look for other signs that your child is sick.

By itself, fever is not harmful. It may even help the body fight infection. Children tend to get higher fevers than adults do. Although high fevers are uncomfortable, they do not often cause medical problems. A very fast-rising temperature can cause a fever seizure, but this is not very common. See page 161.

The body limits a fever caused by infection from going above 106°F. But if there is heat from an outside source, like sun on a parked car, the body temperature can go above 107°F. This can cause brain damage.

Home Treatment

It can be hard to know when to call your doctor when your child has a fever, especially during the cold and flu season. How high a fever is may not be a good measure of how sick your child is. The way your child looks and acts is a much better guide.

Most children will be less active when they have a fever. If your child is comfortable and alert, eating well, drinking enough fluids, urinating normal amounts, and seems to be improving, home treatment is all that is needed.

◆ Give your child extra fluids, or let him or her suck on frozen juice pops.

◆ Dress the child lightly. Do not wrap your child in blankets.

If your child has a fever and feels bad:

◆ Give an over-the-counter medicine like acetaminophen (Tylenol) or ibuprofen (Advil, Motrin). Read and follow all instructions on the label. Do not give aspirin to anyone younger than 20.

◆ Urge your child to drink extra fluids, and watch for signs of dehydration. See page 31.

Taking a Rectal Temperature

Taking a rectal temperature gives you the most accurate reading in a child. Rectal temperature is about 0.5°F to 1°F higher than an oral temperature.

To take a rectal temperature in a baby or small child:

◆ Clean the thermometer. Use only a rectal thermometer to take a rectal temperature.

◆ Put Vaseline or another lubricant on the bulb.

◆ Hold the child bottom-up across your lap.

◆ Hold the thermometer about an inch from the bulb, and gently insert it into the child's rectum no more than 1 inch. Hold the thermometer right at the anus so it can't slip in any farther. Do not let go.

◆ Wait until the thermometer beeps, and then remove it. (Glass thermometers containing mercury are no longer advised. If you have one, call your local health department to learn how to get rid of it safely.)

Fever, Age 12 and Older

When to Call a Doctor

The temperatures listed in this topic are oral.

◆ You have a fever of 104°F or higher.

◆ You have diabetes or a weak immune system (from HIV, steroid use, cancer treatment, or an organ transplant) and have a fever of 101°F or higher.

◆ You have a fever of 103°F to 104°F that does not come down after 12 hours of home treatment.

◆ You have a fever that lasts a while. Many viral illnesses cause fevers of 102°F or higher for short periods of time (up to 12 to 24 hours). Call a doctor if the fever stays high for more than 2 days.

◆ Body temperature rises to 102°F or higher, all sweating stops, and the skin is hot, dry, and red. These may be signs of heatstroke. See page 39.

◆ You have a fever with signs of a wound infection, such as increased pain, redness, swelling, or warmth; red streaks; or pus.

◆ You have a fever with a very stiff neck, headache, vomiting, and confusion. These may be signs of a serious illness. See page 161.

◆ You have a fever and are short of breath and coughing. See page 216.

◆ You have a fever with pain above your eyes or cheekbones. See page 232.

◆ You have a fever with pain or burning when you urinate. See page 251.

◆ You have a fever with belly pain, nausea, and vomiting. See Appendicitis on page 69 and Food Poisoning on page 167.

◆ A person has a fever and seems confused, is not alert, acts strangely, or has other troubling symptoms.

◆ You get a fever after you start a new medicine.

For fever in children age 11 and younger, see page 158.

A fever is a high body temperature. By itself, a fever is not dangerous unless it gets too high. In fact, it can help your body fight illness and infection. Most healthy adults can handle a fever as high as 103°F to 104°F for a short time without problems.

Home Treatment

◆ Drink plenty of water and other fluids.

◆ Take an over-the-counter medicine like acetaminophen (Tylenol) or ibuprofen (Advil, Motrin) to lower a fever. Read and follow all instructions on the label. Do not give aspirin to anyone younger than 20.

◆ Take and record your temperature every 2 hours and whenever symptoms change.

◆ Take a sponge bath with warm (not too hot or cold) water if you ache.

◆ Watch for dehydration. See page 31.

◆ Dress lightly.

◆ Eat light foods that are easy to digest, such as soup.

◆ If you have classic flu symptoms, try home treatment for flu and see how you are doing in a day or two. See page 165.

Encephalitis and Meningitis

Encephalitis is an inflammation of the brain. It may happen after you have a virus like chickenpox, flu, measles, mumps, mono, or herpes (the types that cause cold sores, genital herpes, or shingles). You can also get it from ticks or mosquitoes (see page 16).

Meningitis is an inflammation of the lining of the brain and spinal cord. It may follow an ear or sinus infection or other illness. It may also occur even if you have not been sick.

Either illness can be quite serious. The symptoms are:

◆ Fever with a bad headache, stiff neck, and vomiting.

◆ Trouble staying awake, confusion, or seizures.

◆ A rash that develops quickly and looks like bruises or tiny purple or red blood spots under the skin.

Call your doctor right away if you get these symptoms, especially if you have recently been ill, been around someone with encephalitis or meningitis, or been bitten by mosquitoes.

Fever Seizures

When to Call a Doctor

Call 911 if:

◆ The child stops breathing for longer than 15 to 20 seconds or has severe trouble breathing.

◆ A seizure lasts longer than 3 minutes, or the child has a second seizure.

◆ Seizure occurs with fever, vomiting, severe headache, sleepiness, not being alert or active, stiff neck, or a bulging soft spot on a baby's head.

Call a doctor if:

◆ It is the child's first seizure, or you have not discussed with your doctor what to do if there is another one.

◆ A child younger than 6 months or a child 5 years or older has a seizure.

◆ The seizure affects only one side of the body.

◆ A seizure occurs without fever.

See pages 158 and 160 for when to call a doctor because of fever.

More

Fever seizures are uncontrolled muscle spasms that can happen while a child's temperature rises quickly. Sometimes the seizure occurs before you even know the child has a fever.

A child having a fever seizure may faint. The child's muscles will get stiff, and his or her teeth will clench. Then the arms and legs will start to jerk. The child's eyes may roll back, and he or she may stop breathing for a few seconds and turn slightly blue. The child might also vomit, urinate, or pass stools. Seizures usually last 1 to 5 minutes.

Fever seizures are scary, but in children ages 6 months to 5 years they usually are not serious and do not cause harm. Some children in this age group just seem to get fever seizures for no clear reason. About one-third of children who have a fever seizure will have another one in the future.

Home Treatment

During a seizure

- ◆ Try to stay calm. This will help calm the child.

- ◆ Protect the child from injury. Ease the child to the floor, or hold a very small child facedown on your lap. Do not restrain the child.

- ◆ Turn the child onto his or her side. This will help clear the mouth of any vomit or spit and will keep the airway open so the child can breathe.

- ◆ Do not put anything in the child's mouth to prevent tongue biting, because it may injure the child.

- ◆ Time how long the seizure lasts, if you can.

After a seizure

- ◆ If the child is having trouble breathing, turn his or her head to the side. Use your finger to gently clear the mouth of any vomit or spit so the child can breathe.

- ◆ Check for injuries.

- ◆ Give an over-the-counter medicine like acetaminophen (Tylenol) or ibuprofen (Advil, Motrin) and lukewarm sponge baths. Read and follow all instructions on the label. Do not give aspirin to anyone younger than 20.

- ◆ Put the child in a cool room to sleep. Feeling drowsy is common after a seizure. Check the child often. The child should return to his or her normal behavior and activity level within 1 hour after the seizure.

Fibromyalgia

When to Call a Doctor

◆ You have severe joint or muscle pain, swelling, or weakness.

◆ You feel sad, helpless, or hopeless; lose interest in things you used to enjoy; or have other symptoms of depression. See Are You Depressed? on page 156.

◆ You think you have injured a muscle or joint, and the pain does not go away in a few days.

Fibromyalgia is a painful condition that can make you ache all over and feel tired and weak. You also have tender spots at specific points of the body that hurt only when you press on them. You may have trouble sleeping. These problems can upset your work and home life.

Symptoms tend to come and go, though they may never go away completely. Fibromyalgia does not harm your muscles, joints, or organs.

Fibromyalgia is not very well understood by anyone. Its cause is unknown. Your doctor may suggest prescription medicines to help with some of your symptoms.

Home Treatment

◆ Get regular exercise, such as walking, biking, or swimming. This is the best thing you can do for fibromyalgia. It may help with pain and sleep problems and help you feel better.

◆ Try to get a good night's sleep every night. Go to bed and get up at the same time each day, whether you feel rested or not. Make sure you have a good mattress and pillow. See page 237 for more tips.

◆ Reduce stress. Avoid things that cause you stress, if you can. If not, work at making them less stressful. Learn to use biofeedback, meditation, or other methods to relax. See page 320.

◆ Use a heating pad set on low or take warm baths or showers for pain. Using cold packs for up to 15 minutes at a time can also relieve pain. Put a thin cloth between the cold pack and your skin.

◆ Take an over-the-counter medicine like acetaminophen (Tylenol) or ibuprofen (Advil, Motrin) for pain. Read and follow all instructions on the label.

◆ Think about joining a support group with others who have fibromyalgia to learn more and get support.

Some people with fibromyalgia also use acupuncture, massage, or other treatments to help manage their symptoms.

Fifth Disease

When to Call a Doctor

◆ Your child seems very sick.

◆ Your child feels weak and tired, and his or her skin is pale.

◆ Your child has a rash with high fever. See the fever guidelines on pages 158 and 160.

◆ You are pregnant and think you may have been exposed to a child with fifth disease. Although fifth disease is harmless in children, there is a small chance that it could harm your unborn baby.

◆ You are pregnant and get a rash that looks like fifth disease ("slapped cheeks" rash on the face, or a lacy, pink rash on the arms, legs, torso, and buttocks).

Fifth disease causes a rash and, in some cases, mild flu-like symptoms. It mostly affects children, though adults can get it too.

A child with fifth disease may have:

◆ A red rash on the face that looks like slapped cheeks.

◆ A lacy, pink rash on the torso, buttocks, and backs of the arms and legs.

Most children will have only the rash. But some may get a low fever, runny nose, sore throat, headache, and achy joints 7 to 10 days before the rash appears.

The rash may come and go for several weeks in response to changes in temperature and sunlight.

Sneezing and coughing spread the illness. A child with fifth disease is most likely to give it to others the week before the rash appears, when there is a fever. By the time the rash appears, the child can no longer spread the illness.

Home Treatment

Rest and fluids are the main treatment for fifth disease. Keep your child comfortable, and watch for signs that he or she is getting worse and needs a doctor's care.

If the rash itches, try the tips in Relief From Itching on page 142.

Flu

Flu (influenza) is a viral illness that tends to occur in the winter and often affects many people at once. If you have the flu, you may feel very tired and have fever and shaking chills, lots of aches and pains, headache, and a cough.

The flu is not the same as the common cold.

◆ The symptoms are worse and come on faster.

◆ It lasts for up to 10 days, and you feel pretty bad the whole time.

For most people, the flu does not usually lead to more serious problems. But flu can be dangerous, especially for babies, older adults, pregnant women, and people with health problems like diabetes, asthma, or heart disease.

Antiviral medicine is advised for some of these high-risk people. The medicine can make the illness shorter and less severe if you take it before you have symptoms or within 48 hours after they appear. Even those who are not at high risk may want to take these medicines so that they feel better faster.

 Should you take antiviral medicine? For help deciding, go to the Web site on the back cover and enter **q891** in the search box.

Antibiotics will not help you get over the flu. Home treatment will help you feel a little better until the illness ends.

More

Should You Get the Flu Vaccine?

The flu vaccine helps prevent the flu. It is not foolproof, because there is more than one flu virus, and it can change from year to year. But the flu vaccine gives you the best chance of avoiding the illness.

Get the flu vaccine every year. The vaccine is recommended for all children and adults ages 6 months and older.

There are two types of the flu vaccine: a shot, and a nasal spray that you breathe in through your nose. Anyone can get the flu shot. Some people can also get the nasal spray vaccine. Check with your doctor or local health department to find out which type of vaccine is best for you.

Home Treatment

- Stay home from work, school, and public places for several days after you get sick so you don't give the flu to anyone else.
- Rest.
- Drink plenty of water to replace fluids lost from fever and to ease a scratchy throat. Other good choices are hot tea with lemon, plain water, fruit juice, and soup.
- Take an over-the-counter medicine like acetaminophen (Tylenol) or ibuprofen (Advil, Motrin) to relieve fever, headache, and muscle aches. Read and follow all instructions on the label. Do not give aspirin to anyone younger than 20.
- Before you use cough or cold medicines, check the label. They may not be safe for young children or for people with certain health problems.
- Do not smoke or let others smoke around you.

Stay Well During Flu Season

- Wash your hands often!
- Keep your hands away from your nose, eyes, and mouth.
- Keep up your resistance to infection by eating a healthy diet, getting plenty of rest, and getting regular exercise.
- Consider getting the flu vaccine before flu season starts.

Food Poisoning

When to Call a Doctor

Call 911 if:

◆ You have signs of severe dehydration. These include feeling very dizzy or lightheaded, fast breathing and heartbeat, or not feeling or acting alert.

◆ You think you may have food poisoning from a canned food, and you have symptoms of botulism (blurred or double vision, trouble swallowing or breathing, muscle weakness).

Call a doctor if:

◆ There are signs of moderate dehydration. These include little or no urine for 8 hours; sunken eyes, no tears, and a dry mouth and tongue; or skin that sags when you pinch it.

◆ Severe diarrhea (large, loose stools every 1 to 2 hours) lasts longer than 2 days in an adult.

◆ Vomiting lasts longer than 1 day in an adult.

◆ Symptoms of mild dehydration (dry mouth, dark urine, not much urine) get worse even with home treatment.

◆ You have severe belly pain.

Food poisoning may occur when you eat food that has harmful bacteria in it. Meats, dairy foods, sauces, and spreads like mayonnaise are often the source of the problem. Bacteria can grow in these foods if they are not handled right, cooked well, or stored at a temperature below 40°F.

You may start to feel sick as soon as 1 or 2 hours or as late as 2 days after you eat the food. Nausea, diarrhea, and vomiting are the most common symptoms.

Suspect food poisoning when:

◆ Others who ate the same food now have the same symptoms.

◆ Symptoms start after you eat foods that were left out (at a party, picnic, or buffet).

Botulism is a rare but often deadly type of food poisoning. It is most often caused by improper home canning methods for low-acid foods like beans and corn. Bacteria that survive the canning process may grow and produce poisons in the jar. Symptoms include blurred or double vision and trouble swallowing or breathing.

Home Treatment

◆ Symptoms of food poisoning often go away in a day or two. Good home care can help you get well faster. For adults and older children, see Diarrhea on page 138 and Vomiting and Nausea on page 261. For babies and young children, see pages 137 and 259.

◆ Watch for and treat early signs of dehydration. See page 31. Older adults and young children can quickly get dehydrated from diarrhea and vomiting.

Food Safety

◆ If food looks or smells spoiled, throw it out.

◆ Keep hot foods hot and cold foods cold.

More

- Follow the 2-40-140 rule. Do not eat meat, dressings, salads, or other foods that have been kept between 40°F and 140°F for more than 2 hours.

- Use a thermometer to check your refrigerator. It should be between 34°F and 40°F.

- Defrost meats in the refrigerator or microwave, not on the counter.

- Keep your hands and your kitchen clean. Wash your hands, cutting boards, and counters with hot, soapy water. After you touch raw meat, especially chicken, wash your hands and utensils very well before you prepare other foods.

- Cook meat until it's well done. Use a meat thermometer to make sure you have cooked meat, chicken, and fish to a safe temperature. What the safe temperature is depends on the meat.

- Never eat undercooked hamburger. It's the main source of *E. coli* infection. All of the pink should be gone, and all of the meat (not just the surface) should have reached at least 160°F.

- Do not eat raw eggs or uncooked dough or sauces made with raw eggs.

- Throw away cans or jars with bulging lids or leaks.

- Follow home canning and freezing instructions carefully. Contact your county agricultural office for advice.

Hepatitis A

Hepatitis A is a virus that affects the liver. It is spread mainly by oral contact with stool that contains the virus. If the stool gets into the water or food supply, the virus may infect anyone who drinks the water or eats the food.

The United States does not tend to have this problem with its water and food supply. But sometimes a large group of people who eat at the same restaurant get infected. This usually happens when an employee with hepatitis A does not wash his or her hands well after using the bathroom and then prepares food.

- Symptoms of hepatitis A may not appear for 2 to 7 weeks after you are exposed.

- You may have fatigue, nausea, fever, sore muscles, headaches, and pain in your upper right belly. Your skin and the white part of your eyes may turn yellow. Symptoms usually last less than 2 months.

- Hepatitis A usually goes away on its own and does not cause long-term liver problems.

If you or someone in your home has hepatitis A, take care not to spread it to others. Always wash your hands well after you use the bathroom, after you change a baby's diaper, and before you prepare or eat food.

If you live in an area where hepatitis A is common or you are at high risk, you may want to get the hepatitis A vaccine. See page 326.

Fungal Infections

When to Call a Doctor

- You have signs of a worse infection, such as increased pain, redness, swelling, or warmth; pus; and fever.

- You have diabetes or peripheral artery disease and get athlete's foot.

- You have sudden hair loss, along with flaking, broken hairs, and redness of the scalp, or others in your household start losing hair.

- Ringworm is severe and spreading or is on the scalp. You may need prescription medicine.

- A fungal infection does not improve after 2 weeks or clear up after 1 month even with home treatment. You may want to ask your doctor about prescription medicine.

Fungal skin infections most often affect the feet, groin, scalp, or nails. Fungi grow best in warm, moist areas, such as between the toes, in the groin, and in the area just beneath the breasts.

Home Treatment

- For athlete's foot and jock itch, use a nonprescription antifungal powder or lotion, such as Lamisil, Lotrimin AF, or Micatin. Always wash and dry the area well before you apply the powder or lotion. Use the medicine for 1 to 2 weeks after the symptoms clear up so the infection doesn't come back. Do not use hydrocortisone cream on a fungal infection.

- For ringworm on the body, use one of the antifungals listed above.

- Keep your feet clean, cool, and dry. Dry well between your toes after you swim or shower. Use antifungal powder such as Desenex or Zeasorb in your shoes and socks and on your feet to prevent reinfection.

- Wear leather shoes or sandals that let your feet "breathe," and wear cotton socks to absorb sweat. Give shoes 24 hours to dry before you wear them again.

- Wear flip-flops or shower sandals in public pools and showers.

- Keep your groin area clean and dry. Shower or bathe soon after you exercise, or at least change out of sweaty clothes. Wear cotton underwear, and avoid tight pants and panty hose.

- Do not share hats, combs, brushes, or towels.

More

Common Fungal Infections	Symptoms	Comments
Athlete's foot	Itching and cracked, blistered, peeling areas between the toes and on the soles of the feet	Often comes back; needs to be treated each time
Jock itch	Severe itching and moistness in groin and on upper thighs; red, scaly raised areas that may ooze pus or fluid	Similar to athlete's foot
Ringworm of the skin	Patches that are clear in the center and red, peeling, or bumpy on the edges; itching	Can spread quickly to other areas
Ringworm of the scalp and beard	Bald patches that are scaly, red, crusty, or swollen with small bumps	Hair or beard may have flakes that look like dandruff
Nail infections	Discolored (often yellow), cracking, thickened, or softened nails	Hard to treat
Thrush of the mouth (yeast infection)	White coating inside the mouth that looks like milk but is hard to remove	Common in babies; may occur after taking antibiotics

Gallstones

When to Call a Doctor

If you have not been diagnosed with gallstones, see When to Call a Doctor on page 68 in Abdominal Pain.

Call your doctor if you know that you have gallstones and:

◆ You have sudden, severe belly pain. Severe belly pain can be a sign of a serious or even life-threatening problem.

◆ You develop a yellow tint to your skin and the white part of your eyes, dark yellow-brown urine, or light-colored stools.

◆ You have belly pain along with fever and chills.

◆ You have another attack of gallstone symptoms.

Gallstones are stones (made of cholesterol and other substances) that form in the gallbladder or bile duct. The gallbladder stores bile, which helps you digest fats. Gallstones may be as small as a grain of sand or as large as a golf ball.

Most people who have gallstones do not have any symptoms, but sometimes stones can irritate the gallbladder. When this happens, you may have:

◆ A steady aching or cramping pain that starts in the upper right or upper middle of your belly, just below your breastbone (see the picture on page 69). It may spread to your right upper back or shoulder blade.

◆ Sudden, severe pain that lasts several hours and then quickly fades.

◆ Fever and vomiting.

Symptoms often occur at night, usually at about the same time every night. Pain may or may not be related to a meal.

Gallstones can block the opening of the gallbladder, which can then get infected. If this happens, you will need antibiotics and surgery.

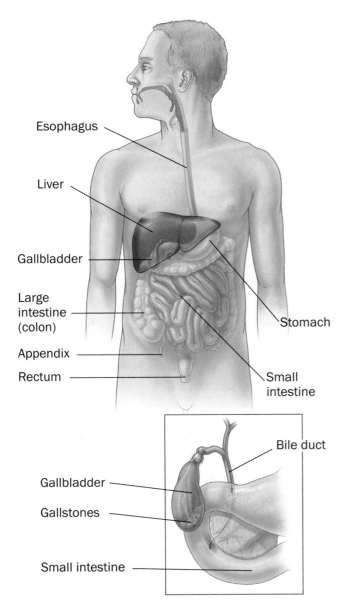

The digestive tract (your gallbladder is in the upper right part of your belly)

Home Treatment

There is no home treatment for gallstones. You may be able to avoid more gallstones if you:

◆ Stay at a healthy weight. If you need to lose weight, see page 300. Crash diets may increase your risk of gallstones.

◆ Eat a healthy, low-fat diet. Avoid foods that cause symptoms.

◆ Get regular exercise.

Do You Need Gallbladder Surgery?

People who have frequent or severe pain from gallstones often have surgery to remove the gallbladder.

◆ If your first attack of gallstone pain is mild, it is often safe to wait and see if you have another attack before you get treatment. You may not need surgery if gallstones do not cause you problems.

◆ Besides the pain of gallstones, you may need surgery for other medical reasons.

◆ Surgery costs a lot and has some risks. If you don't need it, don't have it.

 For help deciding whether surgery is right for you, go to the Web site on the back cover and enter **g126** in the search box. Then talk to your doctor.

Glaucoma

When to Call a Doctor

Call 911 if:

◆ You have sudden vision loss or blurring that does not clear.

◆ You have sudden, severe eye pain.

Call your doctor if:

◆ You have blind spots in your side vision.

◆ Your vision has gotten worse.

◆ You have a family history of open-angle glaucoma, you are age 40 or older, and you have not had an eye exam in the past year.

Glaucoma is an eye disease that damages the optic nerve at the back of the eye. (The optic nerve carries signals from the eye to the brain, which turns them into images that you see.) The damage is often related to increased pressure in the eye.

Open-angle glaucoma is the most common form. It tends to affect side (peripheral) vision. It's often painless and can develop slowly over many years without your knowing. You may not notice any vision changes until a lot of damage has occurred.

Closed-angle glaucoma is not common but can be very serious. It occurs when the flow of fluid in the eye gets blocked. This can cause a quick rise in eye pressure that causes sudden vision changes and severe pain. You can lose vision within just a few hours.

Home Treatment

◆ Use eyedrops and medicines for glaucoma as directed.

◆ Make sure your other doctors know you have glaucoma. You may need to avoid certain medicines, such as antihistamines. Check with your doctor before you take any medicines, including ones you buy without a prescription.

Lens
Cornea
Optic nerve
Retina

Glaucoma damages the optic nerve at the back of the eye.

Finding Glaucoma Early

Untreated glaucoma is a leading cause of blindness in adults. But the disease can be found in an eye exam. It responds well to treatment if you find it early.

Talk with your doctor about how often to have a glaucoma test. This may be based on your age and risk factors.

Grief

When to Call a Doctor

Normal grieving can last for days, weeks, months, or years. Only you know how much grieving is reasonable for you. But if your grief continues and you have any of the following problems, you may need to get some help.

Call a counselor or doctor if:

◆ You feel hopeless and cannot stop yourself from thinking about death or suicide. **Call 911 or the national suicide hotline at 1-800-273-8255.**

◆ You are starting to do things that hurt you physically or financially or that hurt others.

◆ You cannot control your anger toward people you blame for the loss.

◆ You are overwhelmed by guilt.

◆ You feel more and more isolated from other people.

◆ You have been grieving longer than you think is good for you.

Grieving is a natural healing process that lets you adjust to a major change or loss. Grief hurts, but it also helps you heal.

Grief can affect your body as well as your emotions. You may feel tired or restless, have trouble sleeping, get headaches, and not feel like eating. You may feel sad, angry, guilty, or depressed.

No person or book can tell you what your grief should be like. We each have our own ways of grieving. And grief doesn't stick to a schedule.

Although you may not get over a major loss, you can find ways to get through it. Your life may never be the same as it was before. But a time will come when you feel better and more at ease.

Home Treatment

There is no formula for getting over grief. Some of these ideas may help:

◆ Take as much time as you need to grieve.

◆ Let yourself cry. Don't fight the emotions you feel. Look at photos and read old letters.

◆ Try to cut back on some of your usual responsibilities for a little while. Do not make major decisions while you're grieving unless you have no choice.

◆ Talk to friends who will listen and who will encourage you to reconnect with the world. Join a support group, or talk to a counselor or clergy member.

◆ Find ways to express your grief. Keep a journal. Paint or draw.

◆ Take care of yourself. Get enough rest and eat nourishing foods.

◆ Exercise. Move around. Take a walk. It's a good way to relieve stress.

◆ As you start to move past your grief, renew old interests and pursue new ones. Do things that give you a sense of control and hope.

Hair Loss

When to Call a Doctor

- Hair loss is sudden or severe.
- You have patchy hair loss, or hair falls out in clumps.
- You have hair loss after starting a new medicine.
- Hair loss occurs with a scalp rash or any other skin change on your scalp.
- You are losing your hair bit by bit and want to talk about treatment.

Many people lose hair as they age. While men tend to lose hair from the hairline and crown of the head, women's hair gets thinner all over. This hair loss is natural and tends to run in families. It increases your risk of sunburn and skin cancer of the scalp, but you can avoid both of these by wearing sunscreen and a hat.

Bald spots are not the same as baldness.

- Wearing tight braids or having a habit of tugging or twisting your hair may cause bald spots.
- Ringworm is a fungal infection that causes scaly bald spots. See page 169.
- Alopecia areata causes patchy hair loss that may need treatment with medicines. Alopecia universalis can cause total hair loss, including the eyelashes and eyebrows.

Thinning hair can be a sign of problems such as thyroid disease or lupus. Mental or physical stress can cause short-term hair loss all over the head. So can hormone changes during pregnancy or menopause.

Treatment for Hair Loss

If you are thinking about medicine (such as minoxidil) or surgery for hair loss, make sure you understand the risks of treatment, how many treatments you will need, what it costs, and how long the results will last.

 For help deciding about medicine, go to the Web site on the back cover and enter **w704** in the search box.

Hand-Foot-and-Mouth Disease

When to Call a Doctor

◆ Your child has a high fever. See the fever guidelines on pages 158 and 160.

◆ Your child is dehydrated and has a fever with blisters in the mouth or a blistering rash on the hands and feet. See page 31.

Hand-foot-and-mouth disease is a viral illness that most often affects children under age 10. It usually occurs during the summer and fall.

Fever, a sore throat or mouth, and loss of appetite are early symptoms. Within 2 days, mouth and tongue blisters appear. Children often get a blistering rash on the fingers, palms of the hands, and soles and sides of the feet. There may be blisters on the buttocks.

The virus that causes hand-foot-and-mouth disease spreads easily through saliva, mucus from the nose, and stools. Children should not go to school or day care while they have symptoms. They are most contagious in the first 7 to 10 days, but they may be able to spread the disease for a few weeks. Good hand-washing can help prevent this.

Home Treatment

◆ Give your child an over-the-counter medicine like acetaminophen (Tylenol) or ibuprofen (Advil, Motrin) to reduce fever and mouth pain. Read and follow all instructions on the label. Do not give aspirin to anyone younger than 20.

◆ Have your child drink plenty of fluids.

◆ Give your child soft, bland foods and cool or warm (not hot) drinks if the mouth is sore. Frozen juice pops may also help.

◆ If the rash hurts or itches, put calamine lotion on it.

◆ Wash hands well after blowing a runny nose or changing a diaper. This will help prevent spreading the illness to others.

Headaches

When to Call a Doctor

Call 911 if:

◆ You have a sudden, severe headache unlike any you have had before. The headache may seem to "explode" out of nowhere.

◆ You have a headache with signs of a stroke. These may include sudden weakness, numbness, inability to move, loss of vision, slurred speech, confusion, behavior changes, or seizure. See page 53.

Call a doctor if:

◆ You have a headache with stiff neck, fever, vomiting, drowsiness, or confusion. You may have a serious illness. See page 161.

◆ You have had a recent head injury, and your headaches are getting a lot worse.

◆ You have a headache with severe eye pain. This may be a sign of a serious problem. See page 172.

◆ You often have severe headaches with no clear cause.

◆ You think your headaches are migraines, but you have not talked to your doctor about it. There may be medicine that can help prevent them.

◆ You have a lot more headaches than you used to, or they are worse than they used to be.

◆ You often get headaches during or after exercise, sex, coughing, or sneezing.

◆ Headaches wake you from a sound sleep or are worse first thing in the morning.

◆ You are using pain medicine to control headaches more than once a week, or you need help dealing with your headaches.

◆ You have a headache with dizziness and vomiting, and others in your household have the same symptoms. Get everyone out of the house. These may be signs of **carbon monoxide poisoning**.

If your headache seems unusual or occurs with other symptoms, you may want to check the chart on page 62.

Most headaches are **tension headaches**, which get worse when you are under stress. You may have tightness or pain in the muscles of your neck, back, and shoulders with the headache. A past neck injury or arthritis in the neck can also cause tension headaches.

A tension headache may cause pain all over your head, pressure inside your head, or a feeling that you have a tight band around your head. Some people feel a dull, pressing, burning sensation above the eyes. With a tension headache, you can rarely point to an exact spot where it hurts.

Are your headaches migraines?

They may be if:

◆ The pain is severe, throbbing, or piercing.

◆ Headaches occur with nausea and vomiting, or sound seems too loud or light too bright when you get a headache.

◆ The pain is on one side of the head.

◆ You have an "aura"—flashing lights, blind spots, numbness or tingling, strange smells or sounds—about an hour before you get the headache. (Some people may have less noticeable symptoms like hunger or mood changes a day or two before the headache.)

◆ Headaches seem to be related to your menstrual period.

Tracking Your Headaches

If you have headaches often, keep a record of your symptoms. This record will help your doctor know if you need to be checked or treated. It may also help you take control of your headaches, especially if they are migraines.

Write down:

1. The date and time each headache starts and stops.

2. Anything that could have triggered the headache. This might be food, smoke, bright light, stress, or activity.

3. Where the pain is. Is it in one spot or all over your head?

4. What kind of pain you have. Is it throbbing, aching, stabbing, or dull?

5. How bad the pain is. Rate it from 1 to 10 (10 is the worst).

6. Any other symptoms you have, such as nausea, vomiting, vision changes, or sensitivity to light or noise.

7. (Women only) Any link between your headaches and your menstrual cycle, birth control pills, or hormone therapy.

Preventing Headaches

◆ Reduce emotional stress. Take time to relax before and after you do something that has caused a headache in the past. Try relaxation techniques such as meditation or progressive muscle relaxation. See page 320.

◆ Reduce physical stress. Try to relax your jaw, neck, shoulder, and upper back muscles.

◆ Use good posture at work. When you sit at a desk, change positions often and stretch for 30 seconds each hour. See page 213.

◆ Exercise throughout the week. It can help reduce stress and muscle tension.

◆ Get regular massages. Some people find them very helpful in relieving tension.

◆ Limit caffeine to 1 or 2 drinks a day. People who drink a lot of caffeine often get a headache several hours after they have their last caffeine drink. Or they may wake with a headache that does not go away until they drink caffeine. Cut down slowly to avoid caffeine-withdrawal headaches.

Know your triggers

You may find that certain foods, events, medicines, or activities tend to "trigger" your headaches. Learning what your triggers are and finding ways to limit or avoid them can help you prevent headaches. Tracking your headaches is one thing that can help.

 For help figuring out what triggers your headaches, go to the Web site on the back cover and enter **u300** in the search box.

More

Cluster Headaches

Cluster headaches occur in "clusters" over a period of days or months and then disappear for months or even years. During a cluster period, you may have several headaches each day.

These headaches cause sudden, very severe, sharp, stabbing pain on one side, usually in the temple or behind the eye. The eye and nostril on that side may be runny, and the eye may be red. The headaches often start at night and may last from a few minutes to about an hour.

To prevent headaches during a cluster period:

◆ Avoid alcohol.

◆ Get regular sleep. Go to bed and wake up at the same time every day. Don't take naps.

◆ Avoid certain foods like aged cheeses and processed meats.

If you think you are having cluster headaches, talk to your doctor.

Home Treatment

◆ If you get migraines and your doctor has prescribed medicine for them, take it at the first sign that you're getting a migraine.

◆ Stop what you're doing, and sit quietly for a moment. Close your eyes, and breathe slowly. If you can, go to a quiet, dark place and relax. If you have a migraine, sleeping may help.

◆ Take an over-the-counter medicine like acetaminophen (Tylenol) or ibuprofen (Advil, Motrin) for headache pain. Using these medicines too often may make headaches worse or more frequent when the medicine wears off. This is called a **rebound headache**. Read and follow all instructions on the label.

◆ Put a cold pack on the painful area or on your forehead. Put a thin cloth between the cold pack and your skin.

◆ Gently massage your neck and shoulder muscles. Try the neck exercises on page 212.

◆ Put a heating pad on painful or tight muscles, or take a hot shower. But do not use heat if you have a migraine.

◆ Try a relaxation exercise such as progressive muscle relaxation. See page 320.

Headaches in Children

People often start getting migraine headaches during childhood or the teen years. Migraines are the most common headaches in children. Home treatment for migraines in children is the same as for adults, although some of the medicines may be different.

Children's headaches can also be caused by:

◆ Stress about school, sports, relationships, or peer pressure. Even fun activities can be overdone. Many times, just talking about a problem with your child may help.

◆ Hunger. A healthy breakfast and after-school snack may prevent headaches.

◆ Eyestrain. Have your child's eyes checked.

◆ Lack of sleep. Set bedtimes and enforce them. Make sure your child gets enough rest.

◆ Colds, sinus problems, and other illnesses.

When Your Child Has a Headache

◆ See When to Call a Doctor on page 176.

◆ If your doctor has prescribed a specific treatment for your child's headaches, start treatment as soon as your child says he or she has a headache.

◆ For mild headaches that occur only once in a while, let your child rest quietly in a dark room with a cool, wet cloth on his or her forehead. If rest does not help, try an over-the-counter medicine like acetaminophen (Tylenol) or ibuprofen (Advil, Motrin). Read and follow all instructions on the label.

◆ If your child often gets mild headaches, encourage him or her to go on with normal activities. Do not let your child avoid chores, homework, or other things unless the pain is bad. It helps to practice what you preach in this area. When you have a headache, deal with it in a calm, matter-of-fact way, and try to keep up your own usual activities. Your child may follow your example.

◆ Talk to your child. Let him or her know you care. Extra attention and quiet time may be enough to relieve the headache.

Hearing Problems

This topic covers two common hearing problems:

◆ Hearing loss

◆ Ringing in the ears (tinnitus)

Protect Your Hearing

◆ Avoid harmful noise. The noise from machines, guns, snowmobiles, motor-cycles, lawn mowers, power tools, appliances, loud music, and other sources can damage your hearing.

◆ Use hearing protectors such as earplugs or earmuffs when you have to be around harmful noise. These can greatly reduce the noise that reaches the ear. Cotton balls or tissues stuffed in the ears do not help much.

◆ Control the volume when you can. Don't buy noisy toys, appliances, or tools when there are quieter choices. Turn down the stereo, the TV, the car radio, and per-sonal music players with earphones.

◆ Never use cotton swabs, hairpins, or other objects to remove earwax or to scratch your ears. They can damage the ear. See page 148 to learn how to remove earwax safely.

◆ Ask your pharmacist if any medicines you take can affect your hearing. For example, antibiotics, blood pressure medicines, ibuprofen (Advil, Motrin), naproxen (Aleve), and large doses of aspirin can cause hearing loss.

◆ Control diseases that can affect blood flow, such as heart disease, high blood pressure, and diabetes. Some hearing loss may be caused by less blood flow to the inner ear.

◆ During air travel, swallow and yawn a lot when the plane is coming down. If you have a cold, the flu, or a sinus infection, take a decongestant a few hours before the plane lands. Before you use a decon-gestant, check the label. It may not be safe for young children or for people with certain health problems.

◆ If you scuba dive, learn how to dive safely.

More

Hearing Loss

When to Call a Doctor

◆ Hearing loss occurs suddenly (within a matter of days or weeks).

◆ You have hearing loss in one ear only.

◆ You develop a hearing problem since you started taking medicine, including aspirin, ibuprofen (Advil, Motrin), or naproxen (Aleve).

◆ Hearing loss occurs with vertigo (you feel like the room is spinning) or loss of movement in your face.

◆ You think your hearing is slowly getting worse.

◆ You wonder if you need a hearing aid.

◆ You think your baby or child may not be hearing well.

Millions of people cope with reduced hearing. In adults, the most common causes are:

◆ **Noise.** Over time, the noise you are exposed to at work, at play (such as listening to very loud music), or even during common chores (like mowing the lawn) can lead to hearing loss. Your hearing usually gets worse over many years.

◆ **Age.** Changes in the inner ear that occur as you grow older cause a gradual but steady hearing loss. This is called **presbycusis**.

Other causes of hearing loss include earwax buildup, an object in the ear, injury to the ear or head, ear infection, and other ear problems. Some common medicines—aspirin, ibuprofen (Advil, Motrin), naproxen (Aleve), antibiotics, blood pressure medicines—can affect your hearing. Check with your pharmacist. Sometimes hearing loss can be a sign of a serious health problem.

Home Treatment

Hearing loss can affect your work and home life. It can make you feel lonely, depressed, or helpless. But there are things you can do to hear better and feel connected to others.

◆ Protect the hearing you have. Always use hearing protectors around loud noises. Avoid loud noise when you can.

◆ Learn to pay close attention to a speaker's face, posture, gestures, and tone of voice. These clues can help you understand what a person is saying. Face the person you're talking to and have him or her face you. Make sure the lighting is good so that you can see the other person's face clearly.

◆ Consider a hearing aid. See an expert who can help you pick one that fits. Be sure to have your hearing tested and the hearing aid adjusted over time.

◆ Use other helpful devices, such as:

  ❖ Telephone amplifiers.

  ❖ Hearing aids that can connect to a TV, stereo, radio, or microphone.

  ❖ Devices that use lights or vibrations to alert you to the doorbell, a ringing phone, or a baby monitor.

  ❖ TV closed-captioning that shows the words at the bottom of the screen. Most new TVs have this option.

  ❖ TTY (text telephone), which lets you type messages back and forth on the phone instead of talking or listening. These devices are also called TDD.

Ringing in the Ears

When to Call a Doctor

◆ Tinnitus starts suddenly and affects only one ear.

◆ You have new tinnitus with hearing loss, vertigo (you feel like the room is spinning), loss of balance, nausea, or vomiting.

◆ Ringing in your ears does not stop or change.

◆ You get tinnitus after an injury to your head or ear.

◆ Tinnitus lasts longer than 2 weeks, even with home treatment. There may be no cure, but your doctor can help you learn how to live with the problem.

Most people have ringing, roaring, hissing, or buzzing in their ears from time to time. The sound usually lasts only a few minutes. If it does not go away or it happens often, you may have a problem called tinnitus.

Tinnitus is most often caused by being around too much loud noise. But it can have other causes like ear infections, dental problems, and medicines (especially antibiotics and large amounts of aspirin). Be sure to discuss it with your doctor. Drinking alcohol or lots of caffeine can add to the problem.

Home Treatment

◆ Cut back on alcohol and caffeine.

◆ Limit your use of aspirin, ibuprofen (Advil, Motrin), and naproxen (Aleve).

◆ If you have an earwax problem, remove the wax safely. See page 148.

Looking for the **Heart Failure** topic? See page 291.

Heart Palpitations

When to Call a Doctor

Call 911 if you have chest pain or pressure, or a strange feeling in your chest, especially if it occurs with other symptoms of a heart attack (sweating, shortness of breath, nausea or vomiting, feeling dizzy or lightheaded). See page 38.

Call your doctor if:

◆ Heart palpitations occur with:

  ❖ Weakness or fatigue.

  ❖ Confusion.

  ❖ Feeling lightheaded.

◆ It feels like your heart skips beats or beats unevenly all the time.

◆ Heart palpitations are new or different than before and do not go away with home treatment.

More

Heart palpitations are an uncomfortable feeling that your heart is beating very fast or in an odd rhythm. You may feel like:

◆ Your heart is pounding, or there is a fluttering in your chest.

◆ Your heart is doing a "flip-flop" or is skipping a beat.

◆ Your heart is racing, or there is an extra heartbeat.

◆ Your heart is beating in your neck.

Palpitations may be caused by a heart problem. But they also occur because of:

◆ Stress or fatigue.

◆ Too much alcohol, caffeine, or nicotine.

◆ Illegal drugs like meth and cocaine.

◆ A high thyroid level.

◆ Medicines, including diet pills, antihistamines, decongestants, and some herbal products.

Nearly everyone has heart palpitations from time to time. There is usually no reason to worry.

But if you are at higher risk for heart disease (for example, if you smoke or are not very active, or if you have high blood pressure, high cholesterol, a lot of stress, or a family history of heart disease), see your doctor for a checkup. Finding and treating heart problems early is the best way to prevent serious illness.

Home Treatment

◆ Take deep breaths and try to relax.

◆ If you start to feel like you may faint, lie down so that you don't fall.

◆ Write down the date and time, your pulse rate, what you were doing when the problem started, how long it went on, and any other symptoms. Having a record can help you and your doctor figure out the cause of the problem.

To prevent further problems:

◆ Do not smoke. If you need help quitting, see page 316.

◆ Cut down on caffeine and alcohol.

◆ Check with your pharmacist or doctor to see whether any of your medicines can cause heart palpitations.

◆ Reduce stress. See page 318. If you have problems with anxiety, see page 80.

◆ Get regular exercise. If you often have heart palpitations, talk to your doctor before you start an exercise program.

Heartburn

When to Call a Doctor

Call 911 if:

◆ You have pain in your upper belly with chest pain or pressure or other symptoms of a heart attack. See page 38.

◆ You vomit a lot of blood or what looks like coffee grounds.

Call your doctor if:

◆ There are streaks of blood in your vomit.

◆ It often hurts when you swallow, or you have trouble swallowing.

◆ You are losing weight, and you don't know why.

◆ You think a medicine may be causing heartburn. Antihistamines, antianxiety medications, and anti-inflammatories, including aspirin, ibuprofen (Advil, Motrin), and naproxen (Aleve), can sometimes cause heartburn.

◆ Heartburn lasts more than 2 weeks, even with home treatment. Call sooner if your symptoms are severe or do not improve at all with antacids or acid reducers. Also see Ulcers on page 249.

Heartburn occurs when stomach juices flow backward into the esophagus, the tube that leads from the mouth to the stomach. The backflow, called **reflux**, causes a feeling of burning, warmth, or heat beneath the breastbone. You may feel it spread in waves up into your neck and get a sour taste in your mouth.

Heartburn can last up to 2 hours or longer. It gets worse when you lie down or bend over and improves when you sit or stand up.

Don't worry if you have heartburn now and then. Nearly everyone does. Use the home treatment tips to get relief.

But if you have heartburn often, you may have **gastroesophageal reflux disease (GERD)**. GERD can lead to other health problems. You need to see a doctor if you have frequent heartburn and home treatment does not help.

If you have GERD, go to the Web site on the back cover and enter **L457** in the search box to learn what you can do to control your symptoms.

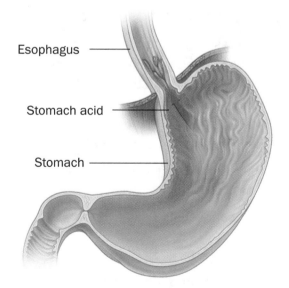

Esophagus

Stomach acid

Stomach

You get heartburn when stomach acid flows up (refluxes) into the esophagus.

More

Home Treatment

◆ Eat smaller meals, and avoid late-night snacks. After eating, wait 2 to 3 hours before you lie down.

◆ Avoid foods that bring on heartburn. These may include citrus fruits and juices (orange, tomato), chocolate, fatty or fried foods, peppermint- or spearmint-flavored foods, alcohol, carbonated drinks, and coffee and other drinks with caffeine.

◆ Do not smoke or chew tobacco.

◆ If you get heartburn at night, raise the head of your bed 6 to 8 inches by putting the frame on blocks or placing a foam wedge under the head of your mattress. (Adding extra pillows does not work well.)

◆ Take a nonprescription product for heartburn. For mild heartburn, an antacid, such as Maalox, Mylanta, or Tums, may help. Or try an acid reducer, such as Pepcid AC, Tagamet HB, or Zantac. You can also buy an acid blocker, such as Prevacid 24HR or Prilosec OTC, without a prescription. Ask your pharmacist to help you choose one of these medicines.

◆ Do not wear tight clothing around your middle.

◆ Do not take aspirin, ibuprofen (Advil, Motrin), or naproxen (Aleve). These can cause heartburn or make it worse. If you need something for pain, try acetaminophen (Tylenol). Read and follow all instructions on the label.

◆ Lose weight if you need to. Losing just 5 to 10 pounds can help.

Heat Rash

When to Call a Doctor

◆ Heat rash occurs with a fever of 100.4°F or higher in a baby younger than 3 months, and the fever does not come down within 20 minutes after you take off some of the baby's clothing. Also see pages 158 and 160.

◆ The rash looks infected or lasts longer than 3 days.

◆ Your baby seems sick.

Heat rash is a rash of tiny red dots on a baby's head, neck, and shoulders. Some people call it prickly heat.

Heat rash often develops when parents dress their baby too warmly or when the weather is hot. Your baby needs, at the most, one more layer of clothing than you do.

The skin should feel warm—not hot and not too cool. Place your hand between the baby's shoulder blades. If the skin is hot or moist, the baby is too warm.

Home Treatment

◆ Keep the baby's skin cool and dry.

◆ Keep the baby's sleeping area comfortable—not too hot, not too cool.

◆ Dress your baby lightly during hot weather. Just a diaper may be fine. Be sure to protect the skin from sunburn.

Heel Pain and Plantar Fasciitis

Heel pain is often caused by **plantar fasciitis**. The plantar fascia is a thick band of tissue that connects your heel bone to your toes and supports the arch of your foot. If it gets irritated, it causes pain in your heel.

Plantar fasciitis is common in athletes, middle-aged people, and those who are overweight. It can result from:

◆ Standing for long periods of time.

◆ Doing repeated, high-impact movements such as running and jumping.

◆ "Overpronating" when you walk or run. This means that the foot rolls too far inward when you take a step. Wearing shoes that are worn out or have poor arch support, having tight calf muscles, or running downhill or on uneven surfaces can make your foot roll inward even more.

Heel pain is often caused by an irritated plantar fascia.

You may get a **heel spur** if calcium builds up where the plantar fascia attaches to the heel bone. Heel spurs usually do not cause pain and do not need to be treated. (Rarely, a painful heel spur may need to be removed.) Many people think their heel pain is caused by heel spurs. But in most cases, it's caused by plantar fasciitis.

More

185

Achilles tendon problems can cause pain in the back of the heel. See Bursitis and Tendon Injury on page 111. If you think you may have torn your Achilles tendon, see Strains, Sprains, and Broken Bones on page 50.

Achilles tendon

Heel bone

Problems with the Achilles tendon can cause pain in the back of the heel.

Home Treatment

Start treating heel pain as soon as you feel it. If you ignore it until it gets bad, it may take a lot longer to get better.

- Cut back on all weight-bearing activities to the point that you do not have any pain. For exercise, try something that gets you off your feet, such as cycling or swimming. You may need to check with your doctor about when you can gradually get back to high-impact activities like running.

- Stretch your Achilles tendon and calf muscles several times a day. See page 314.

- Put ice on your heel at least once a day. Always put a thin cloth between the ice and your skin. See Ice and Cold Packs on page 243.

- Don't go barefoot. Wear shoes or sandals with good cushioning and good arch support anytime you will be standing up or walking. If you get up at night to go to the bathroom, put on shoes.

- Replace shoes that are worn out. Pick new ones with good arch support and a cushioned sole. Or try nonprescription arch supports.

- Take an over-the-counter medicine like acetaminophen (Tylenol) or ibuprofen (Advil, Motrin) for pain. Read and follow all instructions on the label.

- For Achilles tendon problems or plantar fasciitis, try heel lifts or heel cups in both shoes. Use them only until the pain is gone.

 If you have plantar fascia problems, there are special exercises and stretches that may help. To learn how to do them, go to the Web site on the back cover and enter **k148** in the search box.

Your doctor may also suggest other treatments for plantar fasciitis, such as taping, heel splints, shoe inserts, or steroid shots. Surgery is usually done only as a last resort when other treatments have not worked.

Hemorrhoids and Rectal Problems

When to Call a Doctor

Call 911 if you have severe rectal bleeding. Severe means that you are passing a lot of stool that is maroon or mostly blood.

Call your doctor if:

◆ You have severe rectal pain.

◆ Your stools are black or tarry or have streaks of blood.

◆ Rectal bleeding lasts for more than 1 week or happens more than once.

◆ Stools are narrower than usual (they may be as thin as a pencil).

◆ You still have rectal pain after a full week of home treatment.

◆ Any unusual material or tissue seeps or sticks out of the anus.

◆ A lump near the anus gets bigger or more painful, and you get a fever.

Hemorrhoids

Hemorrhoids are enlarged and inflamed veins that may form inside or outside the anus. Straining to pass hard stools, being overweight or pregnant, and sitting or standing for long periods can all cause hemorrhoids.

Hemorrhoids usually last several days and often come back. You may have:

◆ Bright red streaks of blood on stools or toilet paper, or blood dripping from the anus.

◆ Mucus leaking from the anus.

◆ Irritation or itching.

◆ The feeling that you cannot complete a bowel movement.

◆ Tissue or a lump sticking out of the anus.

Pain is not usually a symptom, unless a blood clot forms in a hemorrhoid or the blood flow to a hemorrhoid is cut off (strangulated). A clotted hemorrhoid may be very painful, but it is not dangerous. But a strangulated hemorrhoid may need emergency care.

Hemorrhoids may get better with home treatment. If you have hemorrhoids that bleed a lot, are painful, or make it hard to keep your anal area clean, you may want to talk to your doctor about surgery or other procedures. For help deciding what treatment is right for you, go to the Web site on the back cover and enter **v666** in the search box.

Other Rectal Problems

The rectum is the lower part of the large intestine (see the picture on page 171). At the end of the rectum is the anus, where stools pass out of the body.

Most people have anal itching, pain, or bleeding at some time. These problems are often minor and will go away on their own or with home treatment.

More

Anal itching can have many causes.

◆ Skin around the anus may be irritated by stool. But trying to keep the area too clean by rubbing it with dry toilet paper or using harsh soap may damage the skin.

◆ Itching can be a sign of pinworms, especially in homes with children. See page 215.

◆ Caffeine and spicy foods can irritate the anus.

An **anal fissure** may cause pain during bowel movements and streaks of blood on stools. A fissure is a long, narrow sore that may form when the tissue near the anus is torn during a bowel movement.

Rectal bleeding, recent changes in bowel habits, and rectal pain are also symptoms of **colorectal cancer**. If you have these symptoms, see your doctor to find out if you need tests (see page 127). This is especially important if you are over 50 or have a family history of colon cancer.

Home Treatment

◆ Take warm baths. They are soothing and cleansing, especially after a bowel movement. Warm baths with just enough water to cover the anal area—called sitz baths—can help with hemorrhoids but may make anal itching worse.

◆ Wear cotton underwear and loose clothing to decrease moisture in the anal area.

◆ Put a cool, wet cloth on the anus for 10 minutes, 4 times a day.

◆ Ease itching and irritation with zinc oxide, petroleum jelly, or hydrocortisone (1%) cream. Use a suppository such as Preparation H to ease pain and moisten the rectum. Ask your doctor before you use any product that has an anesthetic (these products end with "-caine" in the name or ingredients). These products cause allergic reactions in some people.

◆ To keep your stool soft, drink plenty of water and eat lots of fresh fruits, vegetables, and whole grains. You may need to use a nonprescription stool softener until you are better. See Constipation on page 130.

◆ Try not to strain when you pass stools. Never hold your breath.

◆ Avoid sitting or standing too much. Take short walks to increase blood flow in your pelvic region.

◆ Keep the anal area clean, but be gentle when you clean it. Use water and a mild soap, such as Ivory, or use baby wipes or Tucks pads.

Hernia

When to Call a Doctor

- A testicle swells and is painful, especially in a child or teen. This could be very serious. See page 246.

- You have a known hernia and you have sudden, severe pain in your groin or scrotum, along with nausea, vomiting, and fever.

- Mild groin pain or an unexplained bump or swelling in the groin lasts for more than 1 week.

- The skin over a hernia or bulge in the groin or belly changes color.

- You cannot push a hernia back into place with gentle pressure when you are lying down.

Most hernias occur when tissue bulges through a weak spot in the belly wall into the groin. These are called inguinal hernias. They are more common in men than in women. In men, inguinal hernias often bulge into the scrotum.

Hernia

Scrotum

A hernia can cause a bulge or lump in the groin or scrotum.

If you have a hernia:

- You may have the sense that something has "given way."

- You may have a tender bulge in your groin or scrotum. The bulge may appear slowly over time, or it may form suddenly after heavy lifting, coughing, or straining. The bulge may flatten when you lie down.

- You may have groin pain that extends into the scrotum. Pain may get worse with bending or lifting. But not all hernias cause pain.

A hernia can form anywhere there is a weakness in the belly wall. Besides the groin, common places for this are the belly button and the site of an incision from a past surgery. Some people are born with a weak spot in the belly wall.

Once in a while, tissue may get trapped in the hernia. If the blood supply to the tissue is cut off, the tissue will swell and die. Sometimes it can get infected. Rapidly increasing pain in the groin or scrotum is a sign that this may have happened and that you need medical care now.

Home Treatment

These tips will also help prevent hernias:

- Use proper lifting techniques. See page 90. Do not lift anything that is too heavy for you.

More

◆ Lose weight if you need to. See page 300.

◆ Avoid constipation, and don't strain when you pass stools or urinate. See page 131 for tips on adding more fiber to your diet and avoiding constipation.

◆ Stop smoking, especially if you have a long-term cough. If you need help quitting, see page 316.

Hiatal Hernias

A hiatal hernia occurs when part of the stomach bulges into the chest cavity. Sometimes this will cause a backflow of stomach acid, which can cause heartburn and a sour taste in the mouth.

See Heartburn on page 183.

High Blood Pressure

When to Call a Doctor

Call 911 if you have high blood pressure and get a sudden, severe headache. See page 53.

Call your doctor if:

◆ Your high blood pressure is usually under control but suddenly rises much higher than normal.

◆ You take your blood pressure, and it is 180/110 or higher.

◆ You have high blood pressure and get new chest pain or discomfort or shortness of breath. See Chest Pain on page 119.

◆ Your blood pressure is higher than 140/90 on two or more occasions.

◆ You have any problems with your blood pressure medicine.

Blood pressure is a measure of the force of blood against the walls of your arteries. Blood pressure readings include two numbers, such as 130/80. (Say "130 over 80.")

◆ The first (or top) number in the reading is the systolic pressure. This is the force of blood when the heart beats.

◆ The second (or bottom) number is the diastolic pressure. This is the force of blood between heartbeats, when the heart is at rest.

Despite what a lot of people think, high blood pressure usually does not cause headaches or make you feel dizzy or faint. Often called the "silent killer," it usually has no symptoms.

Blood Pressure Level	Systolic (Top Number)	Diastolic (Bottom Number)
Normal for adults	119 or below	79 or below
Borderline-high (prehypertension)	120 to 139	80 to 89
High (hypertension)	140 or above	90 or above

But it does increase your risk for heart attack, stroke, and kidney and eye damage. Your risk goes up as your blood pressure goes up. The longer your blood pressure stays high, the higher your risk.

If you have high or borderline-high blood pressure, changes in your lifestyle may help lower your blood pressure. Some people also need medicines to get their blood pressure under control.

Should you take medicine for high blood pressure? It's not always easy to decide. For help, go to the Web site on the back cover and enter **c041** in the search box.

Home Treatment

If your blood pressure is normal, the steps below will help you keep it that way. If you have borderline-high or high blood pressure, these steps may help you lower your blood pressure or keep it from getting worse.

◆ Try to reach and stay at a healthy weight. This is especially important if you put on weight around the waist rather than in the hips and thighs. Losing even 10 pounds can help lower your blood pressure. See page 300.

◆ Exercise for a total of at least 2½ hours each week. For example, you can do blocks of 10 minutes or more a few times each day to reach your goal. See Exercise and Health on page 311.

◆ Limit alcohol to no more than 2 drinks a day for a man and 1 drink a day for a woman.

◆ Limit salt. To learn how to reduce salt in your diet, see page 292.

◆ Eat a low-fat diet rich in fruits, vegetables, whole grains, and low-fat dairy products.

◆ Limit saturated fats. Saturated fat is found in animal products such as milk, cheese, and meat. Limiting these foods will help you lose weight and lower your risk for heart disease. See page 307 for tips on how to cut down on them.

◆ If you smoke, quit. Smoking increases your risk for heart attack and stroke. If you need help quitting, see page 316.

Are You at Risk for High Blood Pressure?

You are more likely to have high blood pressure if:

◆ You smoke.

◆ You are overweight.

◆ Others in your family have high blood pressure.

◆ You are African American.

◆ You don't get regular exercise.

◆ You drink too much alcohol.

◆ You eat a lot of salt or do not eat enough fruits, vegetables, whole grains, or dairy products.

◆ You use decongestants, anti-inflammatory drugs (such as ibuprofen or naproxen), or steroids on a regular basis. Aspirin and acetaminophen (Tylenol) do not increase your risk for high blood pressure.

More

If you know you have high blood pressure:

◆ Take any prescribed blood pressure medicines as your doctor tells you. If you stop taking them, your blood pressure may quickly go back up, which is dangerous.

◆ Talk to your doctor about taking an aspirin each day to reduce your risk of heart attack or stroke. Do not start taking aspirin before you have talked to your doctor about it.

◆ See your doctor at least once a year.

◆ If you take blood pressure medicine, talk to your doctor before you take decongestants or anti-inflammatory drugs, such as ibuprofen (Advil, Motrin) or naproxen (Aleve). Some of these can raise blood pressure.

◆ Check your blood pressure at home regularly. To learn how, go to the Web site on the back cover and enter **c887** in the search box.

Go to Web

High Cholesterol

When to Call a Doctor

◆ Your cholesterol is over 200, and your doctor does not know about it (for instance, if you had a cholesterol test at a health fair or at a work-related event).

◆ You are over age 30 and have never had your cholesterol checked. This is especially important if your family has a history of heart disease, diabetes, or high cholesterol.

Cholesterol is a kind of fat your body makes. You also get it from foods that come from animals, such as meat, milk and dairy foods, eggs, chicken, and fish.

Your body needs some cholesterol. But when you have too much, it can build up in your arteries and make it harder for blood to flow through them. This problem is called **atherosclerosis**. It is the starting point for most heart and blood flow problems, including heart attacks and strokes.

Good and Bad Cholesterol

Your body has a few kinds of cholesterol.

◆ **LDL** is the "bad" cholesterol. For LDL, a lower number is better. High LDL increases your risk for heart disease, heart attack, and stroke.

◆ **HDL** is the "good" cholesterol. For HDL, a higher number is better. Raising your HDL may reduce your risk for heart disease, stroke, and a blood flow problem called peripheral artery disease.

◆ **Triglycerides** are another type of fat in the blood. High triglycerides may increase your risk of heart disease and stroke.

What Do the Numbers Mean?

The numbers in the chart on page 193 are for people who are at average risk for heart disease. If you have diabetes or heart disease or are at higher risk for heart disease, your doctor may use lower numbers for what your cholesterol should be.

Total cholesterol

Best: Less than 200

Borderline-high: 200 to 239

High: 240 and above

LDL ("bad" cholesterol)

Best: Less than 100

Near-best: 100 to 129

Borderline-high: 130 to 159

High: 160 to 189

Very high: 190 and above

HDL ("good" cholesterol)

Best: 60 or higher

Good: 40 or higher

Too low: Less than 40

Triglycerides

Normal: Less than 150

Borderline-high: 150 to 199

High: 200 to 499

Very high: 500 and above

When to Have Cholesterol Tests

You and your doctor can decide how often you should be tested, based on your risk for heart disease.

It's a good idea to have your cholesterol checked often if:

◆ Your total cholesterol was over 200 in a past test.

◆ Your family has a history of early heart disease.

◆ You smoke.

◆ You have high blood pressure or take blood pressure medicine.

◆ You have diabetes or high blood sugar.

◆ Your HDL was below 40 or your triglycerides were over 150 in a past test.

These all increase your risk for heart disease. That's why you need to have your cholesterol checked often.

Basic cholesterol tests are easy, quick, and cheap. Call your local health department to find out where you can get a free or low-cost test.

How to Reduce Your Cholesterol

◆ Eat a heart-healthy diet that is low in cholesterol and saturated and trans fats.

  ❖ Eat less total fat, especially saturated and trans fats. See the tips for eating less fat on page 307. Your total fat intake can be up to 35 percent of total calories, as long as most of it is unsaturated fat.

  ❖ Ask your doctor or a dietitian about the TLC (Therapeutic Lifestyle Changes) diet. This diet will help you lower saturated fat to 7 percent or less of your total calories and your cholesterol from food to less than 200 mg a day.

  ❖ Eat at least 2 servings of fruits and at least 3 servings of vegetables each day.

  ❖ Eat at least 2 servings (4 ounces) of baked or broiled fish each week.

  ❖ Eat more fiber (fruit, beans and peas, whole grains). See page 308.

More

- Exercise for a total of at least 2½ hours each week. For example, you can do blocks of 10 minutes or more a few times each day to reach your goal. Exercise may raise your HDL level. It can also help you lose weight and lower your blood pressure. If you need help getting started, see page 311.

- If you smoke, quit. Smoking increases your risk of heart attack and stroke. If you need help quitting, see page 316.

- Lose weight if you need to. Losing even 5 to 10 pounds can lower triglycerides and raise HDL. Your LDL may fall as well. Exercise and a healthy diet can help you keep the weight off. See page 300.

Start with these changes. Regular activity and a diet low in saturated and trans fats are often all it takes to lower cholesterol.

 Some people also need to take medicines. They may have very high cholesterol or diabetes, be at high risk for heart disease, or have other health problems. For help deciding if you should take medicines for high cholesterol, go to the Web site on the back cover and enter **x194** in the search box.

You can do everything right and still have high cholesterol. A lot of cholesterol comes from food, but your body makes cholesterol too. Your cholesterol goes up as you age, no matter how healthy you are. But healthy habits can help you avoid some of the problems related to cholesterol, like heart attack, heart disease, and stroke.

Hives

When to Call a Doctor

Call 911 if hives occur with dizziness, wheezing, trouble breathing, tightness in the chest, or swelling of the tongue, lips, or face.

Call a doctor if:

- You get hives soon after you start a new medicine.

- Hives cover all or most of your body.

- You still have hives after a full day of home treatment.

Hives are raised, red, itchy, often fluid-filled patches of skin that may come and go at random. Some people call them wheals or welts. Hives may last a few minutes or a few days. They can range in size from less than ¼ inch to more than 3 inches across.

An insect sting may cause a single hive. You may get many hives in response to a medicine, food, or infection. Other causes include plant allergies, inhaled allergens, stress, makeup, and exposure to heat, cold, sunlight, or rubber latex. Often you cannot find the cause.

Home Treatment

◆ If you know what caused the hives, avoid it. If it was a food, don't eat it again. If it was makeup, don't wear it again. If it was a medicine, tell your doctor, and do not take it again.

◆ Use cool, moist cloths to help relieve itching. For more tips, see page 142.

◆ Take an oral antihistamine (such as Benadryl or Chlor-Trimeton) to treat the hives and relieve itching. Some types (Alavert, Claritin, Zyrtec) are less likely to make you sleepy. Before you use these medicines, check the label. They may not be safe for young children or for people with certain health problems. Once the hives go away, decrease the dose of the medicine slowly over 5 to 7 days.

Impetigo

When to Call a Doctor

◆ You think you might have impetigo.

◆ Your face is swollen or tender, especially near the nose and lips or around the eyes.

◆ You get a fever, or you have increased pain, swelling, warmth, or redness near the sores.

Impetigo is an infection that causes oozing, honey-colored, crusty sores. It often appears between the upper lip and nose after a cold or at the corner of the mouth. Impetigo is much more common in children than in adults.

Home Treatment

◆ Do not scratch. Scratching can spread impetigo to other areas.

◆ Soak the area in warm water for 15 to 20 minutes to remove crusts. For the face, put a warm, wet washcloth on the sores. Then scrub gently with a washcloth and antibacterial soap. Pat dry. Do this several times a day, using a clean washcloth each time.

◆ If your doctor prescribed medicine, take it as directed.

◆ Apply an antibiotic ointment. Cover the area with gauze taped well away from the sores. This will help keep the infection from spreading and prevent scratching.

◆ Men should shave around the sores, not over them. Use a clean blade each day. Do not use a shaving brush.

◆ Do not share towels, washcloths, or bathwater.

◆ If your child has a runny nose, keep the area between the child's upper lip and nose clean.

Ingrown Toenail

You can get an ingrown toenail if:

◆ You cut your toenail so that the nail cuts into the skin at the edge of the nail. Always cut your toenails straight across, not curved.

◆ You wear shoes that are too tight.

Because the nail can easily get infected, it needs prompt care.

Cut toenails straight across.

Home Treatment

◆ Soak your foot in warm water for 15 minutes each day to soften the skin around the nail. (This may also relieve swelling and pain while the nail grows out.) You may want to add Epsom salt to the water.

◆ To keep the nail from cutting the skin, wedge a small piece of wet cotton under the corner of the nail to cushion it and lift it slightly. Repeat each day until the nail has grown out and you can trim it.

Cotton

Use a piece of wet cotton to cushion and lift the nail.

◆ Cut the toenail straight across. Leave it a little longer at the corners so that the sharp ends don't cut into the skin.

◆ Wear roomy shoes, and keep your feet clean and dry.

Irritable Bowel Syndrome

When to Call a Doctor

- Your symptoms get worse, start to disrupt your usual activities, or do not respond as usual to home treatment.

- You are more and more tired all the time.

- Your symptoms often wake you.

- Your pain gets worse when you move or cough.

- You have belly pain and a fever.

- You have belly pain that does not get better when you pass gas or stools.

- You are losing weight, and you don't know why.

- Your appetite has decreased.

- There is blood in your stools, or your stools look black and tarry.

Irritable bowel syndrome (IBS) is one of the most common problems of the digestive tract. Symptoms often increase with stress or after you eat and include:

- Bloating, belly pain, and gas.

- Mucus in the stool.

- The feeling that you cannot complete a bowel movement.

- Changes in bowel movements. You may go back and forth between constipation and diarrhea. Stools may be hard sometimes and be loose and watery at other times.

People can have IBS for many years. An episode may be worse than the one before it, but the disorder itself does not get worse over time or lead to more serious diseases such as cancer. Symptoms tend to get better over time. Medicines can help control constipation and diarrhea caused by IBS. Home treatment can help too.

If you have frequent digestive problems but have not been diagnosed with IBS, try to rule out other reasons for your stomach upset, such as new foods, stress, or the flu. Try home treatment for 1 to 2 weeks. If it does not help, call your doctor.

There are no tests that can diagnose irritable bowel syndrome, but your doctor may want to do tests to rule out other problems. Be sure to think about and discuss how much testing is right for you. This may depend on your age, your symptoms, your response to treatment, and your chances of having a more serious problem.

 Tests come with risks and costs, and the results may or may not change your treatment. For questions to think about as you decide about testing, go to the Web site on the back cover and enter **h696** in the search box.

More ➤

Home Treatment

If constipation is your main symptom:

◆ Eat more fruits, vegetables, beans, and whole grains. Add these fiber-rich foods to your diet slowly so they do not make gas or cramps worse.

◆ Add unprocessed wheat bran to your diet. Start by using 1 tablespoon a day, and slowly increase to 4 tablespoons a day. Sprinkle bran on cereal, soup, and casseroles. Drink extra water to avoid bloating.

◆ Try a fiber supplement, such as Citrucel, FiberCon, or Metamucil. Start with a dose or less each day (check the label), and drink extra water to prevent bloating.

◆ Use a laxative only if your doctor suggests it.

◆ Get some exercise every day. Exercise helps the digestive system work better.

If diarrhea is your main symptom:

◆ Try the diet tips for relieving constipation. Fiber-rich foods and wheat bran can sometimes help relieve diarrhea.

◆ Avoid foods that make diarrhea worse. Try cutting out one food at a time, and then add it back bit by bit. If a food does not seem to be related to symptoms, you do not need to avoid it. Many people find that the following foods or ingredients make their symptoms worse:

   ❖ Alcohol, caffeine, and nicotine

   ❖ Beans, broccoli, cabbage, and apples

   ❖ Spicy foods

   ❖ Foods high in acid, such as citrus fruit

   ❖ Fatty foods, including bacon, sausage, butter, oils, and anything deep-fried

◆ Avoid dairy products that have lactose (milk sugar) if they seem to make symptoms worse. But be sure to get enough calcium in your diet from other sources. See Lactose Intolerance on page 139.

◆ Avoid sorbitol, which is an artificial sweetener, and olestra, which is a fat substitute used in some processed foods.

◆ Add more starchy food (whole-grain breads, rice, potatoes, pasta) to your diet.

◆ If diarrhea does not stop, a nonprescription medicine such as loperamide (in products such as Imodium) may help. Check with your doctor if you are using loperamide more than 3 times a week.

To reduce stress:

◆ Keep a record of the life events that occur with your symptoms. This may help you see any link between stress and your symptoms.

◆ Get regular, brisk exercise, such as swimming, cycling, or walking.

◆ Learn and use a relaxation technique. See page 320.

Look for more tips in Dealing With Stress on page 318.

Jaw Pain and Temporomandibular Disorder

When to Call a Doctor

Call 911 if you have jaw pain along with chest pain or pressure or other signs of a heart attack. See page 38.

Call a doctor if:

◆ Jaw pain is severe.

◆ You have jaw pain or other problems after an injury to the jaw.

◆ Your jaw locks.

◆ A jaw problem has not improved after 2 weeks of home treatment.

◆ You have noticed a change in the way your teeth fit together when you close your mouth.

The temporomandibular joint connects the lower jawbone to the skull. When you have pain in this joint and in the jaw muscles, you may have a problem called **temporomandibular (TM) disorder**. You may also hear it called TMJ, TMD, or TM problems.

◆ You may feel pain in one or both jaws when you chew or yawn.

◆ You may have painful clicking, popping, or grating in the jaw joint.

◆ Your jaw may lock, or you may not be able to open your mouth wide.

◆ You may often have headaches or pain in your neck, face, or shoulders.

The most common cause of TM disorder is tension in the jaw, neck, and shoulder muscles. Stress or habits such as clenching or grinding your teeth can cause a lot of tension in these muscles. TM disorder can also occur if there is a problem in the jaw joint itself, such as arthritis.

Home treatment can relieve most TM problems. Your doctor may also suggest a plastic mouth plate or physical therapy to help you not clench your teeth. Surgery is rarely needed and may make things worse.

TM disorder causes pain in the shaded areas.

Home Treatment

The key to treating TM disorder is to reduce tension in your jaw.

◆ Try not to clench or grind your teeth. Do not bite your nails, tuck the phone receiver between your shoulder and jaw, or yawn too widely.

◆ At the first sign of pain in your jaw muscles, stop chewing gum, ice, hard candy, or tough foods. Eat softer foods, and use both sides of your mouth to chew.

More

199

◆ Use good posture. Poor posture may disturb the way the muscles and bones in your face work together.

◆ Rest your jaw, keeping your teeth apart and your lips closed. (Keep your tongue on the roof of your mouth, not between your teeth.)

◆ Put either an ice pack or moist heat on your jaw for 15 minutes several times a day if it makes your jaw feel better. You can also switch back and forth between heat and cold. Gently open and close your mouth while the ice pack or heat is on. Do not use heat if your jaw is swollen.

◆ Take an over-the-counter medicine like acetaminophen (Tylenol) or ibuprofen (Advil, Motrin) for pain. Read and follow all instructions on the label.

◆ Relax. If you have a lot of stress in your life, try some relaxation techniques. See page 320. Get help if you are under severe stress or suffer from anxiety or depression.

Kidney Stones

When to Call a Doctor

◆ You think you have a kidney stone. Symptoms include:

  ❖ Sudden pain in your side, groin, or genital area that gets worse over 15 to 60 minutes until it is steady and severe.

  ❖ Nausea and vomiting.

  ❖ Blood in the urine.

  ❖ Feeling like you need to urinate often or having pain when you urinate.

  ❖ Not being able to find a comfortable position.

◆ You have fever or chills and increasing pain in your back, just below your rib cage.

◆ You pass a stone, even if there was little or no pain. Save the stone, and ask your doctor whether it needs to be tested.

Kidney stones can form from the minerals in urine. The most common cause is not drinking enough water.

As long as they stay in the kidneys, kidney stones usually cause no problems. But if a stone moves into the ureter, which is the tube that leads to the bladder (see the picture on page 251), it may block the flow of urine and cause severe pain. In fact, it may be the worst pain you have ever had.

When the stone moves into the bladder, the pain may vanish suddenly. But it can hurt again when the stone passes out of the body.

Most small kidney stones pass without your needing treatment other than pain medicine. In rare cases, you may need surgery or a procedure that uses sound waves to break the stones into small pieces.

Home Treatment

◆ Drink enough water to keep your urine clear—about 8 to 10 glasses a day. This can help prevent future stones.

◆ Take an over-the-counter medicine like acetaminophen (Tylenol) or ibuprofen (Advil, Motrin) for pain. Read and follow all instructions on the label.

◆ Use heat on sore areas in your back or belly for 20 minutes at a time. Moist heat (a hot pack or a hot bath or shower) works better than dry heat.

Knee Problems

When to Call a Doctor

◆ Your knee gives out or will not bear weight.

◆ You felt or heard a "pop" in your knee at the time of an injury.

◆ Your knee swells a lot within 30 minutes of an injury.

◆ You have signs of damage to the nerves or blood vessels, such as numbness, tingling, a pins-and-needles feeling, or pale, bluish, or cool skin below the injury.

◆ Your knee has an odd shape.

◆ You cannot straighten or bend your knee, or the joint locks.

◆ Your knee is red, hot, swollen, or painful to touch.

◆ The pain is bad enough that you are limping, or it does not improve with 2 days of home treatment.

The knee is a joint that can get hurt easily. It is simply three long leg bones held together with ligaments and muscles. Problems can occur when you overstress your knee. Four common ones are:

◆ **Sprained knee ligaments.** (Ligaments connect bone to bone.) Sprains are usu- ally the result of the knee bending or twisting too far in a direction that it's not supposed to go. Sometimes a ligament tears.

◆ **Cartilage tear.** Cartilage is tissue that cushions the joint. If you tear cartilage in your knee, you feel pain and may feel like your knee is locking.

◆ **Kneecap pain**, also known as patello- femoral pain. This is pain around or behind the kneecap. You may have it when you walk or run downhill, when you go up or down stairs, or after you sit for long periods of time.

◆ **Jumper's knee**, also known as patellar tendinosis. This affects the tendon that attaches your kneecap to your shinbone and causes pain right below your knee. It's common in basketball and volleyball players.

Also see Strains, Sprains, and Broken Bones on page 50 and Bursitis and Tendon Injury on page 111.

More

If knee pain is not related to exercise or a recent or past injury, see Arthritis on page 82.

To learn more about the type of injuries and conditions that may cause knee problems, go to the Web site on the back cover and enter **a001** in the search box.

Thighbone (femur)

Kneecap (patella)

Meniscus

Ligament

Meniscus

Ligament

Fibula

Shinbone (tibia)

You can have knee problems when the structures that support the joint are injured or inflamed.

Home Treatment

◆ Rest and protect your knee. Take a break from anything that causes pain. After several days of rest, you can start gentle exercises and stretching.

◆ Put ice or a cold pack on your knee for 10 to 15 minutes at a time. Always put a thin cloth between the ice and your skin. See Ice and Cold Packs on page 243.

◆ Prop up your leg on a pillow when you ice your knee or anytime you sit or lie down during the next 3 days. Try to keep your leg at or above the level of your heart. This will help reduce swelling.

◆ Take an over-the-counter medicine like acetaminophen (Tylenol) or ibuprofen (Advil, Motrin) for pain. Read and follow all instructions on the label.

◆ Ask your doctor about wearing a brace or an elastic or neoprene sleeve. This may help ease pain during activity. You can buy one at a drugstore or sporting goods store.

Preventing Knee Problems

◆ Strengthen and stretch the leg muscles evenly, especially those in the front of the thigh (called the quadriceps) and the back of the thigh (called the hamstrings). See page 314. This is the best way to prevent knee problems.

◆ Do not do deep knee bends. Imagine a line that starts at the tip of your toes and goes straight up. When you do knee bends, your knees should not pass that line.

◆ Do not run downhill unless your muscles are well trained and strong enough for it.

◆ Wear shoes with good arch supports. Replace running shoes every 3 months or 500 miles.

◆ Do not wear shoes with cleats when you play contact sports.

◆ Do not wear high-heeled shoes.

Laryngitis

When to Call a Doctor

◆ You are hoarse or have lost your voice, and you have a high fever. See the fever guidelines on pages 158 and 160.

◆ You have symptoms of a worse infection, such as fast or shallow breathing, a cough that brings up colored or bloody mucus from the lungs, or pain, fever, and fatigue that are getting a lot worse.

◆ You are hoarse for more than 2 to 3 weeks.

Laryngitis is an infection or irritation of the voice box (larynx). If you have laryngitis, you may be hoarse, lose your voice, and feel like you need to clear your throat a lot. You may also have fever, throat pain, and a cough and feel more tired than usual.

You can get laryngitis because of:

◆ A virus, such as a cold.

◆ Allergies.

◆ Lots of talking, singing, or yelling.

◆ Cigarette smoke.

◆ Backflow (reflux) of stomach acid into the throat.

Your voice box will usually heal in 5 to 10 days. Medicine does not help much.

If you drink a lot of alcohol or smoke, you may reach a point where your throat and voice box are irritated all the time.

Home Treatment

◆ If a cold makes you hoarse, treat the cold (see page 124). You may be hoarse for up to a week after a cold goes away.

◆ Rest your voice. Try not to talk much or clear your throat.

◆ Do not smoke, and avoid other people's smoke. If you need help to quit smoking, see page 316.

◆ Use a humidifier in your bedroom or your whole house. Or try standing in the steam from a hot shower.

◆ Drink extra water and other fluids.

◆ To soothe your throat, gargle with warm salt water (1 teaspoon of salt in 8 ounces of water). Or drink weak tea or hot water with honey or lemon juice in it. Do not give honey to children younger than 1 year of age.

◆ If you think that problems with stomach acid reflux may be the cause, reducing heartburn may help. See page 184.

Leg Pain and Muscle Cramps

When to Call a Doctor

- You have sudden leg pain, and the skin of your lower leg, foot, or toes is cold, pale, or blue-black. This could be a serious problem.

- You have swelling, redness, and pain in the leg or calf. You may also have a fever. These may be signs of phlebitis (see the chart on page 205).

- Leg pain always starts after you walk a certain distance and then goes away when you stop walking. This may be a sign of a blood flow problem.

- Home treatment does not relieve your muscle cramps.

Leg pain and muscle cramps ("charley horse" or "a stitch") are common. They often occur at night or during exercise, especially if the weather is hot or humid. Dehydration, low levels of potassium, or using a muscle that is not stretched well may cause cramps.

Home Treatment

- If you have pain, swelling, or heaviness in only one of your legs, or if you have other symptoms that cause you to suspect phlebitis, call your doctor before you try home treatment.

- Warm up well and stretch before exercise. Also stretch after you exercise. If a muscle cramps, gently stretch and massage it.

- Drink plenty of fluids. Drink extra fluids before and during exercise, especially if the weather is hot or humid.

- Get plenty of potassium in your diet. Bananas, orange juice, and potatoes are good sources.

- If leg cramps wake you at night, take a warm bath and do some stretches before you go to bed. Keep your legs warm while sleeping.

- For shin splints, put a cold pack on your leg for 10 to 15 minutes at a time. You can also take an over-the-counter medicine like acetaminophen (Tylenol) or ibuprofen (Advil, Motrin) for pain. Read and follow all instructions on the label. Take 1 to 2 weeks of rest from high-impact activities like running. Return to exercise slowly.

- To avoid stomach muscle cramps ("side stitch") during exercise, do side stretches before you start. Try to take deep, even breaths.

Growing Pains

Children ages 6 to 12 often have harmless "growing pains" in their legs at night. Unless your child's pain is severe, you don't need to worry about these. A heating pad or gentle massage may help. An over-the-counter medicine like acetaminophen (Tylenol) or ibuprofen (Advil, Motrin) may also help. Read and follow all instructions on the label.

Common Causes of Leg Pain	Symptoms	Comments
Muscle cramps	Sudden cramping pain, usually in lower leg; leg may feel like it is in "knots"	Often happens at night or during exercise
Shin splints	Pain in front of lower leg	Often caused by overuse or high-impact exercise (such as running on a hard surface), especially if you are not used to it
Arthritis	Pain in leg joints (knees, ankles, toes)	See Arthritis, p. 82.
Sciatica (a back problem)	Leg pain that extends from buttock down back of leg and into foot	See Sciatica, p. 88.
Phlebitis (an inflamed vein)	Pain and swelling in one calf; common after surgery, bed rest, and extended air travel	Can be serious if blood clot forms, breaks loose, and travels to lungs
Decreased blood flow (intermittent claudication)	Cramping pain in the calf that starts after you walk a certain distance and goes away when you rest; leg pain and cold, pale skin	

Lice and Scabies

When to Call a Doctor

◆ You have severe nighttime itching that does not go away after a few days.

◆ You see live lice or new nits after you have used a nonprescription lice medicine. Your doctor can prescribe a stronger medicine.

Lice are tiny insects that may live on the skin, hair, or clothing. They feed by biting the skin and sucking blood. Scabies are tiny mites that dig under the skin and lay eggs.

Both cause an allergic rash and itching. And both are common in children who go to day care or school.

More

Common Questions	Lice	Scabies
Where are they found?	In hair on the head (head lice); on clothes (body lice); in groin area, underarms, and eyelashes (body or pubic lice)	Between folds of skin on fingers, toes, wrists, underarms, knees, elbows, and groin
How are they spread?	By close contact with an infested person or his or her clothes, hats, bedding, towels, brushes, or combs; pubic lice by sexual contact	By close contact with an infested person or his or her bedding, clothes, or towels
How do you get rid of them?	Medicine for lice. Wash clothes, bedding, and towels.	Medicine applied to the entire body and left on overnight. Wash clothes, bedding, and towels. Itching may last for several weeks.

Home Treatment

◆ To get rid of lice, try a nonprescription medicine such as Nix or RID. Follow the directions on the label exactly. After you use the medicine, comb the hair well with a fine-toothed nit comb to remove all lice eggs, called nits. You can buy nit combs at most drugstores and supermarkets.

◆ To get rid of scabies, you will need prescription medicine. Call your doctor.

◆ On the day you start treatment for lice or scabies, wash all dirty clothes, bedding, and towels in hot water. Iron or dry-clean items that cannot be washed, or freeze them for 24 hours.

◆ Call your pharmacist or health department for more information about treatment and prevention.

When Can My Child Go Back to School?

Some schools have a "no nits" policy stating that children may not return to school until they are free of lice nits.

Children who have scabies can go back to school as soon as they complete the prescription medicine.

Menopause

When to Call a Doctor

◆ Your periods are longer, heavier, or harder to predict than usual.

◆ You have new bleeding between periods.

◆ You have bleeding after your periods have stopped for 6 months.

◆ You have vaginal dryness, and a lubricant does not help. Your doctor may prescribe an estrogen cream, suppository, or ring.

◆ Your symptoms are disrupting your life, even with home treatment.

◆ You have unexplained bleeding (different from what your doctor told you to expect) while you are taking hormones.

Menopause occurs when the body does not make as much of the female hormones estrogen and progesterone. This happens between ages 45 and 55 for most women and may take several years to complete.

Having both ovaries removed (oophorectomy) also causes menopause, though you can take hormones to treat the symptoms.

Hormone changes may cause:

◆ **Irregular periods.** Your flow may be lighter or heavier than usual. The time between periods may get shorter or longer. You may have spotting. Some women have regular periods until their periods stop suddenly. Others have irregular periods for a long time.

◆ **Hot flashes.** These cause intense heat, sweating, and flushing that can last from a few minutes to an hour. A hot flash usually starts in the chest and spreads out to the neck, face, and arms. If hot flashes often wake you up at night, you may feel tired and distracted because you're not sleeping enough.

◆ **Vaginal dryness.** Your vagina may become drier, thinner, and less stretchy. These changes can make sex hurt. And they may increase your risk for infections (see page 255) and bladder control problems (see page 100).

◆ **Mood changes.** Some women feel nervous, moody, or depressed as they go through menopause. You may lack energy or have trouble sleeping.

You may also need to think about some other issues:

◆ **Osteoporosis.** Loss of estrogen may weaken your bones and make them more likely to break. Hormone therapy can help prevent this but may cause other health problems. To learn more, see page 214. Be sure to get plenty of calcium and vitamin D.

◆ **Birth control.** Until you have finished menopause, your body will continue to release eggs (ovulate). This means that you could get pregnant. If you don't want to get pregnant, use birth control until your doctor confirms that you have finished menopause or until you have not had a period for 12 months.

◆ **Heart disease.** Women who are at the age to start menopause are more likely to get heart disease. Work with your doctor to learn what you can do to prevent it.

More ▶

Hormone Therapy

Your doctor may prescribe hormone therapy to treat symptoms of menopause. There are two types:

◆ Estrogen replacement therapy (ERT). ERT is estrogen alone. Because ERT may increase the risk of uterine cancer, it is usually used only for women who have had their uterus removed (hysterectomy).

◆ Hormone replacement therapy (HRT). HRT is estrogen and progestin, another female hormone. Progestin helps protect against uterine cancer.

Hormone pills are taken every day. You can get some forms of hormone therapy as skin patches, vaginal creams, or vaginal rings.

Benefits of therapy

◆ Reduces hot flashes and vaginal dryness

◆ Helps keep bones strong and lowers your risk of osteoporosis. (But there are other medicines that can help with this too.)

Risks of therapy

◆ May increase your risk for certain health problems such as breast cancer, stroke, and blood clots in your legs and lungs

◆ May cause bloating, sore breasts, vaginal bleeding, and other side effects

◆ Not advised for women who have had breast cancer, uterine cancer, blood clots, heart attack, stroke, liver disease, or who have undiagnosed uterine bleeding

For some women, the short-term benefit of reducing menopause symptoms may outweigh the risks. Using hormone therapy for 1 to 2 years may help with symptoms while they are at their worst, with less chance of causing the long-term side effects.

 Talk with your doctor about whether hormone therapy is a good idea for you. For help with your decision, go to the Web site on the back cover and enter **t747** in the search box.

If you already take hormones, talk with your doctor each year about whether it is still the right thing for you.

Home Treatment

◆ For hot flashes:

❖ Keep your home and workplace cool, or use a fan.

❖ Dress in layers that are easy to take off. Wear natural fibers like cotton and silk.

❖ Drink cold drinks, not hot ones.

❖ Limit caffeine and alcohol, and do not smoke.

❖ Get regular exercise. Women who exercise regularly have fewer problems with hot flashes.

❖ Try a relaxation technique. See page 320.

◆ For vaginal dryness and pain during sex, use a water-soluble lubricant, such as Astroglide or K-Y Jelly. Do not use Vaseline or other oil-based products.

◆ Keep a written record of your periods. You may need to discuss them with your doctor.

◆ Make exercise a part of your life. Regular exercise can ease stress, keep your bones strong, and reduce your risk of heart disease and other health problems.

◆ Get support if you need it. Talking with other women may help.

◆ Try to stay relaxed about menopause. Being tense may make you feel worse.

Menstrual Cramps

When to Call a Doctor

◆ You have severe pain in your pelvis or belly, with or without menstrual bleeding.

◆ You have cramps and a fever.

◆ Menstrual cramps have recently gotten worse.

◆ Pelvic pain does not seem related to your menstrual cycle.

◆ Cramps start 5 to 7 days before your period or continue after your period stops.

◆ Cramps do not respond to home treatment for three cycles, or they keep you from your normal activities.

◆ You think your copper IUD is causing cramps, and the pain is more than you can stand or worse than what your doctor told you to expect.

Many women have painful periods. It's common to have:

◆ Cramping in the lower belly, back, or thighs.

◆ Headaches.

◆ Diarrhea, constipation, or nausea.

◆ Dizziness.

These problems are often caused by normal hormone changes. Pain and cramps can also be related to endometriosis (a problem with the lining of the uterus), pelvic infections, or noncancerous growths (fibroids) in the uterus.

If you tend to get symptoms other than cramping (such as weight gain, headache, and tension) before your period starts, you may have PMS. See page 219.

IUDs and Cramps

If you get a copper IUD (intrauterine device) for birth control, you may have bad cramps for the first few months of use.

If cramping does not stop, you may need to have the IUD removed and use other birth control. See page 96. Birth control pills or the hormonal IUD (Mirena) can reduce cramping.

Home Treatment

◆ Take ibuprofen (Advil, Motrin) or naproxen (Aleve) the day before your period starts or at the first sign of pain. These medicines may ease cramps better than aspirin or acetaminophen (Tylenol).

◆ Exercise. It makes cramps less severe.

◆ Use a heating pad or take a hot bath to relax tense muscles and relieve cramps.

◆ Try herbal teas, such as ginger, chamomile, or mint. These may help soothe tense muscles and anxious moods.

Missed or Irregular Periods

When to Call a Doctor

◆ You have lower belly pain and think you could be pregnant.

◆ A home pregnancy test says you are pregnant, or you think you're pregnant even though the test says you are not.

◆ You have missed two regular periods and don't know why.

◆ You miss two periods while taking birth control pills, and you have not skipped any pills.

◆ You have not had your first period by age 16.

◆ You have not developed breasts or pubic hair by age 14.

Many women miss periods now and then. Missed or irregular periods have many possible causes, such as:

◆ Pregnancy. This is usually the first thing to consider.

◆ Stress or travel.

◆ Weight loss or weight gain.

◆ Increased exercise. Missed periods are common in endurance athletes.

◆ Birth control pills or implants, the Mirena IUD, or Depo-Provera shots. These may cause lighter, less frequent, or skipped periods.

◆ Menopause. See page 207.

◆ Medicines, including steroids, tranquilizers, diet pills, and illegal drugs.

◆ Menarche (the start of menstrual periods). Periods may be irregular for the first few years.

◆ Hormone imbalance or problems in the pelvic organs.

◆ Breast-feeding.

◆ An untreated thyroid problem.

If you have skipped a period, try to relax. Unless you're pregnant, chances are your cycle will return to normal next month.

Home Pregnancy Tests

If you get pregnant, it's important to find out right away so you can take good care of yourself and your baby. The quickest way to know is with a home pregnancy test. Some tests can tell that you are pregnant within a few days of your first missed period.

Tests are cheap and very accurate when you use them right. Choose a test that has simple instructions, and follow them exactly. Mistakes can cause false results.

If the test shows that you are pregnant, see your doctor to confirm it. Even if the test says that you are not pregnant, it's a good idea to see your doctor to be certain.

If you are sexually active and don't want to get pregnant, you need to use birth control. You may also want to get emergency birth control in case you need it. See page 97.

Home Treatment

◆ If you had sex during the past month, take a home pregnancy test. See page 210. Treat yourself like you are pregnant until you know for sure.

◆ Avoid fad diets that greatly restrict calories and food variety, and avoid quick weight loss.

◆ Increase exercise slowly. If you are an endurance athlete, cut back on training, and talk with a doctor about hormone and calcium supplements to protect against bone loss.

◆ Try relaxation techniques to deal with stress. See page 320.

Neck Pain

When to Call a Doctor

Call 911 if:

◆ Neck pain occurs with chest pain or other symptoms of a heart attack (see page 38).

◆ You think you may have a serious injury to your neck. See page 49.

◆ You suddenly lose bowel or bladder control, even if you were not injured.

Call your doctor if:

◆ A stiff neck occurs with fever and a severe headache. You may have a serious illness. See page 161.

◆ You have new weakness or constant numbness in your arms or legs.

◆ Neck pain goes down one arm, or you have numbness or tingling in your hands.

◆ A blow or injury to your neck causes new pain.

◆ You cannot control your pain with home treatment.

◆ Pain has not gotten better after 2 weeks of home treatment.

Most people have pain, stiffness, or a kink in the neck from time to time. Neck pain is most often caused by tension, strain, or spasm in the neck muscles or inflammation of the ligaments, tendons, or joints in the neck. This can happen when:

◆ You stay too long in a position that stresses the neck. Some examples are cradling the phone between your ear and shoulder, sleeping on your stomach or with your neck twisted, or looking up or down at a computer screen all day.

◆ You repeat movements that stress the neck. You might do this during exercise or sports, on the job, or at home.

Arthritis or damage to the discs in the neck can cause a pinched nerve. With this problem, the pain usually spreads down one arm. Your arm or hand may tingle or feel numb or weak. If you have symptoms of a pinched nerve, you need to see your doctor.

More

Neck Exercises

These exercises make your neck stronger and more flexible and help you avoid neck problems. You do not need to do every exercise. Do the ones that help the most. Go slow, and stop any exercise that hurts. Do the exercises twice a day.

Dorsal glide

Sit or stand tall, looking straight ahead (a "palace guard" posture). Slowly tuck your chin as you glide your head backward over your body. Hold for about 6 seconds; then relax for about 10 seconds. Repeat 8 to 12 times. This stretches the back of the neck. If you feel pain, do not glide so far back.

Dorsal glide

Chest and shoulder stretch

Sit or stand tall, and glide your head backward as in the dorsal glide. Raise both arms so that your hands are next to your ears. As you exhale, lower your elbows down and back. Feel your shoulder blades slide down and together. Hold for about 6 seconds; then relax for about 10 seconds. Repeat 8 to 12 times.

Hands on head

Move your head backward, forward, and side to side against gentle pressure from your hands. Hold each position for about 6 seconds; then relax for about 10 seconds. Repeat 8 to 12 times.

Chest and shoulder stretch

Home Treatment

Much of the home treatment for back pain also works for neck pain. See page 86. These tips may also help:

- Try ice or a cold pack on your neck for 10 to 15 minutes several times a day. This can help reduce pain. But always put a thin cloth between the ice and your skin. If the problem is near your shoulder or upper back, it often helps more to ice the back of your neck.

- You can also try putting heat on the sore area for 20 minutes at a time. Or try switching back and forth between ice and heat. Do what works best for you.

- Take an over-the-counter medicine like acetaminophen (Tylenol) or ibuprofen (Advil, Motrin) for pain. Read and follow all instructions on the label.

- Try to get back to your daily activities or take some easy walks as soon as you can. These may help you feel better faster.

- Once the pain starts to get better, try the neck exercises on page 212.

If neck pain occurs with a headache, see page 176.

Preventing Neck Pain

You can prevent most neck pain by using good posture, getting regular exercise, and not stressing your neck too much or too often. You can strengthen and protect your neck by doing neck exercises. See page 212.

Reducing stress may help too. See the relaxation exercises on page 320.

To avoid pain at the end of the day, be careful how you sit, stand, and move during the day.

- Sit straight in your chair with your lower back supported. Do not sit for long periods without getting up or changing positions. Take mini-breaks several times each hour to stretch your neck.

- If you work at a computer, have the top of the screen at eye level. Use a document holder that puts the copy at the same level as the screen.

- If you use the phone a lot, use a headset or speakerphone.

To avoid neck stiffness in the morning, you may need better neck support when you sleep. (Morning neck pain may also be the result of things you did the day before.)

- Fold a towel lengthwise into a 4-inch-wide pad and wrap it around your neck. Pin the ends together for good support.

- You may need a special neck support pillow. Look for a pillow that supports your neck comfortably when you lie on your back and on your side (try before buying). Do not use pillows that push your head forward when you are on your back.

- Do not sleep on your stomach with your neck twisted or bent.

Osteoporosis

When to Call a Doctor

◆ You think you have a broken bone, or you cannot move a part of your body.

◆ You have sudden, severe pain or cannot put weight on a body part.

◆ One of your arms or legs is not its normal shape. This may mean you have a broken bone.

◆ You are concerned about your risk for osteoporosis.

Also see Strains, Sprains, and Broken Bones on page 50.

Osteoporosis means that your bones are thin and weak and can break easily. The problem affects millions of older adults, especially older women.

Osteoporosis is more common after menopause, when the body makes less estrogen. Too much thyroid hormone can also weaken your bones.

You are at highest risk for osteoporosis if:

◆ Other people in your family have had it.

◆ You do not get much weight-bearing exercise and have not done much in the past.

◆ You have a slender body frame.

◆ You smoke, or you drink a lot of alcohol.

◆ You drink a lot of dark sodas, such as cola.

◆ You take certain medicines that cause bone thinning. These include some used to treat chronic lung disease, thyroid problems, or prostate cancer.

◆ You are of Asian or European heritage.

Osteoporosis usually develops over many years without symptoms. The first sign may be a broken bone, a loss of height, a slowly forming curve or hump in the upper back, or back pain.

A special X-ray called a **DEXA scan** measures bone thickness (density) and can tell you how much bone loss you have. If you are at high risk for osteoporosis, a bone density test may give you and your doctor information that can help you decide whether you need treatment. This test is recommended for anyone at risk for osteoporosis, and especially for women starting at age 65.

For help deciding whether you are at risk and need this test, go to the Web site on the back cover and enter **m508** in the search box.

What You Can Do

Weakening bones are a natural part of growing older. But if you start healthy habits early in life, you may be able to delay the problem. If you already have osteoporosis, these same habits can help slow the disease process and may reduce your risk of broken bones.

◆ Get plenty of weight-bearing exercise. Walking, jogging, dancing, lifting weights, and other exercises make bones stronger.

◆ Eat a healthy diet with lots of calcium and vitamin D. You need both of these to build strong, healthy bones.

  ❖ Get calcium from yogurt, cheese, milk, and dark green vegetables.

- ❖ Get vitamin D from eggs, fatty fish, and fortified cereal and milk.

- ❖ Talk to your doctor about taking a calcium and vitamin D supplement if you think you might need one.

- ◆ If you smoke, quit. If you need help quitting, see page 316.

- ◆ Limit alcohol to no more than 1 drink a day for a woman and 2 drinks a day for a man.

- ◆ Cut down on dark sodas, such as cola. This includes diet kinds. They may make your bones thinner.

There are medicines that can help prevent osteoporosis. Hormone therapy is one choice, but it has other risks. Talk with your doctor about what's right for you. Also see Hormone Therapy on page 208.

If you have osteoporosis, medicines can help slow bone loss and build bone strength. Bisphosphonates (such as Actonel, Boniva, or Fosamax) are medicines used most often.

If you know your bones are weak, be extra careful to avoid falls. See page 332 for tips on how to make your home safer.

Pinworms

When to Call a Doctor

- ◆ You or your child has itching in the anal area (especially at night), but you have not seen any worms. If this is the first infection, see a doctor to make sure that pinworms are the problem.

- ◆ You or your child vomits or has pain after taking pinworm medicine.

- ◆ You or your child still has anal itching after treatment. You may need another round of treatment or a stronger medicine.

- ◆ You or your child has pinworms and has any of these symptoms:

  - ❖ Fever or belly pain

  - ❖ Redness, tenderness, swelling, or itching in the genital area

  - ❖ Pain when urinating

Pinworms are tiny worms that infect the digestive tract. They are most common in school-age children, but anyone can get them.

Pinworms lay their eggs just outside the anus. This makes the area itch. Itching is often worse at night. When a child scratches and then later sucks a thumb or puts a finger in his or her mouth, the child swallows the eggs, and the cycle starts again.

Pinworms are hard to avoid if you have young children. The problem spreads easily, and the eggs can survive on clothing, bedding, and toys for days. Teach children to wash their hands after they use the toilet and before they eat.

Home Treatment

- ◆ Ask your pharmacist for a nonprescription medicine for pinworms. Do not take the medicine if you are pregnant, and do not give it to a child younger than 2 unless your doctor tells you to.

More

215

◆ Treat every child in the house between the ages of 2 and 10. If there is still a pinworm problem, you may need to treat everyone else in the house as well.

◆ On the first day of treatment, wash all underwear, pajamas, bedding, and towels in hot water and detergent to get rid of any eggs. Clean toys with disinfectant, or wash them. Clean bathrooms and sleeping areas with a strong disinfectant.

◆ Trim your child's fingernails and keep them short.

◆ Wash hands often. Take morning showers, and change and wash pajamas and underwear every day until you finish the treatment.

Pneumonia

When to Call a Doctor

◆ You have fever and a cough that brings up yellow, green, rust-colored, or bloody mucus from your lungs.

◆ You have new pain in your chest that gets worse when you take a deep breath or cough.

◆ You have had a cold, bronchitis, or other viral illness, and you get worse instead of better.

◆ You are short of breath.

◆ Fast, shallow breathing.

◆ Pain in the chest muscles (chest-wall pain) that is worse when the person coughs or takes a deep breath.

◆ A fast heartbeat.

◆ Fatigue that is worse than tiredness from a cold.

Pneumonia can be a serious problem for babies, young children, older adults, and people who have long-term health problems. It's important for these groups to get the pneumococcal vaccine. See page 323.

Pneumonia is an infection or inflammation in the lungs. It sometimes follows a viral illness like a cold, the flu, or bronchitis. Having bronchitis and another lung disease, such as asthma, may make you more likely to get pneumonia.

Pneumonia is usually caused by bacteria, but it can be caused by viruses and other things too. A person who has bacterial pneumonia is usually very sick and may have:

◆ A bad cough that brings up yellow, green, rust-colored, or bloody mucus (sputum) from the lungs.

◆ A fever and shaking chills.

Home Treatment

◆ If your doctor prescribes any medicines, take them as you are told.

◆ Drink extra fluids to stay hydrated.

◆ Take an over-the-counter medicine like acetaminophen (Tylenol) or ibuprofen (Advil, Motrin) to reduce fever and pain. Read and follow all instructions on the label. Do not give aspirin to anyone younger than 20.

◆ Before you use cough or cold medicines, check the label. They may not be safe for young children or for people with certain health problems.

◆ Get lots of rest. It takes time to get well.

Pregnancy Problems

When to Call a Doctor

Call 911 if:

◆ You have heavy vaginal bleeding, and you are in your second or third trimester of pregnancy.

◆ You have severe pain in your belly or pelvis.

◆ You faint.

◆ Fluid gushes or leaks from your vagina, and you know or think the umbilical cord is bulging into your vagina. If this happens, get on your hands and knees, and keep your rear end higher than your head. This will decrease the pressure on the cord until help arrives.

Call your doctor if:

◆ You have sudden swelling of your face, hands, or feet; a severe headache; or new vision problems (dimness, blurring).

◆ You have pain, cramping, or any vaginal bleeding.

◆ You have a fever.

◆ You have 4 or more contractions in 20 minutes or 8 or more in 1 hour, even after you drink water and rest.

◆ You have a sudden release of fluid from your vagina.

◆ You have low back pain or pelvic pressure.

◆ You notice that your baby has stopped moving or is moving much less than normal.

◆ You vomit more than 3 times a day, or you are too sick to eat or drink.

◆ You itch all over your body. You may also have dark urine or pale stools, or your skin or eyes may turn yellow.

Problems can happen during pregnancy no matter how careful you are. But you can increase the chances that your baby will be healthy by following some basic guidelines.

Work With Your Doctor

◆ Go to all your prenatal appointments. At each visit, your doctor will check your blood pressure and check your urine for protein. High blood pressure and protein in the urine are signs of preeclampsia. This problem can be dangerous for you and your baby.

◆ Follow your doctor's advice about activity. Your doctor will let you know how much exercise is safe for you. This may change as you get closer to the end of your pregnancy.

◆ Ask your doctor whether you can have sex. If you are at risk for preterm labor, your doctor may ask you to not have sex after a certain point.

◆ If you take medicine for another health problem, talk with your doctor about whether you can continue your treatment or need to change it.

More

Morning Sickness

Many women have nausea and vomiting during the first few months they are pregnant. This is called morning sickness, though it can occur at any time of day. It is normal but unpleasant.

To avoid or at least reduce morning sickness:

◆ Eat 5 or 6 small meals a day so your stomach is never empty. Eat some protein in each of the meals.

◆ Eat crackers or dry toast before you get out of bed in the morning.

◆ Sip a sports drink when you have trouble with solid food.

◆ Get more vitamin B6 and B12 by eating more whole grains and cereals, wheat germ, nuts, seeds, and legumes. But talk with your doctor before you take any vitamin supplements.

◆ Try ginger tea or ginger candy.

◆ Avoid foods or smells that make you sick.

◆ Get plenty of rest.

Call your doctor if you cannot keep down food or liquids, if you are vomiting more than 3 times a day, or if you are losing weight.

Get Good Nutrition

◆ Eat a balanced diet that has plenty of calcium- and iron-rich foods. Foods high in calcium include milk, cheese, yogurt, almonds, and broccoli. Iron-rich foods include beef, shellfish, chicken and turkey, eggs, beans, raisins, whole-grain bread, and leafy green vegetables.

◆ If you need help paying for food, call your local WIC (Women, Infants, and Children) agency to learn whether you are eligible for help. WIC provides vouchers for nutritious food, nutrition education, and breast-feeding support to pregnant women, women with new babies, and children younger than 5.

◆ Take a daily multivitamin that contains 0.4 mg to 0.8 mg (400 mcg to 800 mcg) of folic acid (folate). Folic acid helps prevent certain birth defects. Other good sources of folic acid are fortified cereal and whole wheat bread.

◆ Drink plenty of fluids. Dehydration can cause contractions.

◆ If you drink coffee, tea, or soda with caffeine, cut back to about 1 cup a day.

Protect Your Baby

◆ Do not smoke.

◆ Do not drink alcohol or use illegal drugs.

◆ If you have a cat, have someone else clean the litter box. Avoid cat feces.

◆ Wash your hands well after you handle raw meat. Fully cook all meat before you eat it.

◆ Avoid all chemical vapors, paint fumes, and poisons.

◆ Avoid getting very hot. Do not use saunas or hot tubs. Don't stay out in the sun in hot weather for long periods.

◆ Do not take any prescription or over-the-counter medicines, herbal supplements, or vitamins (other than your prenatal vitamins) without talking to your doctor or pharmacist first.

◆ Take care to prevent falls. During pregnancy, your joints are loose and your balance is off. After your 25th week, avoid sports with a high risk of falls or injury, such as bicycling, skiing, in-line skating, and horseback or motorcycle riding. Do not dive or scuba dive.

Prepare for Childbirth

Late in your pregnancy, it's a good idea to start getting ready for the birth itself.

◆ Take childbirth classes with your partner or the person you choose to be your "coach."

◆ Learn about early signs of labor so you know what to watch for.

◆ If you have other children, talk to them about the new baby and help them adjust to the idea.

◆ Learn a relaxation exercise or two (see page 320). They can help while you are in labor.

◆ Think about creating a birth plan with your doctor that states what you want and what you expect to happen during labor and delivery. This can cover things like who you want there for the birth and whether you want medicine to help with the pain. But keep in mind that some things may be out of your and your doctor's control.

◆ Learn about breast-feeding, and find resources that can help (such as La Leche League or the Nursing Mothers Counsel). See page 106.

◆ Get plenty of rest, eat well, and be nice to yourself.

Premenstrual Syndrome (PMS)

When to Call a Doctor

◆ You do not feel better within a few days after your period starts.

◆ PMS often keeps you away from work, school, and your normal activities.

◆ You feel out of control because of PMS.

◆ PMS upsets your work, family life, or friendships.

Many women have cramps, tender breasts, and other mild symptoms just before and during the first few days of their periods. This is normal. When the symptoms are so bad that they disrupt your life or affect your relationships, they are called premenstrual syndrome, or PMS.

PMS symptoms are different for each woman. Some of the common ones include:

◆ Breast swelling, bloating, weight gain, and acne.

◆ Mood changes, food cravings, and decreased sex drive.

◆ Cramps, headaches, breast pain, and muscle aches.

◆ Sleep problems and lack of energy.

You may be able to prevent or reduce your symptoms with some of the diet and lifestyle changes and other tips in the Home Treatment section. But it may take a couple of periods before things improve.

More

219

If PMS is severely disrupting your life, see your doctor. Your doctor can prescribe medicines that may help. For help deciding whether these are right for you, go to the Web site on the back cover and enter **z963** in the search box.

A small number of women have premenstrual dysphoric disorder (PMDD), a severe form of PMS that can make you angry or even violent and upset your relationships at work and home. Prescription medicines and self-care can help you get back in control.

Home Treatment

◆ Keep a daily record of your symptoms—what they are, how bad they are, and when you have them. By helping you see patterns in your cycle, this record may help you prevent, reduce, or better cope with PMS. For example, if you know when your cramps usually start, you can start taking medicine just before they begin. This works better than waiting until you are in pain.

◆ Eat small meals every 3 to 4 hours. Include plenty of whole grains, fruits, and vegetables. Limit fats and sweets.

◆ Reduce salt to help limit bloating.

◆ Do not smoke, and reduce alcohol and caffeine.

◆ Exercise.

◆ Try nonprescription PMS medicines such as Midol or Pamprin. These contain several drugs to help relieve cramps, bloating, and headaches.

◆ Reduce stress as much as you can. Try yoga or other relaxation techniques. See page 320.

◆ Find support. Talk with your family, friends, and any others who may be affected by your symptoms. Or join a PMS support group.

Prostate Cancer

When to Call a Doctor

◆ You have blood or pus in your urine, or you have blood in your semen.

◆ You have urinary symptoms that come on quickly, bother you enough that you want help, or last longer than 2 months. (Also see Prostate Enlargement on page 222.)

◆ You already have prostate problems, and you develop back or bone pain.

Prostate cancer is the second leading cause of cancer deaths in men. (See pictures of the prostate on pages 222 and 224.) But it can often be cured if it is found early, before it has spread to other organs. And it tends to grow slowly. Many older men with prostate cancer die of another cause (like heart disease) before the cancer has grown enough to cause problems.

Most men with prostate cancer have no symptoms. In a few cases, the cancer can cause urinary symptoms like those of prostate enlargement. See page 222. If it spreads to bones or other organs, it can cause pain and other symptoms.

Any man can get prostate cancer. But the risk is highest for:

◆ Older men. Most men who get prostate cancer are over 65.

◆ African-American men.

◆ Men who have a family history of prostate cancer.

Should You Be Tested?

Doctors can use one of two simple tests to look for signs of prostate cancer:

◆ Digital rectal exam, in which the doctor puts a gloved finger in your rectum and feels the prostate

◆ PSA blood test

Finding prostate cancer early can save lives in some cases. But in other cases, it never affects a man's life. Talk with your doctor about your risk for prostate cancer and the pros and cons of PSA testing.

To help decide whether testing is right for you, go to the Web site on the back cover and enter **t951** in the search box. Then talk to your doctor.

Should You Be Treated?

If you have prostate cancer, here are a few things you should know:

◆ You may not die any sooner than you would have without the cancer. Prostate cancer tends to occur later in life and usually grows slowly.

◆ If the cancer does not cause symptoms, it may not affect your quality of life.

◆ The younger you are and the larger or more advanced the cancer is, the more serious the disease may be.

◆ Treatment can cause lasting problems with bladder control or erections.

Learn all you can about your treatment options—which may include not treating the cancer. You need to consider your age, your health, and the nature of the cancer itself when you make treatment decisions. For example, if you are older and the cancer is not growing much, it may make sense to take a wait-and-see approach.

To help decide what approach you want to take, go to the Web site on the back cover and enter **r808** in the search box. Your doctor can help you with the decision.

Prostate Enlargement

When to Call a Doctor

- You cannot urinate at all.
- You feel like you cannot empty your bladder completely.
- You have urinary problems along with fever, chills, vomiting, or pain in your back or belly.
- It hurts or burns when you urinate.
- There is blood or pus in your urine.
- You have new or worse urination problems after you start a new medicine.
- You have trouble starting your urine stream.
- Your urine stream has gotten weaker over the past months.

As a man ages, his prostate gland may get bigger. This is called **benign prostatic hyperplasia,** or **BPH**. As the gland gets bigger, it may squeeze or partly block the urethra. This can cause problems with urine flow, such as:

- Trouble getting the urine stream started or fully stopped. This may cause dribbling. But dribbling is very common. It may not mean you have BPH.
- Needing to urinate more often, especially at night.
- A weak urine stream.
- Feeling like you cannot empty your bladder all the way.

BPH is not a serious problem unless you have a lot of trouble urinating or unless backed-up urine causes bladder or kidney problems.

Many men find that they can manage their symptoms with self-care. Sometimes symptoms clear up on their own. In these cases, the best treatment may be no treatment at all.

Bladder

Prostate

Urethra

Urethra

Normal prostate   Enlarged prostate

As the prostate gets bigger, it may squeeze the urethra.

The main factor in deciding how to treat your symptoms is how much you are bothered by them. To take a quiz that scores your symptoms, go to the Web site on the back cover and enter **x253** in the search box.

Go to Web

Some men decide to try medicine, surgery, or other treatments to help with symptoms. For help deciding whether these are right for you, go to the Web site on the back cover and enter **s204** in the search box. Then talk to your doctor.

Home Treatment

◆ Avoid allergy and cold medicines (antihistamines, decongestants, and nasal sprays). They can make urinary problems worse.

◆ If having to get up at night to urinate bothers you, cut down on fluids before bed, especially those with alcohol or caffeine. But drink plenty of water and other fluids during the day.

◆ Take plenty of time to urinate. Turn on a faucet, or try to picture running water. Some men find this helps. Read or think of other things while you wait.

◆ Sit on the toilet to urinate.

◆ Try "double voiding." Urinate as much as you can, relax for a few moments, and then try again.

◆ Herbal products such as saw palmetto help some men with BPH. Talk to your doctor before you take this or any herbal product.

Also see the tips in Bladder Control on page 100.

Prostatitis

When to Call a Doctor

◆ You have urinary problems along with fever, chills, vomiting, or pain in your back or belly.

◆ Your urine is bloody, red, or pink for no clear reason (see page 67).

◆ Pelvic pain or urinary problems last more than 5 days, even with home treatment.

◆ Pelvic pain or urinary problems suddenly change or get worse.

◆ It hurts when you urinate, ejaculate, or pass stool.

◆ There is a strange discharge from your penis. Also see page 229.

Prostatitis is any painful inflammation or infection of the prostate. If you have this problem:

◆ You may often feel the urge to urinate but only be able to pass a little urine each time.

◆ It may burn when you urinate.

◆ You may feel like you can't empty your bladder all the way.

◆ You may have trouble starting to urinate, or you may have a weak urine flow.

◆ You may have to urinate a lot at night.

◆ You may have pelvic pain. You may feel it in your lower back or belly, your scrotum, the area between your scrotum and anus, your upper thighs, or the pubic area.

◆ It may hurt when you ejaculate.

More

A prostate infection caused by bacteria often gets better with home treatment and antibiotics. If the infection comes back, you may need to take more antibiotics.

But most men with prostatitis do not have a bacterial infection. In these cases, home treatment tends to be the best approach.

Home Treatment

◆ Avoid alcohol, caffeine, and spicy foods. They may make your symptoms worse.

◆ Take hot baths to help soothe pain and reduce stress.

◆ Eat plenty of foods that are high in fiber and drink plenty of water to help avoid constipation. Straining to pass stool can hurt when you have prostatitis.

◆ Take an over-the-counter medicine like acetaminophen (Tylenol) or ibuprofen (Advil, Motrin) for pain. Read and follow all instructions on the label.

◆ If your doctor gives you antibiotics, take them as you are told.

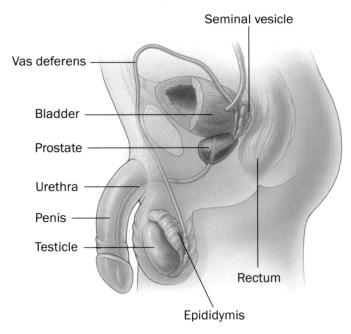

Male pelvic organs
(the prostate is just under the bladder)

Psoriasis

When to Call a Doctor

◆ Psoriasis covers much of your body or is very red. Severe cases often need medical care.

◆ You have signs of skin infection. These may include pain, swelling, warmth, or redness; red streaks leading from the area; pus; and fever.

Psoriasis is a long-term skin problem that causes raised, red patches topped with silvery, scaling skin. The patches are most often on the knees, elbows, scalp, hands,

feet, or lower back. If the problem is severe, your skin may be itchy and tender.

You can treat psoriasis with good care at home and, sometimes, with medicine from your doctor. Your doctor also may suggest ultraviolet light treatments.

Psoriasis does not spread from person to person.

Home Treatment

◆ Keep your skin moist. Use a very mild soap when you bathe. After you bathe, use a moisturizing ointment, cream, or lotion while your skin is still damp. This seals in moisture.

◆ Use hydrocortisone cream on small patches. Other products for psoriasis (lotions, gels, shampoos) may also help, but they may make your skin more sensitive to the sun.

◆ Try to prevent sunburn. Short periods of sunlight reduce psoriasis in most people. But sunburn injures the skin and may make psoriasis worse or cause it to appear in new areas. Use sunscreen on areas that do not have psoriasis.

◆ Avoid harsh chemicals and skin products, such as those that contain alcohol.

◆ Use a vaporizer or humidifier to add moisture to your bedroom.

◆ Try to reduce stress. See page 318. Stress may make psoriasis worse in some people.

Rashes

When to Call a Doctor

◆ You have a rash that develops quickly and looks like bruises or tiny purple or red blood spots under the skin. You may have a serious illness. See page 161.

◆ You have a rash with signs of infection. These may include increased pain, redness, swelling, or warmth; red streaks leading from the rash; pus; and fever.

◆ You get a rash after being bitten by a tick. See page 14.

◆ You get a rash after you start a new medicine.

◆ You have a rash with fever and joint pain.

◆ A rash occurs with a sore throat. See information about scarlet fever on page 239.

◆ You are not sure what's causing a rash.

◆ A rash does not clear up after 2 to 3 weeks of home treatment.

Rashes can be caused by lots of things—illness, allergy, bacteria, heat, and stress, to name a few.

When you first get a rash, ask yourself these questions to help find the cause:

◆ Do you have a rash in an area that came in contact with something new? This could be a plant; soaps, detergents, or shampoos; perfumes, makeup, or lotions; jewelry or fabric; or a new tool, an appliance, or latex gloves. Any of these could irritate your skin.

◆ Have you eaten anything new that you may be allergic to?

◆ Are you taking any new medicines?

◆ Have you been more stressed or upset than usual lately?

◆ Have you been sick?

◆ Is the rash spreading?

◆ Does it itch?

Also see the Skin Problems chart on page 61. If your child has a rash, the Rashes in Children chart on page 227 may help.

More

Poison Ivy, Oak, and Sumac

The leaves of poison ivy, oak, and sumac have an oil that many people react to. If you touch the leaves or the oil, you may get a red, blistered, and very itchy rash. The rash often appears in lines where the leaves brushed against the skin.

You may be able to prevent or reduce the rash if you act fast.

◆ Wash your skin with rubbing alcohol or lots of water within 10 to 15 minutes to get the oil off your skin.

◆ Use soap only after using lots of water.

◆ Wash your clothes, your dog, and anything else that may have touched the plant.

If you get a rash anyway, follow the tips in Home Treatment.

Home Treatment

◆ Wash the area with water. Soap may irritate the rash. Pat dry.

◆ To reduce itching, try these tips. Also see Relief From Itching on page 142.

❖ Use cold, wet cloths.

❖ Try nonprescription antihistamines. Some types, such as Alavert, Claritin, and Zyrtec, are less likely to make you sleepy. Before you use these medicines, check the label. They may not be safe for young children or for people with certain health problems.

❖ Use hydrocortisone cream to provide short-term relief from itching. Do not use it on the face or the genital area.

◆ Keep cool, and stay out of the sun.

◆ Leave the rash open to the air. Baby powder can help keep it dry.

◆ If you have a plant rash, calamine lotion may help. Use it 3 or 4 times a day. A mild lotion like Cetaphil may soothe some rashes.

◆ Do not use products that have caused a rash in the past, such as detergents, skin care products, makeup, clothing, or jewelry.

◆ Use fragrance-free or hypoallergenic soaps, detergents, lotions, and makeup if you often have rashes.

Poison ivy

Poison oak

Poison sumac

Learn what poison ivy, oak, and sumac look like so you can avoid them.

Rashes in Children

Symptoms	Possible Causes
Red spots like pimples that turn to blisters; fever	Chickenpox, p. 121
Rash in diaper area only	Diaper rash, p. 135 Yeast infection, p. 255
Red rash on face that looks like slapped cheeks; pink rash on torso that comes and goes; possible fever	Fifth disease, p. 164
Red or pink dots on head, neck, shoulders; more common in babies	Heat rash, p. 184
Sudden high fever for 2 to 3 days followed by rosy pink rash on torso, arms, and neck after fever goes down	Roseola, p. 228
Fine pink rash that starts on face and covers whole body; swollen glands behind ears	Rubella (rare)
Fever, runny nose, hacking cough; red eyes 2 to 3 days before spotty red rash covers whole body	Measles (rare)
High fever, sore throat, sandpapery rash, and raspberry-textured tongue	Scarlet fever, p. 239
Blisters on mouth and tongue appearing 1 to 2 days after onset of fever and sore mouth or throat; painless, blistering rash on fingers, hands, feet	Hand-foot-and-mouth disease, p. 175

Rosacea

When to Call a Doctor

◆ You think you may have rosacea.

◆ Redness, pimples, and eye irritation get worse even with treatment.

Rosacea is a long-term skin problem that causes:

◆ Red patches, red lines (tiny blood vessels), and small pimples on the face. You may think you have acne.

◆ Burning and soreness in the eyes or eyelids. Rosacea can lead to more serious eye problems if you do not treat it.

◆ Large bumps on the nose and face in severe cases.

You are more likely to get rosacea if you have fair skin and blush easily or if your face stays red and flushed longer than most people's. The problem tends to run in families.

The sooner you start to treat rosacea, the better. If it stays mild, you may be able to control it well. Prescription medicines may help if home treatment is not enough.

More ▶

227

Home Treatment

◆ Find out what triggers redness and pimples for you, and try to avoid those things. They may include:

❖ Very cold or hot weather. In winter, wear a hat and scarf to shield your face from cold and wind. Use a face moisturizer.

❖ Stress. Eat a healthy diet, and get plenty of exercise and sleep.

❖ Alcohol, spicy foods, or very hot drinks.

❖ Getting too hot when you exercise. Try working out for a shorter time. In the summer, exercise during the cool morning hours or in an air-conditioned gym.

❖ Hot showers. Take warm or cool ones instead. Don't use hot tubs or saunas.

◆ Always wear sunscreen on exposed skin.

◆ Use soaps, lotions, and makeup made for sensitive skin that don't contain alcohol, are not abrasive, and won't clog pores.

◆ If you have rosacea on your eyelids, gently wash your eyelids with a product made for the eyes. Use artificial tears if your eyes feel dry.

◆ Talk to your doctor about antibiotic creams and other medicines that can help with pimples and redness. In advanced cases, laser treatment can reduce redness.

Roseola

When to Call a Doctor
See the fever guidelines on page 158.

Roseola is a mild viral illness in young children that often starts with a sudden high fever (103°F to 105°F). The fever lasts 2 to 3 days. As the fever drops, a rosy pink rash appears on the torso, neck, and arms. The rash may last 1 to 2 days. Most babies feel fine when they have roseola.

Since the fever is quite high and comes on quickly, some children may have fever seizures. See page 161.

Roseola is most common in children from 6 months to 2 years old. It's rare after age 4.

Home Treatment

◆ If your child has a fever and feels bad, give an over-the-counter medicine like acetaminophen (Tylenol) or ibuprofen (Advil, Motrin). Read and follow all instructions on the label. Do not give aspirin to anyone younger than 20.

◆ Give your child plenty of liquids.

Sexually Transmitted Infections (STIs)

When to Call a Doctor

All sexually transmitted infections (STIs) need to be diagnosed and treated. Your doctor or a health professional at your local health department can help with testing and treatment.

Call your doctor if:

◆ You think you may have been exposed to an STI. Your sex partner(s) may also need to be treated, even if they have no symptoms. Without treatment, you and your partner(s) may reinfect each other or have serious complications.

◆ You have any unusual discharge from your vagina, penis, or anus; burning when you urinate; or any sores, redness, or growths on your genitals or anus.

◆ Your or your partner's behavior puts you at risk for HIV.

◆ You are pregnant and have any reason to think you may have been exposed to an STI, especially HIV.

◆ You have symptoms such as fatigue, weight loss, fever, diarrhea, cough, or swollen lymph nodes that do not go away after a short time and do not seem to be related to any illness.

◆ You are HIV-positive and you have:

❖ A fever of 101°F or higher.

❖ Increased outbreaks of cold sores or any unusual skin or mouth sores.

❖ Severe numbness or pain in your hands and feet.

❖ Unexplained weight loss.

❖ Unexplained fever and night sweats.

❖ Severe fatigue.

❖ Diarrhea or other bowel changes.

❖ Shortness of breath and a frequent dry cough.

❖ Swollen lymph nodes in your neck, armpits, or groin.

❖ Personality changes, trouble concentrating, confusion, or severe headache.

Sexually transmitted infections (STIs), also called sexually transmitted diseases, are passed from person to person through sex, genital contact, and contact with fluids such as semen, vaginal fluids, and blood (including menstrual blood). Some of these infections can also be spread by sharing drug needles, razors, and other items that may have infected blood or fluids on them.

You can get an STI from any kind of sexual contact. This includes:

◆ Vaginal sex.

◆ Anal sex.

◆ Oral sex.

Preventing STIs is a lot easier than treating them or living with them. To learn how to protect yourself, see Safe Sex on page 321.

Some of the most common STIs are described in the chart on page 230. If you think you may have been exposed to any

More

Sexually Transmitted Infections

Symptoms	Infection	Treatment	Other Concerns
Discharge from vagina or penis; pain or burning when you urinate; for women, pain and bleeding during or after sex	**Chlamydia, gonorrhea, trichomoniasis**	Antibiotics for all partners. Do not have sex until you and your partner(s) have finished treatment and have no symptoms.	If not treated, can lead to pelvic inflammatory disease and fertility problems. Gonorrhea can spread to joints, causing arthritis.
Red, painless sore in genital or rectal area or on mouth about 3 weeks after exposure Two months later: Rash, patchy hair loss, fever, flu-like symptoms	**Syphilis**	Antibiotics for all partners. Do not have sex until you and your partner(s) have finished treatment and have no symptoms.	If not treated, can cause serious health problems and death.
Painful sores or blisters in genital or anal area 2 to 7 days after exposure; fever, swollen lymph nodes, headache, and muscle aches	**Genital herpes**	No cure. Medicine can reduce pain and speed healing during an outbreak.	Those with frequent or severe outbreaks may take medicine daily to help prevent them. Couples should avoid sex during an outbreak. Pregnant women should tell their doctor immediately if they have an outbreak.
Small, fleshy bumps or flat, white patches in genital or anal area	**Genital warts and HPV (human papillomavirus)**	No cure for HPV. Warts can be removed but may return. Infection may go away on its own.	Some types of HPV can increase a woman's risk for cervical cancer, but there is an HPV vaccine that can help prevent it. Talk to your doctor about whether to get the vaccine.
Yellowing of skin and whites of eyes; flu-like symptoms; steady pain in upper right belly, under rib cage; diarrhea or constipation; muscle aches and joint pain; skin rash	**Hepatitis B virus**	No treatment for short-term (acute) hepatitis; most people get better in 6 to 8 weeks. Medicine for long-term (chronic) hepatitis, but no cure.	Can become chronic and lead to liver damage or cancer. If you are at risk for hepatitis B, get the vaccine. See page 326.
Flu-like symptoms soon after infection; then no symptoms for years until disease progresses	**HIV (human immunodeficiency virus)**	No cure. Medicine slows progress of disease, delays AIDS, and prolongs life.	Weakens immune system, leading to AIDS and in many cases death. See page 231.

of them, use the chart to check your symptoms and learn more.

HIV: Should You Get Tested?

HIV (human immunodeficiency virus) is a virus that attacks your immune system. This makes it hard for your body to fight infection and disease. AIDS is the last and most severe stage of HIV infection.

Are You at Risk?

All kinds of people get HIV—men and women, gay and straight, all ages, all races. If you or your partner does things that could expose you to HIV, you are at risk.

HIV spreads through contact with body fluids such as semen, vaginal fluids, and blood (including menstrual blood). The behaviors that spread HIV include:

◆ Having more than one sex partner.

◆ Having unprotected sex. Unprotected sex means having sex without properly using a condom. This is especially risky if you are a man who has sex with men, but it is a risk for everyone. Sex without condoms is not safe unless both you and your partner are sure that neither of you has HIV and that neither of you is having sex with anyone else.

◆ Sharing needles or other drug supplies with someone who is HIV-positive.

◆ Having a sex partner who does any of the above.

You will not get HIV from touching, hugging, or lightly kissing someone who is HIV-positive. HIV is not spread by mosquitoes, toilet seats, donating blood, or being touched or coughed on by someone who is HIV-positive or who has AIDS.

STIs During Pregnancy

Many STIs can be spread from an infected mother to her unborn baby. These include chlamydia, gonorrhea, hepatitis B, herpes, HIV, and syphilis.

The good news is that getting treated while you are pregnant can prevent the spread of many of these infections to your child.

If you are infected with or think you may have been exposed to an STI, talk to your doctor about how you can protect your baby before and after he or she is born.

Getting Tested

If you do things that put you at risk for HIV infection, be sure to have an HIV test every 6 months. Here's why:

◆ Medicine for HIV can help delay or prevent AIDS and helps you live longer and better. The sooner you find out whether you have HIV and start getting checked, the better your chances of staying healthy. Regular checks of your immune system will help you and your doctor know when you need to start medicine.

◆ A blood test is the only way to know whether you have HIV. You may not feel sick or notice any symptoms for years. But inside your body, the virus is growing.

◆ If you have HIV and do not know it, you may spread the infection to others.

More

◆ If you are pregnant, getting tested is the most important thing you can do for yourself and your baby. If you are HIV-positive, medicine during pregnancy can greatly reduce the chance that your baby will be born with HIV.

All it takes is a simple, cheap blood test. The test checks for HIV antibodies in your blood. If HIV antibodies are found, you are considered HIV-positive. If HIV antibodies are not found, you may need to be tested again. This is to make sure HIV antibodies do not appear at a later time. It can take up to 6 months after you are first exposed to HIV for antibodies to appear.

You can have the test in your doctor's office or at the local health department.

If you find out you are HIV-positive, work with your doctor to get the right treatment and stay as healthy as you can. Many people live with HIV for years or even decades before they develop AIDS.

If you need help dealing with HIV or AIDS, or if you just want to learn more, call the CDC-INFO hotline at 1-800-232-4636.

Sinusitis

When to Call a Doctor

◆ Cold symptoms last longer than 10 to 14 days or get worse after the first 7 days.

◆ You have a severe headache that is different from a "normal" headache, and nonprescription medicines do not help.

◆ You have swelling in your face, or your vision changes or gets blurry.

◆ The mucus from your nose changes from clear to yellow or green after 5 to 7 days of a cold, and pain and fever get worse. If the mucus is colored from the start of a cold, call if it lasts longer than 7 to 10 days.

◆ You have face pain (especially in the sinus area or above your cheekbones) after 2 days of home treatment.

◆ You have finished your antibiotics and still have symptoms.

Sinusitis is an inflammation or infection of the sinuses and nasal passages. The sinuses become blocked, which causes pain and pressure in the face.

Sinusitis most often follows a cold. Sinus problems can also be caused by allergies, an infected tooth, air pollution, and other things.

Is It Sinusitis or a Cold?

Colds and sinusitis have some of the same symptoms, like a stuffy nose and cough. But if you have a sinus problem, you may also have:

◆ Pain above your cheekbones and upper teeth.

◆ Pain in your forehead over your eyebrows.

◆ Pain around or behind your eyes.

Along with the pain, you may have a headache, swelling around your eyes, a fever, or mucus draining down the back of your throat. Face pain and these other symptoms are not likely with just a cold. Children can get sinusitis too.

The sinuses are hollow spaces in the head.

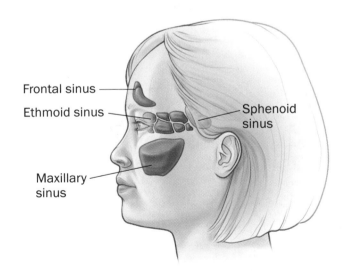

Frontal sinus

Ethmoid sinus

Sphenoid sinus

Maxillary sinus

Do You Need Antibiotics?

Sinusitis usually gets better with good self-care. If you try the tips in Home Treatment, you may be able to avoid antibiotics and a trip to the doctor.

But if your symptoms are severe or last more than 10 to 14 days, you may need antibiotics. If you do not treat a bad sinus infection or it does not respond to treatment, it can lead to long-term sinus problems that are harder to treat.

There are good reasons not to use antibiotics unless you really need them:

◆ Antibiotics can cost a lot.

◆ You will probably have to see the doctor to get a prescription. This costs you time and money.

◆ Antibiotics can have harmful side effects, such as diarrhea, vomiting, and skin rashes.

◆ You could be allergic to the antibiotics.

◆ The most important reason of all: If you take antibiotics when you don't need them, they may not work when you do need them. Each time you take them, you are more likely to carry some bacteria that were not killed by the medicine. Over time, these bacteria get tougher and can cause longer and more serious infections. To treat them, you may need different, stronger, and more costly antibiotics.

More

233

Home Treatment

◆ Drink plenty of water and other fluids to stay hydrated.

◆ Put a warm, damp towel or gel pack on your face several times a day for 5 to 10 minutes at a time.

◆ Breathe warm, moist air from a steamy shower, a hot bath, or a sink filled with hot water.

◆ Use a humidifier in your home, or at least in your bedroom. Avoid cold, dry air.

◆ Use decongestant pills or liquids, a decongestant nose spray, or a cough medicine that has guaifenesin. Do not use a decongestant nose spray for more than 3 days in a row.

◆ Do not take antihistamines unless your symptoms may also be caused by allergies.

◆ Before you use decongestants or antihistamines, check the label. They may not be safe for young children or for people with certain health problems.

◆ Take an over-the-counter medicine like acetaminophen (Tylenol) or ibuprofen (Advil, Motrin) for face pain and headache. Read and follow all instructions on the label. Do not give aspirin to anyone younger than 20.

◆ Do not smoke, and avoid other people's smoke.

◆ If you see streaks of mucus in the back of your throat, gargle with warm water.

◆ Blow your nose gently. Do not block one nostril when you blow your nose.

◆ A saltwater (saline) wash can help clear out mucus and bacteria. You can use a nonprescription saline nose spray, or you can make your own saline wash at home.

❖ Use a bulb syringe to gently squirt the liquid into your nose. Or snuff it from the palm of your hand, one nostril at a time.

❖ Blow your nose gently when you are done.

❖ Repeat 2 to 4 times a day.

Saline Nose Sprays

Nonprescription saline nose sprays (such as NaSal and Ocean) are cheap and easy to use. They will keep tissues in the nose moist and help clean out mucus and bacteria. Unlike other kinds of nose sprays, they do not cause swelling inside the nose.

You can also make a saline nose wash at home. Mix ½ teaspoon of salt, ½ teaspoon of baking soda, and 1 cup of distilled water or water that has been boiled and then cooled. Keep the saltwater mix in a clean bottle with a dropper. After 3 days, throw out the mix and make a fresh one.

Using a bulb syringe

Skin Cancer

When to Call a Doctor

- A mole is itchy, tender, or painful.

- A mole starts to get bigger or changes color or shape.

- A mole scales, oozes, or bleeds, or its color spreads into surrounding skin.

- You notice a new bump or nodule on a mole or any change in how the mole looks.

- You have a sore that does not heal.

- You have any irritated or unusual skin growth.

If your moles do not change over time, there is little reason to worry about them. If you have a family history of malignant melanoma, let your doctor know. You may be at greater risk.

Skin cancer is the most common type of cancer. Most skin cancer is caused by sun damage, so it tends to occur on areas that get the most sun, such as the face, neck, and arms. Light-skinned, blue-eyed people are more likely to get skin cancer. Dark-skinned people have less risk.

Most of a person's harmful sun exposure occurs by age 20, so keep your children protected. (See Don't Get Sunburned on page 56.) Repeated sun exposure (including sunlamps) and severe sunburns can greatly increase your risk of skin cancer.

Most skin cancers are **nonmelanoma** skin cancers. These include basal cell and squamous cell carcinomas. Nonmelanoma skin cancer is rarely life-threatening. But it is still best to find and treat it promptly. It is usually easy to treat.

Melanoma is a more serious type of skin cancer. It may affect only the skin, or it may spread to other organs and bones. Melanoma can be deadly if it is not found and treated early. Early removal of thin melanomas can cure the disease in most cases.

Watch for Skin Changes

Once a month, examine all areas of your skin with a mirror (or have someone help you). Look for odd moles, spots, bumps, or sores that will not heal. Pay extra attention to areas that get a lot of sun: hands, arms, back, chest, back of the neck, face, and ears. Report any changes to your doctor.

Skin cancers differ from other skin growths in these ways:

- They tend to bleed more and are often open sores that do not heal.

- They tend to grow slowly. But melanoma may appear suddenly and grow quickly.

Also watch for any of these **ABCDE changes** in a mole or other growth:

- **A**symmetry: One half does not match the other half.

- **B**order: The edges are ragged, notched, or blurred.

- **C**olor: The mole changes color, has shades of red and black, or has a red, white, and blue blotchy appearance.

More ▶

235

◆ **D**iameter (size): A mole grows larger than a pencil eraser.

◆ **E**volving: The mole looks different from your other moles or is changing in size, shape, or color.

NCI Visuals Online. Skin Cancer Foundation.

| Asymmetry | Border irregularity | Color | Diameter of ¼ inch |

Evolving

Watch for these "ABCDE" mole changes.

Sleep Problems

When to Call a Doctor

◆ You regularly take sleeping pills and cannot stop taking them.

◆ You think a medicine or a health problem is causing sleep problems.

◆ You or your partner snores loudly and often feels extremely sleepy during the day.

◆ You, your partner, or your child often stops breathing, gasps, and chokes during sleep.

◆ Your child snores, has trouble breathing while asleep, sleeps restlessly and wakes up often, or is very sleepy during the day.

◆ You often wake up because your legs move or get cramps.

◆ A full month of self-care does not solve your sleep problem.

Insomnia can mean:

◆ Having trouble getting to sleep (taking more than 45 minutes to fall asleep).

◆ Waking up often and not being able to fall back asleep.

◆ Waking up too early in the morning when you do not want to.

None of these are problems unless you feel tired all the time. If you are less sleepy at night or wake up early in the morning but still feel rested and alert, there is little need to worry.

Short-term insomnia, lasting from a few nights to a few weeks, is usually caused by worry or stress. Long-term insomnia, which can last months or even years, is often caused by frequent or constant anxiety, medicines, long-term pain, depression, or other health problems.

Sleep apnea is a problem usually caused by a blockage in your airways. When airflow through the nose and mouth is blocked, you repeatedly stop breathing for 10 to 15 seconds or longer while you are asleep. People who have sleep apnea often snore loudly and are very tired during the day. They are not aware of waking up at night but do have very restless sleep.

Changing some of your pre-bedtime habits may help cure mild insomnia or sleep apnea. More severe insomnia or sleep apnea may need medical treatment.

Tips for Better Sleep

Try this seven-step formula for 2 weeks:

1. Do relaxing activities in the evening. Read (but not in bed). Take a warm bath. Or do some slow, easy stretches.

2. Use your bed for sleeping and sex only. Do not eat, watch TV, read, or work in bed.

3. Sleep only at bedtime. Do not take naps, especially in the late afternoon and evening.

Snoring

Up to half of all adults snore once in a while; about 1 in 4 adults snores regularly. Snoring is caused by blockage of the airways in the back of the mouth and nose. The airways can be blocked for many reasons, such as excess neck tissue caused by being overweight or a stuffy nose caused by allergies or a cold. Some people who snore have sleep apnea.

Snoring can disrupt your sleep patterns, which may leave you sleepy and less alert during the day. It can also disrupt the sleep of family members or roommates.

Tips for people who snore

◆ Exercise daily to stay at a healthy weight and improve muscle tone. Don't exercise within 3 to 4 hours of bedtime (it may make it harder to fall asleep).

◆ Avoid heavy meals, alcohol, sleeping pills, and antihistamines before bedtime.

◆ Try to sleep on your side instead of your back. (Sew a pocket onto the back of your pajama top, and put a tennis ball in the pocket. This will keep you off your back.)

◆ Go to bed at the same time every night, even on weekends.

◆ Let a bedmate or roommate who does not snore fall asleep first.

If snoring is a problem for you or affects your household, see a doctor. You may need an exam of your nose, mouth, and neck.

 Treatment will depend on what is making you snore. Your doctor may want to do a sleep study to see if sleep apnea is one of the reasons why you snore. For help deciding whether you want this kind of testing, go to the Web site on the back cover and enter **y240** in the search box.

More

4. Go to bed only when you feel sleepy.

5. If you lie awake for more than 15 minutes, get up, leave the room, and do something relaxing.

6. Repeat steps 4 and 5 until it is time to get up.

7. Get up at the same time every day, even on weekends.

These tips may help too:

◆ Keep your bedroom dark, quiet, and cool. Try using a sleep mask and earplugs. Or play relaxing music or sounds, like sounds of the ocean.

◆ Get regular exercise. But don't exercise within 3 to 4 hours of bedtime (it may make it harder to fall asleep).

◆ Avoid alcohol and smoking before bedtime. Limit caffeine, and avoid it after noon.

◆ Avoid foods that upset your stomach.

◆ Drink warm milk at bedtime. But don't drink more than one glass of fluid before you go to bed, or you may have to get up in the night.

◆ Review all your prescription and nonprescription medicines with a pharmacist to rule out side effects that affect your sleep.

You may want to read about anxiety on page 80 or depression on page 156. Either problem can upset your sleep.

What About Sleeping Pills?

Prescription and nonprescription sleep medicines may give you fast relief from insomnia. But use them only for a short time, and stop taking them as soon as you can. They can cause daytime confusion, memory loss, and dizziness. You can also get addicted to some of them.

Continued use of sleeping pills actually makes sleep problems worse in many people.

If you want to try sleeping pills, check with your doctor first, and don't take them for long. For help deciding if sleeping pills might help you, go to the Web site on the back cover and enter **n719** in the search box.

Sleep Habits in Babies

Babies have sleep cycles that go from light to deep or heavy. Each sleep cycle may be about 60 minutes of light sleep, 60 to 90 minutes of deep sleep, and another 30 minutes of light sleep. At the end of this cycle, the baby is semi-alert and can be wakened easily.

You can help your baby sleep through the night by helping the baby learn to soothe himself or herself back to sleep during periods of light sleep.

For babies age 4 to 6 months:

◆ Put the baby in the crib when he or she is drowsy but still awake.

◆ Make middle-of-the-night feedings short. Do not turn them into playtime.

◆ As the baby gets older, delay the middle-of-the-night feeding, and stop it sometime after age 6 months.

Always put your baby to sleep on his or her back. This is the best way to prevent sudden infant death syndrome (SIDS).

Sore Throat

When to Call a Doctor

- You have trouble breathing or swallowing because of a sore throat, or you drool a lot because you cannot swallow.

- You get a severe sore throat after being exposed to someone with strep throat.

- You have a sore throat with at least 2 of these 3 symptoms of strep throat:

  - Fever of 101°F or higher

  - White or yellow coating on the tonsils

  - Swollen lymph nodes in the neck, armpits, or groin (see the picture on page 245)

- A rash occurs with a sore throat. Scarlet fever is a rash you may get because of strep throat. Like strep throat, scarlet fever is treated with antibiotics.

- You have a sore throat that's not related to a cold, allergies, smoking, overuse of your voice, or any other clear reason.

- A mild sore throat lasts longer than 2 weeks.

- Your child has had at least 4 to 6 episodes of tonsillitis in the past year, even with treatment with antibiotics.

- Your child breathes through his or her mouth a lot of the time, often snores, or has a very nasal- or muffled-sounding voice a lot of the time. These are signs of a problem with the adenoids.

Most sore throats are minor and go away with home treatment. You may get a sore throat because of:

- A cold or other virus.

- Smoking, air pollution, or dry air.

- Yelling.

- Breathing through your mouth when you sleep. People who have stuffy noses from allergies or colds often do this.

- Backflow (reflux) of stomach acid into the throat. If you think this may be the cause of your throat pain, see Heartburn on page 183.

Tonsillitis

In children, sore throats are often caused by inflammation of the tonsils (tonsillitis) or adenoids (adenoiditis). This is usually caused by a virus.

Along with a sore throat, your child may have a fever, swollen lymph nodes, tiredness, and symptoms like a cold, such as a runny nose and cough. It may hurt to swallow. The tonsils are often bright red, spotted with pus, and swollen.

More

Location of tonsils

Location of adenoids

Adenoiditis can also cause headache and vomiting. If the adenoids are inflamed a lot of the time, they can swell and block the tubes that connect the throat and the ears. This can lead to ear infections. See page 145.

Strep Throat

Strep throat is a sore throat caused by streptococcal bacteria. It is most common in children 3 to 15 years old. You can get strep throat even if you have had your tonsils taken out.

Most sore throats are not strep throat. The more you feel like you have a cold, the less likely it is that you have strep. Strep throat causes some or all of these symptoms:

◆ Severe and sudden sore throat

◆ Fever of 101 °F or higher

◆ Swollen lymph nodes

◆ White or yellow coating on the tonsils

Antibiotics are used to treat strep throat and prevent rheumatic fever, a rare but serious problem that can occur if strep is not treated.

Mono

Mono (mononucleosis) is a viral illness that can cause a severe, long-lasting sore throat. It is most common in older teens and young adults.

Mono may also cause fever, body aches, and swollen lymph nodes in the neck, armpits, and groin. You may feel tired and weak. The upper left part of your belly may hurt (because your spleen is enlarged).

Most people recover from mono after several weeks. But it may take a few months to get your energy back, and lymph nodes may stay swollen for up to a month (see page 245).

There is no treatment for mono except rest, plenty of fluids, saltwater gargles for throat pain, and an over-the-counter medicine like acetaminophen (Tylenol) or ibuprofen (Advil, Motrin) for body aches. Before you use one of these medicines, read and follow all instructions on the label. Do not give aspirin to anyone younger than 20.

Home Treatment

◆ Gargle with warm salt water several times a day to reduce throat swelling and pain. Mix 1 teaspoon of salt in 8 ounces of water.

◆ Drink extra fluids to soothe your throat. Honey and lemon in hot water or in weak tea may help. Do not give honey to children younger than 1 year.

◆ Do not smoke, and avoid other people's smoke. If you need help quitting, see page 316.

◆ Take an over-the-counter medicine like acetaminophen (Tylenol) or ibuprofen (Advil, Motrin) to relieve pain and reduce fever. Read and follow all instructions on the label. Do not give aspirin to anyone younger than 20.

◆ Before you use cough or cold medicines, check the label. They may not be safe for young children or for people with certain health problems.

◆ Try nonprescription throat lozenges that have a painkiller to numb your throat, such as Sucrets Maximum Strength. Cough drops or hard candy may also help. But do not give them to children, who may choke on them.

◆ If you have strep throat, stay home from work or school until 24 hours after you have started antibiotics.

◆ If you have mono, do not share eating or drinking utensils, do not kiss anyone, do not play contact sports for 4 weeks, and do not donate blood while you have symptoms.

Tonsils and Adenoids: Should They Be Taken Out?

Your child may need to have his or her **tonsils** removed if:

◆ Your child has had severe tonsillitis caused by strep at least 4 to 6 times in the past year, even after treatment with at least two antibiotics.

◆ Your child has breathing or sleep problems because of swollen tonsils.

◆ There are deep pockets of infection in the tonsils that have not gotten better after treatment with medicine.

Your child may need to have his or her **adenoids** removed if:

◆ The adenoids block the airway and cause breathing trouble and sleep problems.

◆ Your doctor thinks an adenoid problem is causing frequent ear infections that are hard to treat.

If your doctor recommends surgery but your child does not have the problems described above, you may want to get a second opinion to be sure. The benefits need to greatly outweigh the costs, risks, and pain.

 For help deciding, go to the Web site on the back cover and enter **q586** in the search box.

Sports Injuries

When to Call a Doctor

◆ You cannot use a limb or joint at all because of an injury.

◆ A limb or joint has an odd shape.

◆ You do not get better with home treatment.

For a sudden injury like an ankle sprain or a broken bone, see page 50.

Sports injuries are common among active people. Most are caused by either accidents or overuse. Accidents are hard to avoid if you play a sport. But you can avoid overuse injuries if you train properly and use the right equipment.

You can find information on specific injuries on the following pages:

◆ Head injury, page 37

◆ Bursitis and tendon injury, page 111

◆ Tennis elbow and golfer's elbow, page 112

◆ Knee problems, page 201

◆ Achilles tendon problems, page 186

◆ Heel pain and plantar fasciitis, page 185

◆ Shin splints, page 205

◆ Strains, sprains, broken bones, and dislocations, page 50

◆ Stress fractures, page 50

Preventing Injuries

◆ Warm up before you exercise. Cool down and stretch when you are done.

◆ Do not make sudden increases in how hard or how long you exercise. Slow buildups are better. As you get more fit, you will be able to exercise harder without hurting yourself.

◆ Use proper sports techniques and equipment. For example, wear supportive, well-cushioned shoes for running, aerobics, and walking. Use a two-handed tennis backhand stroke. Wear knee pads and wrist guards for in-line skating. Make sure that your bike is adjusted properly for your body. Wear the right kind of helmet for your sport.

◆ Switch between hard workouts and easier ones to let your body rest. For example, if you run, alternate long or hard runs with shorter or easier ones. If you lift weights, do not work the same muscles 2 days in a row.

◆ Try cross-training. This means you do several activities instead of the same one all the time. Cross-training lets you work different muscle groups while the others rest. For example, rotate days of walking or running with biking or swimming.

◆ Do not ignore aches and pains. When you first feel pain, rest or reduce your activity for a few days. Taking care of the problem early with ice and other home treatment may help you avoid a more serious injury.

Ice and Cold Packs

Ice can relieve pain, swelling, and inflammation from injuries and problems like bursitis and arthritis. You can use any of these items to "ice" an area:

◆ A cold pack you buy at the drugstore or grocery store. Store the pack in the freezer.

◆ A homemade cold pack. Seal 1 pint of rubbing alcohol and 3 pints of water in a 1-gallon, heavy-duty, plastic freezer bag. Seal that bag inside a second bag. Mark it "Cold pack: Do not eat," and store it in the freezer.

◆ A bag of frozen vegetables. Peas or corn work well. Do not eat them once you have used them as a cold pack. Label the bag "Do not eat." You can reuse it several times.

◆ An ice towel. Wet a towel with cold water, and squeeze it until it is just damp. Fold the towel, place it in a plastic bag, and freeze it for 15 minutes. Take the towel out of the bag, and use it like a cold pack.

◆ An ice pack. Put about a pound of ice in a plastic bag. Add water to barely cover the ice. Squeeze the air out of the bag and seal it. Wrap the bag in a damp towel, and put it on the sore area.

Ice the area at least 3 times a day. For the first 48 hours, ice for 10 to 15 minutes once an hour. After that, a good pattern is to ice for 10 to 15 minutes, 3 times a day: in the morning, in the late afternoon after work or school, and about half an hour before you go to bed. Also ice after any long periods of activity or hard exercise.

Always keep a thin cloth between your skin and the cold pack so that the cold does not damage your skin. Press the pack firmly so that it touches all parts of the affected area.

Do not use cold for longer than 10 to 15 minutes at a time, and do not fall asleep with ice on your skin.

More ➤

Home Treatment

The biggest challenge for most people with sports injuries is to get enough rest and heal without losing their overall fitness.

◆ Stay fit by cross-training with activities that do not stress the injury. If you have sore knees, try swimming. If you have sore feet or ankles, get on a bike. If your elbows or shoulders hurt, try walking. Do not return too fast to the activity that caused the injury.

◆ Get back to your regular activity gradually. Start with a slow, easy pace, and do the activity for shorter periods of time than usual. If you are lifting weights, use less weight and do fewer reps. Increase the pace, time, and intensity only if you have no pain.

◆ Break down your sport into small steps. Once you can throw a ball a short distance without pain, try throwing it a little farther. If you can walk without pain, try slow jogging. Once you can jog slowly without pain, try running a little faster.

Styes

When to Call a Doctor

◆ Redness and swelling spread to the entire eyelid or the eyeball.

◆ The stye hurts a lot, grows larger quickly, or does not stop draining.

◆ The stye blocks your vision.

◆ The stye does not improve within 1 month of home treatment.

A stye is an infection of the eyelash follicle. It looks like a small, red bump or pimple either in the eyelid or on the edge of the lid. Styes come to a head and break open after a few days.

Styes are very common and are not a serious problem. But they can hurt, and they may blur your vision. Most will go away with home treatment.

Home Treatment

◆ Do not rub your eye, and do not squeeze or open the stye.

◆ Apply a warm, moist cloth for 5 to 10 minutes, 3 to 6 times a day, until the stye comes to a head and drains.

◆ Do not wear eye makeup or contact lenses until the stye heals.

Swollen Lymph Nodes

When to Call a Doctor

◆ The lymph nodes are large, very firm, red, or very tender.

◆ You have swollen lymph nodes and signs of infection in a nearby cut or sore. Signs may include increased pain, redness, swelling, and warmth; red streaks leading from the cut; pus; and fever.

◆ You have swollen lymph nodes after traveling outside the United States or in wilderness areas.

◆ Your lymph nodes swell for no clear reason, and the swelling has not gone away after 2 weeks.

◆ You have swollen lymph nodes in areas other than your neck, armpits, or groin.

The lymph nodes are small glands found all through the body. They swell as the body fights minor infections from colds, insect bites, or small cuts. More serious infections and some types of cancer can make lymph nodes hard, sore, and quite large.

The lymph nodes in the neck are the ones people most often notice. They may swell when you have a cold or sore throat. The lymph nodes in the groin may swell if you have a vaginal or other pelvic infection or if you have a cut or sore on your leg or foot.

Home Treatment

Treat the cold or other infection that is making the lymph nodes large. Use the index in the back of the book or the symptom charts on pages 61 to 67 to find what you need.

Lymph nodes may stay swollen or hard for several weeks after the infection goes away. This is very common in children. If the lymph nodes near the site of the infection are not sore and are not getting larger, you can watch them at home and report them at the child's next doctor visit.

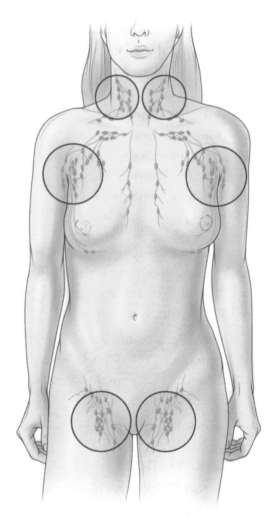

Swollen lymph nodes in the neck, armpits, and groin are usually easy to feel.

Testicle Problems

When to Call a Doctor

◆ You have sudden, severe pain in a testicle or the scrotum. This may be a sign of testicular torsion, which needs urgent medical care.

◆ Pain or swelling in a testicle or the scrotum gets worse over a period of several hours or days or does not go away after a few days.

◆ Pain or swelling occurs with fever.

◆ Pain or swelling starts after exposure to the mumps virus.

◆ You find a lump.

◆ You have a change in the shape, size, or feel of a testicle.

◆ One testicle feels very heavy.

The testicles produce sperm and male hormones. Males normally have two testicles, which are behind the penis inside a sac of skin called the scrotum.

Injury to the Testicles

The location of the testicles makes them an easy target for injury, especially during contact sports. Pain caused by an injury should go away within an hour or so.

To relieve pain after an injury:

◆ Use a pillow to prop up the scrotum, and apply ice or a cold pack for 10 minutes, once an hour. Put a thin cloth between the ice and your skin.

◆ Take an over-the-counter medicine like acetaminophen (Tylenol) or ibuprofen (Advil, Motrin) for pain. Read and follow all instructions on the label.

◆ Wear a jockstrap if it helps.

Testicular Cancer

Testicular cancer is rare and most often affects males between ages 15 and 35. It usually affects only one testicle and responds well to treatment if found early.

Symptoms may include a painless lump or swelling that men find on their own. The testicle may also feel heavier than normal.

How to Do a Self-Exam

After taking a warm bath or shower:

◆ Stand with your right leg on the side of the tub or the toilet seat.

◆ Gently roll your right testicle between the thumb and fingers of both hands. Feel for any hard lumps or swelling. The testicle should feel round and smooth.

Feel each testicle for hard lumps or swelling.

◆ Look for any changes in the size, shape, or feel of the testicle. It is normal for one testicle to be slightly larger than the other.

◆ Repeat the exam on your left testicle.

◆ Tell your doctor about any lumps, swelling, major size differences, or changes in feeling or appearance.

Other Testicle Problems

Problem	Symptoms	Cause	Comments
Epididymitis (inflammation of tube at top of testicle; see the picture on page 224)	Pain and swelling in scrotum that slowly gets worse; scrotum feels hot and tender; fever	Sexually transmitted infection (see page 229); irritation from bladder infection or injury	Call your doctor. You may need antibiotics.
Orchitis (inflammation of a testicle)	Pain and swelling in the scrotum; scrotum feels heavy	Mumps virus; bacterial infection of prostate or epididymis (see the picture on page 224)	Call your doctor. If not treated, orchitis can cause infertility. Make sure your son gets the MMR vaccine to prevent mumps. See page 325.
Torsion (testicle rotates on its spermatic cord, cutting off blood flow)	Sudden, severe pain in the scrotum that may spread to the belly; nausea and vomiting; fever	Unknown; may occur during sleep or after heavy exercise; most common in teenage boys.	**This may be an emergency.** You may need surgery within hours to restore blood flow and prevent permanent damage.

Toilet Training

Every child has his or her own schedule for becoming toilet-trained. Most children are ready to start between 24 and 30 months of age.

Your child may be ready if he or she:

◆ Passes stools at about the same time each day.

◆ Is able to have a dry diaper for at least 2 hours at a time during the day.

◆ Makes certain faces when urinating or passing stools.

◆ Lets you know when a diaper is dirty and asks to have it changed.

◆ Seems eager to please and can follow simple instructions.

◆ Tells you that he or she wants to use the toilet or wear "big kids" underwear.

If you think your child is ready to start toilet training, some of these tips may make it go more smoothly:

◆ Get your child a potty chair. Give him or her time to get used to it. Have your child sit on the chair with a diaper on when he or she is passing stools or urinating.

◆ Let your child watch you or a sibling of the same sex use the toilet. Talk with your child about what you're doing.

◆ Choose clothing for your child that's easy to take off. Elastic waistbands and Velcro or snaps work best. Pull-on diapers can help too.

◆ Reward every success with hugs and praise. Expect some accidents in the first few weeks, and don't get mad when they happen. Keep a relaxed attitude.

Toothache

When to Call a Dentist

◆ You have signs of a tooth or gum infection, such as:

❖ Increased pain, swelling, warmth, or redness.

❖ Red streaks on the skin over the area.

❖ Pus or blood that drains into the mouth or onto the face.

❖ Swollen lymph nodes in the neck.

❖ Fever.

◆ You have a severe toothache that does not improve after 2 hours of home treatment.

◆ You have face pain or swelling.

◆ You have a painful bump near the sore tooth.

◆ A toothache keeps you from sleeping or doing your usual activities.

◆ You have had a toothache off and on for 2 weeks or longer.

You may have teeth that ache or tingle when you touch them or when you eat or drink something hot, cold, sweet, or sour. The pain may come from a worn-down tooth or from gums that have pulled away from the teeth and exposed the roots and inner parts of the teeth.

If you have sharp pain, you may have tooth decay or an infection, have lost a filling, or have a crack in the tooth. Another cause is damage from nervous grinding of your teeth. A tooth that is coming in but cannot break through the gum also can cause a toothache.

A dentist can help find the cause of your toothache and keep your tooth alive.

Home Treatment

◆ Put ice or a cold pack on the outside of your cheek for 10 to 15 minutes at a time. Put a thin cloth between the ice and your skin. Do not use heat.

◆ Take an over-the-counter medicine like acetaminophen (Tylenol) or ibuprofen (Advil, Motrin) for pain. Read and follow all instructions on the label.

◆ Avoid very hot, cold, or sweet foods and drinks if they make the pain worse.

◆ Talk to your dentist about special toothpaste for sensitive teeth. Brush with this toothpaste regularly, or rub a small amount of it on the sensitive area with a clean finger 2 or 3 times a day. Floss gently.

◆ Do not smoke or chew tobacco. It can make gum problems worse. It also makes you less able to fight infection in your gums. If you need help quitting, see page 316.

Ulcers

When to Call a Doctor

Call 911 if:

◆ You have pain in your upper belly with chest pain or pressure or other symptoms of a heart attack. See page 38.

◆ You have been diagnosed with an ulcer and:

❖ You have severe belly pain.

❖ You have severe vomiting.

❖ You vomit a lot of blood or what looks like coffee grounds.

❖ You have severe rectal bleeding. Severe means you are passing a lot of stool that is maroon or mostly blood.

❖ Your belly is hard and swollen.

❖ You faint.

Call your doctor if:

◆ Mild symptoms of an ulcer do not improve after 10 to 14 days of home treatment.

◆ You are losing weight, and you don't know why.

◆ You often vomit or feel nauseated right after you eat.

◆ Belly pain wakes you from sleep.

More ▶

Ulcers

A peptic or gastric ulcer is a sore or crater in the lining of the upper digestive tract. Without treatment, ulcers can cause dangerous health problems, such as bleeding in the stomach and small intestine.

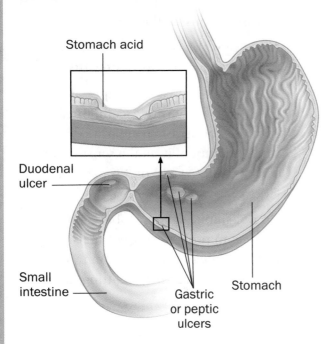

Most ulcers form in the stomach (gastric or peptic ulcers) or in the opening to the small intestine (duodenal ulcers).

The two most common causes of ulcers are:

◆ Infection with *H. pylori* bacteria. Most people who have *H. pylori* in their stomach do not get ulcers, but it does increase the risk.

◆ Frequent or long-term use of aspirin, ibuprofen (Advil, Motrin), naproxen (Aleve), and other anti-inflammatory medicines.

Your risk of an ulcer is higher if you smoke or if you drink a lot of alcohol.

Symptoms of an ulcer may include a burning or gnawing pain between your belly button and breastbone. The pain often occurs between meals and may wake you during the night. Eating something or taking an antacid often relieves the pain. Ulcers may also cause bloating, nausea, or vomiting after meals.

Sometimes people think that they have an ulcer, but they really have heartburn (see page 183).

Home Treatment

◆ Avoid foods that seem to cause symptoms. Spicy or greasy foods are often a problem. You don't need to avoid a food if it doesn't cause problems.

◆ Avoid coffee, tea, cola, and other sources of caffeine. Caffeine often makes pain worse.

◆ Try eating smaller, more frequent meals.

◆ If you smoke, quit. Smoking slows the healing of ulcers and increases the chance that they will come back.

◆ Limit alcohol. Large amounts may slow healing and make symptoms worse.

◆ Do not take aspirin, ibuprofen (Advil, Motrin), or naproxen (Aleve). Try acetaminophen (Tylenol) if you need something for pain.

◆ Try a nonprescription antacid, such as Maalox, Mylanta, or Tums, or an acid reducer, such as Pepcid AC, Tagamet HB, or Zantac 75. Acid blockers, such as Prevacid 24HR and Prilosec OTC, are also sold without a prescription.

  ❖ If you take antacids, you may need frequent, large doses to do the job. Talk with your doctor about the best dose.

  ❖ Your doctor may also suggest that you take a prescription medicine such as Nexium, Prevacid, or Prilosec. These drugs reduce how much acid your stomach produces and can help your ulcer heal.

◆ Learn to relax. See page 318.

Urinary Tract Infections

When to Call a Doctor

- Painful urination occurs with:
  - Fever or chills.
  - Not being able to urinate when you feel the urge.
  - Pain in the back, side, groin, or genital area.
  - Blood or pus in the urine.
  - Unusual discharge from the vagina or penis.
  - Nausea and vomiting.

- Urinary symptoms do not improve after 1 or 2 days, or they get worse even with home treatment. Untreated urinary tract infections (UTIs) can spread, which may lead to kidney infections and other serious problems.
- You are pregnant or have diabetes, and you have symptoms of a UTI.
- You are a man, and you have symptoms of a UTI.
- You think that your child may have a UTI. See page 252.

Urinary tract infections, or UTIs, are usually caused by bacteria that live in the body all the time. Infection can occur in any part of the urinary tract.

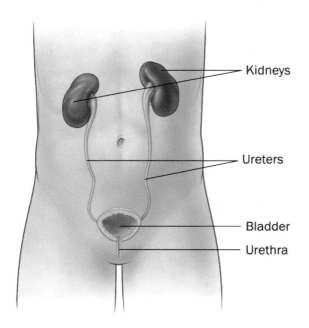

Kidneys

Ureters

Bladder

Urethra

The kidneys filter the blood, and the waste products from the blood become urine. Urine travels through the ureters to the bladder and then leaves the body through the urethra.

Symptoms of a UTI may include:

- Burning or pain when you urinate, as well as itching or pain in the urethra.
- Cloudy or reddish urine with a strange odor.
- Pain in the lower belly or back.
- Often having the urge to urinate but not being able to pass much urine.
- Fever or chills if the infection is bad, especially if it has spread to the kidneys.

Urinary pain or burning may also be a symptom of a sexually transmitted infection. See page 230.

Men with symptoms like those of a UTI may have a prostate infection (see page 223) or epididymitis (see page 247).

More

251

Home Treatment

Start home treatment at the first sign of a UTI. A day or two of self-care may clear up a minor infection.

◆ Drink extra fluids as soon as you notice symptoms and for the next 24 hours.

◆ Urinate often, and follow the other tips in Preventing UTIs.

◆ Watch for fever. A fever may mean you have a more serious infection.

◆ Use a heating pad or take a hot bath to help relieve pain. Do not use bubble bath or harsh soaps.

◆ Do not have sex until symptoms improve.

Cost-saving tip

If you get UTIs often, ask your doctor whether it would be okay to get an extra prescription to have on hand for the future. That way, the next time you get a UTI, you can start the medicine without having to wait for an appointment.

If your doctor agrees that this is a safe option for you, it may save you time and money. It also lets you treat your UTI right away.

Preventing UTIs

These tips may be especially useful if you tend to get UTIs.

◆ Drink plenty of water and other fluids.

◆ Urinate often.

◆ Females should wipe from front to back after using the toilet. This will reduce the spread of bacteria from the anus to the urethra. Teach young girls this habit when you toilet train them.

◆ Do not use douches, vaginal deodorants, or perfumed feminine hygiene products. Avoid bubble baths.

◆ Do not use a diaphragm for birth control. Choose another method.

◆ Wash your genitals once a day with water and a mild soap. Rinse and dry well.

◆ Drink extra water before you have sex, and urinate right afterward.

◆ Wear cotton underwear, cotton-lined panty hose, and loose clothing.

◆ Avoid alcohol, caffeine, and carbonated drinks.

◆ Drink cranberry and blueberry juice.

UTIs in Children

UTIs in children are of special concern because they can easily spread to the kidneys and cause damage and scarring. Repeated scarring can lead to high blood pressure and kidney problems, including kidney failure. Babies and young children seem to be more likely to have scarring.

UTIs in children usually clear up fast if you treat them right away. But it can be hard to tell that your baby or young child has a UTI. Young children may not have the usual symptoms, and they cannot tell you how they feel.

The only signs of a UTI in a baby or young child may be:

◆ Unexplained fever.

◆ Urine that looks or smells odd.

◆ Not eating.

◆ Vomiting.

◆ Being extremely fussy.

Call your child's doctor today if you suspect your child has a UTI.

Vaginal Bleeding

When to Call a Doctor

Call 911 if:

◆ You have severe vaginal bleeding, and you faint or feel lightheaded. (Severe means passing blood clots and soaking through your usual pads each hour for 2 or more hours.)

◆ You have heavy vaginal bleeding, and you are in your second or third trimester of pregnancy.

Call a doctor if:

◆ You are pregnant and have any vaginal bleeding.

◆ You have pain in your lower belly with unexpected vaginal bleeding.

◆ You have unexpected bleeding and a fever.

◆ Bleeding is heavy.

◆ Bleeding between periods lasts longer than 1 week or happens 3 months in a row.

◆ You bleed after you have sex or douche.

◆ You are over 35 and have any bleeding between periods.

◆ You are over 35, and your periods last longer than 10 days.

◆ You use a hormonal form of birth control (pills, shots, implants under the skin, the patch), and your periods are not like what your doctor told you to expect.

◆ You have any bleeding after menopause.

Bleeding Between Periods

Many women have bleeding or spotting between periods. It does not always mean that you have a health problem.

Common causes of bleeding or spotting include:

◆ Ovulation (when the ovary releases an egg each cycle).

◆ Birth control pills or Depo-Provera shots.

◆ Using an IUD (intrauterine device).

◆ Breast-feeding.

◆ Stress.

In all these cases, if the bleeding is not heavy and occurs only once in a while, you probably don't need to worry. Do not take aspirin. It may make the bleeding last longer.

Less common causes of bleeding are:

◆ Uterine fibroids. These growths are not cancer.

◆ Miscarriage or a problem with a pregnancy (see page 217).

◆ Ectopic pregnancy. This means a fertilized egg has attached somewhere other than the uterus.

◆ Pelvic infection. You may also have a fever, cramping, pain during sex, and a smelly vaginal discharge. See page 255.

◆ A problem with the cervix (the opening of the uterus).

◆ Cervical or uterine cancer (rarely).

More ▶

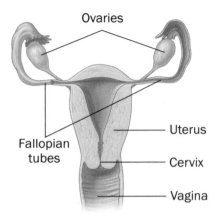

Ovaries

Fallopian
tubes

Uterus

Cervix

Vagina

The female pelvic organs

Bleeding After Menopause

If you have gone through menopause (see page 207) and are not taking hormones, you should not have any vaginal bleeding. If you do, you may have an abnormal growth in your uterus and should see a doctor.

If you are taking hormones, a little bleeding after menopause may be normal. But be sure to tell your doctor about it.

Normal Menstrual Bleeding

The menstrual cycle is the series of changes a woman's body goes through to prepare for a possible pregnancy.

About once a month, the uterus grows a new, thickened lining (endometrium) so that it is ready to receive a fertilized egg. The ovaries release an egg. If the egg does not get fertilized, or if the fertilized egg does not implant in the uterus, the uterus sheds its lining.

The bleeding that results is your monthly period. For most women, the bleeding lasts from 2 to 7 days. It may be heavy or light. Each woman is different. Learn what's normal for you, and watch for changes.

Also see Missed or Irregular Periods on page 210.

Vaginitis and Yeast Infections

When to Call a Doctor

- You have lower belly or pelvic pain, fever, and unusual vaginal discharge.

- You have pain or bleeding during or after sex, and a lubricant does not help.

- Your vaginal discharge smells bad or does not look normal.

- You think you have a yeast infection but are not sure.

- You know you have a yeast infection, and nonprescription medicine does not clear it up in 3 or 4 days.

- You think you may have a sexually transmitted infection. See page 229. Your sex partner(s) may need to be treated too.

- You get yeast infections often and are not taking antibiotics. This can be a sign of diabetes or other problems.

- You are or may be pregnant and have symptoms of a vaginal infection (pain, redness, itching, smelly discharge).

- You have symptoms of a urinary tract infection (pain or burning, frequent urge to urinate). See page 251.

- Your vagina is dry and irritated, and a lubricant does not help.

If you plan to see a doctor, do not douche, use vaginal creams, or have sex for 48 hours before your appointment.

Vaginitis is any infection, inflammation, or irritation of the vagina that changes your normal vaginal discharge.

If it hurts or burns when you urinate and you feel the need to urinate often, you may have a urinary tract infection. See page 251.

Home Treatment

- Follow the tips in Preventing Vaginal Problems on page 256.

- Do not have sex until your symptoms have gone away.

- Do not scratch. Relieve itching with a cold pack or a cool bath. Put a thin cloth between the cold pack and your skin.

- Make sure the cause of vaginitis is not a forgotten tampon or other object.

- If you think you may be pregnant, do a home pregnancy test. See page 210. Infection can be more serious if you are pregnant.

- If you know that you have a yeast infection, try a nonprescription medicine such as Monistat or Gyne-Lotrimin. If you're pregnant, talk with your doctor first.

- Use pads instead of tampons if you are using a vaginal cream or suppository. The tampons can absorb the medicine.

Vaginitis may clear up in a few days. If your symptoms do not go away, be sure to call your doctor.

More

Vaginal Problems

Common Causes	Symptoms	What to Do
Yeast infection	Itching and redness; white, odor-free discharge that looks like cottage cheese; burning when you urinate or have sex	Infection may clear on its own; try nonprescription medicine for yeast infection (Monistat, Gyne-Lotrimin).
Bacterial vaginosis	Thin gray or yellow discharge that smells fishy; pain when you have sex	Call your doctor for treatment, especially if you are pregnant.
Trichomoniasis and other sexually transmitted infections (see page 230)	Redness and irritation; bad odor; a lot of foamy, white or colored discharge; pain when you urinate or have sex	Call your doctor for treatment. Any partner(s) need treatment too.
Atrophic vaginitis (happens after menopause)	Burning, pain, and dryness when you have sex	Try a vaginal lubricant (Astroglide, K-Y Jelly). Ask your doctor about an estrogen cream or ring.

Preventing Vaginal Problems

◆ Do not take antibiotics unless you really need to.

◆ Wash your vaginal area once a day with plain water or a mild, unscented soap. Rinse and dry well.

◆ Do not douche.

◆ Do not use feminine deodorant sprays and other perfumed products. They irritate and dry tender skin.

◆ During your period, change tampons at least 3 times a day, or switch between tampons and pads. Don't leave tampons in for more than 8 hours. And be sure to remove the last tampon you use.

◆ Wipe from front to back after you use the toilet.

◆ Limit how many sex partners you have. Use condoms.

◆ If you think the problems may be related to your birth control (diaphragm, spermicide, condoms), discuss other options with your doctor. See page 96.

◆ Do not wear panty hose or tight nylon underwear.

◆ Try a vaginal lubricant during sex if you have a problem with dryness.

◆ If you have diabetes, keep your blood sugar under control. This can help prevent yeast infections.

Varicose Veins

When to Call a Doctor

◆ You have pain or swelling in your leg. You may have a clot in a deep vein, which could be serious.

◆ The skin over a varicose vein bleeds heavily on its own or after an injury, and you cannot stop the bleeding.

◆ You have an open sore on your leg or foot.

◆ A tender lump appears on your leg for no clear reason (you have not bumped or bruised your leg).

Varicose veins are large, twisted veins near the surface of the skin. They are most common in the legs and ankles.

You get a varicose vein when a vein becomes weak and stretched and can no longer help move blood up and back to the heart. (This is not harmful, because there are so many other veins in the body.) Blood pools in the weak vein, causing it to swell.

Obesity, pregnancy, or standing for long periods of time can cause varicose veins. They also tend to run in the family.

◆ Varicose veins may not cause any symptoms. The blue color of the veins may be the only reason you notice them.

◆ Your legs, feet, or ankles may ache, swell a little, and feel tired.

◆ If the veins get worse, they can cause dry, itchy skin and may break open and bleed, causing open sores.

Some people have tiny varicose veins near the surface of the skin. These are called spider veins. They are not a health problem, but you may not like the way they look if you have them.

Varicose veins usually do not need treatment other than self-care. If they bother you or cause bleeding or skin problems, you may want to think about treatments such as sclerotherapy or surgery. For help deciding whether you want or need treatment, go to the Web site on the back cover and enter **d904** in the search box.

Home Treatment

◆ Wear supportive, full-length elastic stockings. Do not wear knee-highs. For mild symptoms, regular support panty hose may work. Or your doctor can give you a prescription for compression stockings, which you can buy at a drugstore or medical supply store.

◆ Do not wear socks or stockings that leave red marks around your legs. Do not wear tight belts or pants that are tight in the waist or thighs.

◆ Put your feet up when you sit. If you cannot put your feet up, then sit with your feet flat on the floor or crossed at the ankles. Do not cross your legs at the knee. At the end of the day, lie down and prop your legs above the level of your heart.

◆ If you have to sit a lot (at work, for example), get up and walk around often. If you have to stand a lot, move around often, or sit down and put your feet up when you can.

◆ Get regular exercise, such as walking, cycling, swimming, or dancing. Working your leg muscles keeps blood from pooling in the legs.

◆ Lose weight if you need to. See page 300.

Vomiting and Nausea, Age 11 and Younger

When to Call a Doctor

Call 911 if:

◆ Your child faints, or you cannot wake your child.

◆ Your child has signs of severe dehydration. These include feeling very dizzy or lightheaded, fast breathing and heartbeat, not feeling or acting alert, or having trouble waking up.

◆ Your child vomits blood or what looks like coffee grounds.

Call a doctor if:

◆ Vomiting occurs with severe headache, a stiff neck, not acting alert, or having trouble waking up. Your child may have a serious illness. See page 161.

◆ Your child has signs of moderate dehydration. These include sunken eyes, no tears, and a dry mouth and tongue; a sunken soft spot on your baby's head; little or no urine for 8 hours; or skin that sags when you pinch it.

◆ Your child refuses to drink or cannot take in enough liquid to replace lost fluids.

◆ Severe vomiting (vomiting most or all clear liquids and feedings) occurs in a baby younger than 3 months. For older children, call if severe vomiting goes on:

❖ Longer than 4 hours in a baby 3 to 12 months old.

❖ Longer than 8 hours in a child 1 to 11 years old.

◆ Your child vomits now and then, has no other symptoms, and can keep fluids down between vomiting. Call if this goes on longer than 2 days.

◆ Your child has severe belly pain.

◆ Your child has belly pain and vomiting for more than 12 hours but has little or no diarrhea.

◆ Belly pain started several hours before the vomiting and seems like more than just stomach cramps.

◆ Your child has pain in just one part of the belly, especially the lower right belly. See the picture on page 69. It may be hard to tell where the pain is in a small child.

For vomiting and nausea in people age 12 and older, see page 260.

Nausea and vomiting in children is often caused by:

◆ Viral stomach flu. Stomach flu often starts with vomiting that is followed in a few hours (sometimes 8 to 12 hours or longer) by diarrhea. Sometimes there is no diarrhea.

◆ Eating unusual kinds or amounts of food. A baby's digestive system sometimes cannot handle large amounts of juice, fruit, or even milk.

Nausea and vomiting can also be caused by serious illness, though this is not common. In these cases, nausea and vomiting will usually occur with other signs of illness, such as stiff neck, constant crying, and not being alert or active.

Babies and young children need special care when they are vomiting, because they can quickly get dehydrated. This means the body has lost too much fluid. Keep a close watch on how your child looks and acts, and make sure he or she gets enough fluids.

Home Treatment
Babies through 6 months

◆ Do not feed your baby anything for 30 to 60 minutes after he or she has vomited. Watch your baby closely for signs of dehydration (see When to Call a Doctor).

◆ If your baby is breast-fed, offer short but frequent feedings.

◆ If your baby is formula-fed, switch to an oral electrolyte solution, such as Pedialyte. Offer ½ ounce every 10 minutes for the first hour. After the first hour, slowly increase the amount you offer your baby. You can go back to regular feedings after 6 hours have passed without your baby vomiting.

◆ Do not give your baby plain water.

Children 7 months through 12 months

◆ After 1 hour has passed since your child last vomited, give ½ ounce of a clear liquid every 10 minutes for 1 hour. Safe choices are children's oral rehydration solution; clear broth; gelatin dessert, such as Jell-O; and fruit juice mixed to half strength with water.

Children 13 months through 11 years

◆ After 1 hour has passed since your child last vomited, give 1 ounce of a clear liquid every 20 minutes for 1 hour.

In general, for children ages 7 months through 11 years:

◆ Gradually increase the amount of clear liquids that you give as long as your child does not vomit.

◆ Do not use sports drinks (such as Gatorade or All Sport), soda, or full-strength fruit juice. These drinks have too much sugar. Do not offer plain water or diet soda. These lack the calories and minerals your child needs.

◆ After 6 hours with no vomiting, offer your child regular foods. Avoid high-fiber foods (such as beans) and foods with a lot of sugar, such as candy or ice cream.

Vomiting and Nausea, Age 12 and Older

When to Call a Doctor

Call 911 if:

◆ Vomiting occurs with chest pain or pressure or other signs of a heart attack. See page 38.

◆ You have signs of severe dehydration. These include feeling very dizzy or lightheaded, fast breathing and heartbeat, or not feeling or acting alert.

◆ You vomit a lot of blood or what looks like coffee grounds.

Call a doctor if:

◆ You vomit after a head injury. See page 37.

◆ You have signs of moderate dehydration. These include little or no urine for 8 hours; sunken eyes, no tears, and a dry mouth and tongue; or skin that sags when you pinch it.

◆ There are streaks of blood in your vomit.

◆ Symptoms of mild dehydration (dry mouth, dark urine, not much urine) get worse even with home treatment.

◆ Vomiting occurs with any of these signs of serious illness:

❖ Severe headache, sleepiness, or stiff neck. See page 161.

❖ Fever and increasing pain in the lower right belly. See page 69.

❖ Fever and shaking chills.

❖ Swelling in the belly.

❖ Pain in the upper right or upper left belly.

◆ Vomiting and fever last longer than 48 hours.

◆ You think that a medicine may be causing the problem.

◆ Any vomiting lasts longer than 1 week.

For vomiting and nausea in children age 11 and younger, see page 258.

Nausea is a very unpleasant feeling in the pit of your stomach. You may feel weak and sweaty and produce lots of spit. Intense nausea often leads to vomiting, or "throwing up." Good home treatment will help you feel better and avoid dehydration.

Common causes of nausea and vomiting are:

◆ Viral stomach flu or food poisoning. See page 167.

◆ Stress or nervousness.

◆ Medicines, especially antibiotics, aspirin, ibuprofen (Advil, Motrin), and naproxen (Aleve).

◆ Pregnancy and morning sickness. See page 217.

◆ Diabetes.

◆ Migraine headaches. See page 176.

◆ Head injury. See page 37.

Nausea and vomiting can also be signs of other serious problems. Be sure to check the Digestive Problems chart on page 66 if this topic does not meet your needs.

Home Treatment

◆ Watch for and treat early signs of dehydration. See page 31. Older adults and young children who are vomiting can quickly get dehydrated.

◆ After vomiting has stopped for 1 hour, drink 1 ounce of a clear liquid every 20 minutes. Drink more as you feel better and as your body can handle it. Clear liquids include apple or grape juice mixed to half strength with water, rehydration drinks (see page 33), weak tea with sugar, clear broth, and gelatin dessert (such as Jell-O). Avoid orange juice and grapefruit juice.

◆ If vomiting lasts longer than 24 hours, sip a rehydration drink to restore lost fluids and nutrients. See page 33.

◆ When you feel better, try clear soups and liquids and mild foods. Good choices are bananas, rice, applesauce, dry toast, crackers, and gelatin dessert (such as Jell-O). Stick with these mild foods until all symptoms have been gone for 12 to 48 hours.

◆ Rest in bed until you feel better.

Warts

When to Call a Doctor

◆ A wart looks infected.

◆ A plantar wart hurts when you walk, and foam pads do not help.

◆ You have warts in the anal or genital area. See page 230.

◆ You have a wart on your face that you want removed.

◆ You have diabetes or peripheral artery disease and get a wart on your foot.

Warts are skin growths caused by a virus. They can appear anywhere on the body. Plantar warts are on the soles of the feet. Most of the wart lies under the skin surface, and it may make you feel like you are walking on a pebble.

Warts come and go for no clear reason. They can last a week, a month, or even years.

There are several ways to deal with warts:

◆ Do not treat them. If warts don't bother you, there is no reason to spend time and money treating them.

◆ Use home treatment to remove them. There are three methods for this: salicylic acid, tape, and cryotherapy. See Home Treatment on page 262. Home treatment works a lot of the time, but not always.

◆ Have surgery to remove them. If you have a very painful wart that will not go away, or if you have enough warts to bother you, you may want to think about surgery. But you should know that warts may come back after surgery.

 Talk with your doctor about your treatment choices and their pros and cons. For help deciding what's right for you, go to the Web site on the back cover and enter **V098** in the search box.

Home Treatment

- Do not try to remove genital warts. See page 230.

- Do not pick at a wart. It may spread to the skin under your nails.

- Do not try to cut or burn off a wart.

- Do not try to remove a wart if you have diabetes or peripheral artery disease. Talk to your doctor.

To Remove Warts

Try the least costly method first. You may save a trip to your doctor. If you find a treatment that works, stick with it.

If you are sure that your skin growth is a wart, you can treat it with one of three methods:

- **Method 1:** Use a nonprescription salicylic acid product. Over time, this will soften the wart so that you can rub or file it off. Follow the instructions on the label. Salicylic acid works as well as any other treatment for warts. It may take 2 to 3 months to work.

- **Method 2:** Cover the wart with a piece of waterproof tape (such as duct tape), and leave it on for 6 days. After 6 days, remove the tape and soak the wart in water. Then gently rub it with a nail file or pumice stone. (You will need to clean or replace the nail file or pumice stone often.) Leave the tape off overnight. Repeat the process until the wart is gone. But if it has not worked after 2 months, try another method.

- **Method 3:** Use a nonprescription cryotherapy product. You spray medicine into a foam applicator and then hold the applicator to the wart for a few seconds. This "freezes" the wart off. Pregnant or breast-feeding women and children younger than 4 should not use this treatment.

If treatment irritates the area, take a 2- to 3-day break from it.

If you rub the wart with a pumice stone or file to remove dead tissue, do not use the item for any other purpose. It can spread the wart-causing virus. Wash your hands with soap after you touch the debris from the wart or the pumice stone or file.

To Reduce Pain From a Plantar Wart

- Wear comfortable shoes and socks. Don't wear high heels or shoes that put pressure on your foot.

- Cushion the wart with a doughnut-shaped pad or a moleskin patch you can buy at a drugstore. Place the pad around the plantar wart. You may also want to place pads or cushions in your shoes.

Living Better With Chronic Disease

How to Live Better With Chronic Disease

Chronic diseases are long-term health problems. They can last for months or years. Often they last a lifetime.

A minor chronic health problem may not have much of an impact on your life. But for millions of people, coping with a chronic disease is part of their daily lives. The good news is that even if chronic disease is part of your life, it doesn't have to be the only part. No matter what your health problem is, there are things you can do to help control your disease and live better.

1. Get informed. Good information can help you make good health decisions. If this book does not address the health problem you have—or even if it does—go to the Web, your local library, or a hospital library to start learning about your disease.

Don't be afraid to use your doctor as a teacher. See page 3 for tips on how to get the most out of your partnership with your doctor.

If you see more than one doctor, make sure that each doctor knows what health problems you have and what medicines and other treatment you are getting.

2. Get support. For major health problems, support can make a big difference in how well you do and how good you feel. Look for support from:

◆ Family and friends. Let them know how they can help, even if all you need is someone to talk to.

◆ Support groups. People who have the same disease you do can be a great source of emotional and practical help. Look for a support group in your area or online. There are online groups and chat rooms for nearly every health problem. (Be careful with what you learn online, and talk to your doctor before you change your treatment or try any new medicines, vitamins, or herbal products.)

◆ Large organizations focused on specific diseases, like the American Diabetes Association or the American Heart Association.

◆ Counselors and therapists. Living with a chronic disease can be overwhelming at times. If you're feeling depressed or don't feel like you are coping well, talking with an expert might help.

3. Follow your treatment plan. Your doctor can guide your treatment, but whether you stick to the plan is up to you. Depending on the disease, treatment may include things like:

◆ Taking medicines every day, on time, and in the right amount.

◆ Changing your diet. (Maybe you need to eat a low-sodium diet or avoid certain foods.)

◆ Making changes in your lifestyle, like being more active, quitting smoking, or getting more rest. For some health problems, changes like these are not just healthy habits. They're vital to treating the disease.

◆ Doing physical therapy.

◆ Having treatments like radiation, dialysis, or chemotherapy.

Following your treatment plan may be hard sometimes, but it can make a big difference. Talk with your doctor if you have any problems with your treatment. There may be ways to make it easier.

4. Avoid "triggers" when you can. Triggers are things that make your symptoms or disease worse. For example, smoke, dust, and pollution are common triggers for people with breathing problems. For certain diseases, a meal that has a lot of salt or certain nonprescription medicines might trigger symptoms. Stress and lack of sleep are triggers for some health problems.

If you're not sure what your triggers are, it may help to keep a record of your symptoms. Write down when you have them, how bad they are, and what seems to make them worse or better. With time, you may start to see patterns that can help you recognize your triggers. Then you can try to avoid them.

5. Monitor your health. Part of your self-care job may be to regularly test and keep track of some aspect of your disease. People with diabetes need to check their blood sugar. People with asthma have to check their peak flow, which measures how well they are breathing. If you have high blood pressure, you may need to check your own blood pressure often.

Doing these "self-tests" can help you:

◆ Know when there's a problem before it becomes severe. You may be able to stop the problem before it gets worse.

◆ Know when to call your doctor right away rather than wait for your next visit.

◆ Know how well your treatment is working. Your records can help your doctor track your health over time.

6. Know what problems to watch for. Sometimes there may be warning signs that your disease is about to flare up. Or you may need to watch for early signs of complications.

Talk to your doctor about what symptoms you should watch for, and have a plan for how to handle them. Should you go to the hospital? Is there medicine you can take? Get instructions for what to do if you suddenly get worse.

7. See your doctor regularly. Regular visits and, in some cases, tests let you and your doctor check in on your health and know whether your treatment needs to be changed. They can also help your doctor find problems early, when they may be easier to correct.

Agree on a schedule for visits and tests. Once a year? Every 3 months? Work with your doctor to decide what's best for you.

8. Stay as healthy as you can. Chronic disease can become harder to manage when you start to have other health problems too. For most people, healthy lifestyle choices— eating right, not smoking, being active, reducing stress—can make a difference. Remember to take care of your whole self.

Where to Go From Here

The rest of this section covers six common chronic diseases: asthma, COPD, coronary artery disease, depression, diabetes, and heart failure. If you have one of these conditions, read on to learn the basics of how to manage your disease.

If you have a different health problem, check the index at the back of the book or go to the Web, your local library, or a hospital library. With the right information and a little coaching, you can start living better with your disease today.

Living Better With Asthma

If you have asthma, it may help to know just what it is and what it does to your body. Asthma causes inflammation and swelling in the airways (bronchial tubes) that lead to the lungs. This makes the airways narrower, which makes it harder for you to breathe.

How often you have trouble breathing depends on how bad your asthma is and what triggers it. Some people breathe normally most of the time, while others feel as if they are always short of breath. Other people may have trouble breathing only at night or when they exercise.

When you have a lot of trouble breathing, you are having an asthma attack. Your airways are very swollen, and it's hard to get air through them.

Along with the symptoms asthma can cause from day to day, it also can damage your airways and lungs. Even mild asthma can cause long-term problems. Asthma can make illnesses like bronchitis and pneumonia worse.

But asthma does not have to control your life or your future. There are things you can do today and every day to prevent these kinds of problems and to live better with asthma.

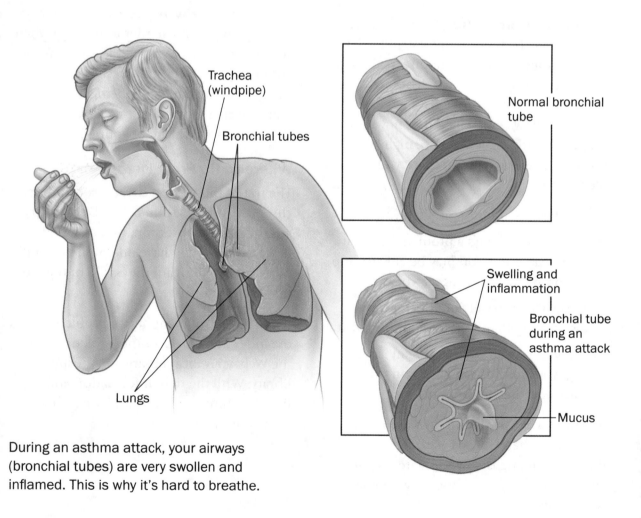

Trachea (windpipe)

Bronchial tubes

Lungs

Normal bronchial tube

Swelling and inflammation

Bronchial tube during an asthma attack

Mucus

During an asthma attack, your airways (bronchial tubes) are very swollen and inflamed. This is why it's hard to breathe.

What You Can Do

◆ Have and follow an asthma action plan. An asthma action plan can give you much of what you need to manage your asthma. See Your Asthma Action Plan on this page.

◆ Take your asthma medicines. If you are not sure how or when to take them, talk to your doctor. See page 268.

◆ Take part in your care. Check your peak flow (see page 269). Keep track of your symptoms. Do not ignore your asthma just because you feel good.

◆ Learn what things make your asthma worse or lead to asthma attacks. Avoid these triggers when you can. See page 269.

◆ See your doctor regularly. How often depends on how bad your asthma is. If you have mild asthma, you may need a checkup every 6 months. If your asthma is out of control, you may need one every 2 to 6 weeks.

◆ If you smoke, quit. Smoking makes your asthma worse, and it raises your risk for lung cancer and other problems. If you need help quitting, see page 316.

Your Asthma Action Plan

An asthma action plan is a written plan that tells you what asthma medicine to take each day and how to treat an asthma attack. It can help you make quick decisions about what to do when your asthma gets worse.

To use an asthma action plan, you need to know a few things:

◆ Your peak flow. Peak flow is how fast you breathe out when you try your hardest. It tells you how well your airways and lungs are working. Checking your peak flow is easy. See page 269 to learn how.

◆ Your personal best peak flow. This number is a baseline for knowing whether you are doing well or getting worse. You find your personal best by taking peak flow readings over 2 to 3 weeks when your asthma is under control.

◆ Your asthma zones. There are three zones: green, yellow, and red. Your action plan tells you what to do when you are in each zone. The zones are based on your peak flow and your symptoms.

An asthma action plan can help you feel better and avoid serious health problems. If you don't have a plan now, ask your doctor to help you make one. For help getting started, go to the Web site on the back cover and enter **f384** in the search box.

More

Take Your Medicines

Asthma medicine helps prevent your symptoms and makes you more able to do the things you want to do. It helps you control your asthma instead of your asthma controlling you.

Most people need two types of asthma medicine:

◆ Controller medicine. Take your controller medicine every day, even when you do not have symptoms. It prevents asthma attacks and helps stop problems before they occur.

◆ Quick-relief medicine. Use this when you have symptoms of an asthma attack. It acts fast to treat an attack before it gets bad. Always have some of this medicine with you.

Using Your Inhaler

Asthma medicine usually comes in an inhaler, a device that lets you breathe the medicine in through your mouth so it goes right to your airways and lungs.

 To get the best results from your medicine, be sure to use the inhaler correctly. For a step-by-step guide (with pictures!), go to the Web site on the back cover and enter **n247** in the search box. You can also ask your doctor or pharmacist for help.

Your doctor may suggest that you use a spacer. A spacer is a piece you attach to the inhaler. It makes using an inhaler easier for many people.

If you still have trouble, tell your doctor. There may be another way you can take your medicine.

Quick-Relief Medicine: For Attacks, Not Daily Use

Since quick-relief medicine helps your breathing problems so fast, you may be tempted to use it often to control your asthma instead of taking your controller medicine.

This is not a good idea. Quick-relief medicine is for times when you cannot prevent symptoms and need to treat them. It is not intended as the daily medicine you take to control your asthma—just like controller medicine is not used to treat an attack (it acts too slowly).

Why does it matter?

◆ The goal is to prevent symptoms before they start. This is the job of controller medicine. Quick-relief medicine does not help as well with this.

◆ Using quick-relief medicine too often can cause your heart to beat too fast or in an odd rhythm.

◆ Needing to take quick-relief medicine on more than 2 days a week may mean that your asthma is not controlled.

Talk to your doctor if you are using quick-relief medicine on more than 2 days a week.

Note: Some people with asthma need to take quick-relief medicine before they exercise. If your doctor has advised this, it is okay to take it as often as you exercise.

Check Your Peak Flow

Peak flow (peak expiratory flow, or PEF) is how fast you can breathe out when you try your hardest. Checking your peak flow regularly can help you:

◆ Know when an asthma attack is coming and treat it before it gets bad. This helps you stay healthy and stay out of the hospital.

◆ Know how well your lungs are working, even if you don't have symptoms.

◆ Find out what things make your asthma worse. For example, if your peak flow is always worse when you are under stress or when you let your dog sleep in your bedroom, it's a good clue that these things are not good for your asthma.

Checking your peak flow is quick and easy. You can do it at home with a simple, low-cost device called a peak flow meter. Here's how:

◆ Take a breath and blow into the tube on the meter as hard and as fast as you can.

◆ Write down the number on the meter. Use a notebook or calendar where you can keep track of your peak flow and asthma symptoms over time.

◆ Do what your asthma action plan (see page 267) says to do based on your peak flow.

Work with your doctor to find out what your peak flow should be and how often to check it. Bring your records of your peak flow readings and symptoms whenever you have a checkup. These can help your doctor know whether you need to change your treatment.

Checking your peak flow is an easy, low-cost step to help you control your asthma and avoid severe attacks. For a complete, step-by-step guide to checking your peak flow, go to the Web site on the back cover and enter **r703** in the search box.

Avoid Asthma Triggers

A trigger is anything that makes your asthma worse and can cause an attack. Smoke, pollution, pollen, pet dander, colds, stress, and cold air are triggers for many people.

You can learn what triggers an asthma attack for you by keeping track of your peak flow and your symptoms. When you get worse or better, think about what may have caused it. Is the pollen count high? Did you spend the evening in a smoky bar? Did you go for a jog in the cold air?

Once you know what your triggers are, try to prevent or avoid them. These tips may help with the most common triggers:

◆ If you smoke, quit. See page 316 if you need help quitting. Stay out of smoky places. Do not use a wood-burning stove or fireplace in your home.

◆ Reduce dust, dust mites, pollen, and mold in your home—especially your bedroom. See page 77 for lots of ideas that can help.

◆ Do not exercise outside when the air is cold and dry. Try an indoor workout at the gym. Walk at the mall. Get an exercise video you can do at home.

More ▶

◆ Keep pets out of the house, or at least out of your bedroom. Have your pet stay in areas that have hard floors. They are easier to clean than carpeted ones.

Avoiding your triggers can help prevent asthma attacks and keep you healthy and out of the hospital. For more help finding out what your triggers are and how to deal with them, go to the Web site on the back cover and enter **z654** in the search box.

If Your Child Has Asthma

Many children have asthma and handle it very well. You can help your child feel better, do more, and avoid emergencies and long-term problems.

◆ Make sure your child takes his or her asthma medicines. This means taking controller medicines every day (or as prescribed) and using quick-relief medicine at the right times. Your child may need some help using an inhaler properly.

◆ Tell teachers, coaches, and the school nurse that your child has asthma. Talk about what to do if your child has an asthma attack.

◆ Make sure your child has quick-relief medicine available at all times.

◆ Help your child check and keep track of his or her peak flow. With a little support, many older children can do this on their own.

◆ Encourage your child to be active, play, and do what other kids do. Asthma does not have to hold your child back.

For parents of teens with asthma

Teens may feel like asthma cuts into their freedom or sets them apart from their friends. There are ways you can help your teen stick with treatment and feel better about it.

◆ Let your teen meet with the doctor alone. This helps your teen take charge of his or her care.

◆ Work out a treatment plan that lets your teen do what he or she likes to do (sports, music, school activities).

◆ Help your teen see that treatment will help him or her lead an active, normal life.

◆ Talk with your teen about the dangers of smoking. Smoking is bad for all teens. It's especially bad for teens with asthma.

◆ Help your teen meet other teens with asthma so they can support each other.

When to Call a Doctor

Call 911 if you have severe trouble breathing.

Call your doctor if:

◆ You have taken your quick-relief medicine and, after 20 to 30 minutes, you do not feel better.

◆ You measure your peak flow, and it is less than 50 percent of your personal best.

◆ Your symptoms do not get better after you have followed your asthma action plan.

◆ You cough up yellow, dark brown, or bloody mucus.

◆ You wake up at night once a week or more because you are coughing or wheezing.

◆ You do not have an asthma action plan, and you want one.

◆ You need to use quick-relief medicine on more than 2 days a week (for reasons other than exercise).

◆ You have any problems with your asthma medicine.

Living Better With COPD

COPD (chronic obstructive pulmonary disease) is a long-term illness that makes it hard to breathe. When you have COPD, air does not flow easily out of your lungs. You may be short of breath, cough a lot, and have a lot of mucus in your airways.

If you have emphysema or chronic bronchitis, you have a form of COPD.

With time, breathing problems get worse, and it gets harder to do everyday activities. COPD can lead to heart problems and to death. But you can make a difference in your health.

The best thing you can do is stop smoking. This is the only sure way to slow the disease. But it may also be the hardest step to take when you have COPD.

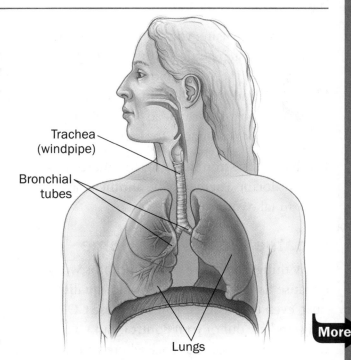

When you have COPD, the lungs and the tubes (trachea and bronchial tubes) leading to the lungs get damaged. This makes it hard to breathe.

More

Talk to your doctor about stop-smoking programs and medicines that can help. Also see Quitting Smoking on page 316.

Other good self-care can help you stay healthier for a longer time. For example, regular exercise, special breathing techniques, and rest breaks during the day may help you feel better from day to day. Taking the medicines your doctor prescribes may help with your breathing.

Take Your Medicines

COPD medicines reduce shortness of breath, control coughing and wheezing, and can prevent or reduce a flare-up. Most people with COPD find that medicine makes breathing easier.

COPD medicines usually come as an inhaler—a device that lets you breathe the medicine in through your mouth so it goes right to your airways and lungs.

Be sure you are using your inhaler correctly. For a step-by-step guide (with pictures!), go to the Web site on the back cover and enter **e492** in the search box. You can also ask your doctor or pharmacist for help.

If you still have trouble using an inhaler, talk to your doctor. There may be another way you can take your medicine.

Breathe Clean Air at Home

Many things can make your symptoms worse or cause flare-ups—smoke, poor air quality, dust, even the weather. Some of these COPD "triggers" are out of your control. But you can make your home a place where you can breathe easier.

◆ Do not let anyone smoke in your home. That means you too.

COPD Flare-Ups

Sometimes your usual shortness of breath will suddenly get worse. You may start coughing more and have more mucus. This is called a COPD flare-up or exacerbation.

Air pollution or a lung infection can cause a flare-up. Sometimes a flare-up may happen after a quick change in temperature or after being around chemicals.

A COPD flare-up can be life-threatening. If you have one:

◆ Use your inhaler medicine first.

◆ If your symptoms do not get better after you use your medicine, have someone take you to the emergency room. Call 911 if you have to.

You may need to be treated in a hospital until you can breathe better on your own. With the right treatment, most people recover from a flare-up, and their breathing is no worse than it was before.

Do everything you can do to avoid flare-ups and stay out of the hospital:

◆ Take your medicines.

◆ Avoid "triggers" like smoke, poor air quality, and chemicals.

◆ Clear mucus from your lungs.

◆ Stay as healthy as you can.

 By taking these steps, you should avoid most flare-ups. To learn more about triggers and ways to clear your lungs, go to the Web site on the back cover and enter **j782** in the search box.

- If you have air-conditioning, use it so you don't have to open the windows. Fresh air may seem like a good idea, but air pollution and other outdoor triggers can make your COPD worse.

- Use an air purifier with a HEPA filter.

- Make sure gas appliances are vented well and have tight-fitting doors. Check flues and chimneys for cracks that could let in fumes. Don't use an open fireplace or wood-burning stove; wood smoke is bad for your breathing.

- Do not use strong chemicals or aerosol sprays in your home, and do not mix cleaning products. Try natural cleaners like vinegar, lemon juice, boric acid, or baking soda.

- Do not keep items for recycling indoors. Newspapers, rags, cans, or bottles can give off fumes.

- Reduce the dust in your house as much as you can. See page 77 for tips.

- Make sure outdoor fresh-air intake vents for heating and air-conditioning systems are above ground. Keep cars, trucks, and other sources of pollution away from the vents.

Breathing Lessons

People with COPD tend to take quick, short breaths. Breathing this way makes it harder to get air into your lungs. But you can learn some other ways to breathe that make it easier.

Use these methods when you are more short of breath than normal. Practice them every day so you can do them well.

Pursed-lip breathing

Breathe in through your nose and out through your mouth while almost closing your lips. Breathe in for about 4 seconds, and breathe out for 6 to 8 seconds.

Pursed-lip breathing helps you breathe more air out so that your next breath can be deeper. It makes you less short of breath and lets you exercise more.

Breathing while bending

Bending forward at the waist may make it easier for you to breathe. It can reduce shortness of breath while you are exercising or resting.

Breathing with your diaphragm

Breathing with your diaphragm helps your lungs expand so that they take in more air.

- Lie on your back or prop yourself up on several pillows.

- With one hand on your belly and the other on your chest, breathe in. Push your belly out as far as you can. You should feel the hand on your belly move out, while the hand on your chest should not move. When you breathe out, the hand on your belly should move in.

Once you can do this while you are lying down, you can learn to do it while sitting or standing.

More ▶

Stay Healthy, Feel Better

There are things you can do that will help you be able to do more and give you more energy.

◆ Stop smoking. This is the most important step you can take to feel better and live longer. See page 316 to get started.

◆ Avoid colds and the flu.

   ❖ Get the flu vaccine each fall. Ask those you live or work with to do the same, so they don't get the flu and infect you.

   ❖ Wash your hands often, especially during cold and flu season.

   ❖ Get a pneumococcal vaccine. Some people need two shots of the vaccine.

◆ Avoid smoke; cold, dry air; hot, humid air; and high altitudes. Stay inside with the windows closed when air pollution is bad.

◆ Try to exercise throughout the week. Walking is a great way to be more active. To learn what other kinds of exercise are great for people with COPD, go to the Web site on the back cover and enter **L228** in the search box.

◆ Ask your doctor whether a pulmonary rehab program would be good for you. Rehab includes exercise programs, education about your disease and how to manage it, help with diet and other changes, and emotional support. Many people with COPD find these programs helpful.

◆ Take short rest breaks when you are doing chores and other activities. This will help your breathing and help you avoid getting too tired.

◆ Eat regular, healthy meals. People with COPD often find it hard to eat because of their breathing problems, but there are some simple ways to make it easier. Go to the Web site on the back cover and enter **k820** in the search box.

What About Oxygen Therapy?

At some point you may need oxygen therapy. By boosting the oxygen in your blood, this treatment helps you breathe easier and gives you more energy. It may also help you live longer and stay out of the hospital.

You can use oxygen therapy while you move around and do daily tasks. You may breathe the oxygen through a flexible plastic tube in your nostrils (nasal cannula), a face mask, or a tube put into your windpipe.

The oxygen can be supplied in several ways. For example, you can get an oxygen gas tank, liquid oxygen that comes in a small container, or an oxygen concentrator. Each has its pros and cons in terms of weight, cost, how much oxygen it holds, and how dangerous it is. (Do not use oxygen around a lit cigarette or an open flame.)

You may need oxygen only when you exercise or when you are asleep. Or you may need it all the time. If you and your doctor decide that you need oxygen to prolong your life, work together to decide what is best for you. Learn how to get the most out of treatment. Go to the Web site on the back cover and enter **q028** in the search box.

Planning for the Future

Over time, your breathing and your over-all health are probably going to get worse no matter what you do. It's normal to feel frightened, angry, hopeless, or even guilty. Talk to your family, friends, or a therapist about how you feel, or join a support group. Talking about your feelings can help you cope.

You may also feel a little more at peace with the future if you plan for it. Talk to your doctor and your family about what you want to happen when your health gets worse. Write out advance directives, including a living will, so that you get to decide what kind of treatment you have at the end of your life.

For help with end-of-life planning, see page 295.

When to Call a Doctor

Call 911 if you have severe trouble breathing.

Call your doctor if:

◆ You have shortness of breath or wheezing that is getting worse.

◆ You are coughing more deeply or more often than usual.

◆ You cough up blood.

◆ Swelling in your legs or belly gets worse.

◆ You have a fever.

◆ Your medicine does not seem to be working as well as it had been.

Living Better With Coronary Artery Disease

Coronary artery disease (CAD) means that the blood vessels that bring blood to the heart have become narrow or blocked. They usually get blocked by **plaque**, which is a buildup of fat and other substances.

When you have CAD, your blood vessels cannot bring as much blood and oxygen to your heart. Poor blood flow can cause chest pain or other symptoms when your heart has to work harder. If the blood flow gets completely blocked, you may have a heart attack.

With poor blood flow over time, your heart may get weaker and not pump as well as it should. This can lead to dangerous heartbeat problems and heart failure.

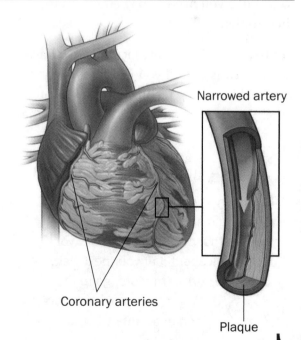

Narrowed artery

Coronary arteries

Plaque

Plaque is a buildup of fat and other substances that can block your arteries.

More

How to Avoid a Heart Attack

For many people with CAD, their biggest fear is a heart attack. To avoid a heart attack and live longer and better, you will need to take steps to improve your health. The good news is that you are in control.

Here are things you can do now to get healthy and stay that way:

◆ If you smoke, quit. See page 277.

◆ Eat healthy food. Eat more fiber, and cut down on cholesterol, saturated and trans fats, and salt. See page 277.

◆ Try to get some exercise throughout the week. Start with short walks or any other activity you enjoy. See page 278.

◆ Take any medicines your doctor prescribes, such as high blood pressure and high cholesterol medicines.

You may not feel sick at all until your heart disease gets a lot worse. Some people have CAD for years without having chest pain or any other symptoms. This may make it hard to feel like you need to pay attention to the problem.

But try not to ignore the fact that you have heart disease, even if you feel fine right now. The goal is to keep feeling good for a long time. You have a better chance of doing that if you start living healthier today. What you do can make a big difference.

Dealing With Angina

Many people with CAD have no symptoms. But others may feel chest pain or pressure or have other symptoms when their hearts have to work harder. These symptoms are called angina.

Angina is a signal that your heart is not getting enough oxygen. The pain or pressure usually is mild at first and gets worse over several minutes. You may feel it in your chest, back, neck, jaw, upper belly, shoulder, or arms.

If you have had angina for a while, you may be able to predict almost exactly how much activity will cause your symptoms. You know what things cause your angina, and you know what to expect and what to do when it happens. This is called stable angina.

Watch for changes in your angina. If your angina is worse or lasts longer than usual, or if you start getting it more often, it could mean that your heart disease is getting worse. Call your doctor right away. You may need a checkup or tests, or your doctor may need to change your treatment.

What to do when you have angina

◆ Stop what you are doing. Sit down and rest.

◆ If your doctor has prescribed a medicine like nitroglycerin, take one dose.

◆ If you are not feeling better within 5 minutes, **call 911**. Stay on the phone. The emergency operator will tell you what to do next.

An Aspirin a Day?

Taking an aspirin each day may help you avoid a heart attack or stroke. If you have not discussed this with your doctor, ask about it at your next visit.

To learn more, go to the Web site on the back cover and enter **d061** in the search box.

If you take nitroglycerin

Nitroglycerin is a medicine that opens blood vessels to improve blood flow. This relieves angina and reduces how hard the heart has to work.

Your doctor will tell you when to use your nitroglycerin. You may need to take it:

◆ To relieve sudden angina.

◆ Before stressful activities that can cause angina, such as exercise or sex.

Do not take erection-producing medicines such as Cialis, Levitra, or Viagra if you are taking nitroglycerin. Taking any of them with nitroglycerin can be very dangerous. If you get chest pain and have taken one of these erection-producing medicines, tell your doctor so that you are not given nitroglycerin or a similar medicine.

Eat a Heart-Healthy Diet

Most experts agree that the best diet for your heart is high in fiber, low in cholesterol and saturated and trans fats, and low in salt.

The tips in the chart below can help you get started. (See page 305 for more about healthy eating.) Your doctor may suggest that you follow the DASH (Dietary Approaches to Stop Hypertension) diet or something similar. To learn what this diet

 is and how it can help you, go to the Web site on the back cover and enter **s309** in the search box.

Stop Smoking

Quitting smoking is one of the best things you can do if you do not want to die of heart disease. Your risk of dying from heart attack or stroke will start to go down very soon after you quit. Within several years, your risk will be no higher than someone who has never smoked.

If you have had angioplasty or bypass surgery to fix blocked arteries, those arteries will be less likely to get blocked again if you quit smoking.

Eating a Heart-Healthy Diet	
Instead of:	**Try this:**
Frying your food	Bake, broil, steam, poach, or grill your food.
Eating convenience foods (canned soups, TV dinners, frozen pizza)	Eat fresh fish, skinless chicken, fruits, and vegetables.
Using butter, shortening, or oil high in saturated and trans fats	Use products low in saturated and trans fats, such as olive oil, vegetable oil, canola oil, or chicken broth.
Using salt, soy sauce, or barbecue sauce	Use salt-free spices.
Eating all of the meat product	Trim fat from meat and skin from chicken.
Eating egg yolks	Eat egg whites or egg substitutes.

More

You will also feel better once you quit smoking. Your angina may get better. You will have more energy and breathe easier. And you may feel more hopeful about your future and have less fear of getting sick or dying suddenly from heart disease.

Smoking is bad for everyone, but it is even worse for people with coronary artery disease.

◆ It makes your blood cells more likely to form clots. This can cause a heart attack or stroke.

◆ It can cause spasms in your coronary arteries, which can reduce the blood flow to your heart.

◆ It can make your heart beat in an odd rhythm.

◆ It lowers "good" cholesterol and lets "bad" cholesterol build up in your arteries more easily.

◆ It reduces how much oxygen your blood can carry. This means your heart (and the rest of your body) may not get enough oxygen.

Quitting smoking is not easy. Many people have to try several times before they quit for good. But the point is that they do finally succeed. And with the right help, so can you.

See Quitting Smoking on page 316 to learn how to get started.

Exercise Your Heart

If you are not active right now, starting to exercise may seem hard. But it is worth it. You do not have to do a lot to make a difference.

Being more active can:

◆ Help you control your weight and blood pressure.

◆ Make your heart stronger and reduce symptoms like chest pain.

◆ Help you avoid heart attack and stroke and live longer.

◆ Reduce stress and give you more energy.

What Is Angioplasty?

Angioplasty is a way to widen a narrow or blocked coronary artery and improve blood flow to your heart without surgery. It is often used during or soon after a heart attack to help relieve chest pain. It can also help prevent a heart attack for some people with coronary artery disease.

During angioplasty, your doctor threads a tiny tube called a catheter into the blocked or narrow artery. At the end of the catheter is a tiny balloon. The doctor inflates the balloon inside the artery to open the blocked area.

The doctor may also put a stent in the artery. A stent is a small, wire-mesh tube that expands and pushes out against the walls of the artery to keep it open. Some stents also release a drug that helps keep the artery open.

Should you have angioplasty? Whether you need it depends on how badly your arteries are blocked, how much chest pain you have, and several other issues. *Go to Web* For help deciding, go to the Web site on the back cover and enter **h780** in the search box.

Walking is a great, easy way to get exercise. If your doctor says it's safe, start out with some short walks, then gradually make the walks a little bit longer.

If you don't enjoy walking, you might try swimming, biking, or water aerobics. Your doctor can help you make a plan.

 The important thing is to try to get some exercise throughout the week. Even a little bit of exercise can help if you have not been active at all. For some ideas that might work for you, go to the Web site on the back cover and enter **x762** in the search box.

You might also ask your doctor about joining a cardiac rehab program. Many people with heart disease find this type of program helpful. To learn more about whether cardiac rehab might be right for you, go to the Web site on the back cover and enter **x867** in the search box.

Be safe when you exercise

See your doctor before you start exercising. He or she may want to do a test to see how much activity your heart can handle.

If your doctor has prescribed nitroglycerin for you, be sure to have it with you whenever you exercise. Stop what you are doing right away if you have any chest pain or start to feel bad.

When to Call a Doctor

Call 911 if:

◆ You have chest pain or pressure, or a strange feeling in your chest, with other signs of a heart attack. These may include:

  ❖ Sweating.

  ❖ Shortness of breath.

  ❖ Nausea or vomiting.

  ❖ Pain, pressure, or a strange feeling in your back, neck, jaw, upper belly, or one or both shoulders or arms.

  ❖ Lightheadedness or sudden weakness.

  ❖ A fast or irregular heartbeat.

  After you call 911, the operator may tell you to chew 1 adult-strength aspirin or 2 to 4 low-dose aspirin (unless you are allergic to it). Do not try to drive yourself to the hospital.

◆ You have been diagnosed with angina, and your angina does not go away with rest or within 5 minutes of taking nitroglycerin.

◆ You faint.

Call your doctor if:

◆ You have been diagnosed with angina and it's getting worse or lasting longer than usual, or you start getting it more often.

◆ You have had any chest pain, even if it has gone away.

◆ You have any problems with your medicines.

Living Better With Depression

If you think you are depressed but you have not seen a doctor about it, see Are You Depressed? on page 156.

Depression is a medical problem, not a character flaw or weakness. Many people do not get help because they're embarrassed or they think they'll get over depression on their own.

If you are depressed, there is no reason for you or your loved ones to suffer. Treatment works very well for most people. With counseling, medicines, good self-care, and a little time, you can feel a lot better. Treatment can also help you avoid future problems with depression.

Seasonal Affective Disorder

Some people feel more depressed during the winter months when there is less sunlight. This is sometimes called seasonal affective disorder (SAD).

It may help to:

◆ Go out in the sun as often as you can. (Remember to protect your skin.)

◆ Get regular exercise, either outdoors or indoors near a sunny window.

◆ Ask your doctor about light therapy. This involves sitting or working in front of special lights for up to several hours a day.

As with other forms of depression, medicine and counseling can also help.

Counseling Can Help

The words "counseling" or "therapy" may make you think of lying on a leather couch and talking about your childhood. But the most common kind of counseling does not look for hidden feelings or memories. It deals with how you think about things and how you act each day. It helps you replace thoughts or behaviors that make you feel bad with ones that make you feel better. Over time, these changes turn into habits.

To treat depression, you may need to see a counselor regularly for several months or longer. Keep going to the appointments even if at first it seems like they aren't helping. Sometimes it takes many meetings before you start to feel better.

Choosing a counselor

Your counselor may be a psychiatrist (a medical doctor), a psychologist, or a licensed counselor. When you choose a counselor:

◆ Be sure the person has experience and training in treating depression. Also make sure that he or she has a license in your state. Some states have strict rules about who can work as a counselor.

◆ Choose someone you like and trust. For counseling to work, you have to talk honestly about your feelings. Having a counselor you feel comfortable with makes this easier. If you meet with someone and don't feel good about it, try someone else.

Antidepressant Medicines

Antidepressant medicines help many people with depression get better. They can help keep the chemicals in your brain in balance. They do not change your personality.

There are many medicines that can help, and there is no evidence that one works better than another. But they have different side effects.

What About St. John's Wort?

St. John's wort is an herbal supplement sold in health food stores and drug-stores. Europeans have used it for centuries to treat depression.

High-quality St. John's wort may help with mild or moderate depression. After talking to your doctor about it, you may want to see if it works for

you. Go to the Web site on the back cover and enter **d183** in the search box to learn more.

Do not take St. John's wort with antidepressants or any other medicines unless your doctor has told you it's safe. It can cause dangerous reactions when you use it with other medicines.

Keep in mind that herbal supplements are not regulated the way medicines are. Always tell your doctor if you're using an herbal product. You could have serious side effects.

Your doctor will consider many things when deciding which drug to give you:

◆ How did you respond to medicines used in the past?

◆ Are you taking medicine for other health problems? Your doctor will not want to give you a drug that will react badly with any other drugs you're taking.

◆ Will the drug make any other illness you have worse or harder to treat?

◆ How old are you? How is your overall health? Older adults may need lower doses.

◆ How much are the side effects likely to bother you?

You may need to take antidepressants for as long as 2 months before you feel completely well. But you may start to feel better in 2 or 3 weeks. Here are things to keep in mind:

◆ Most antidepressants take 4 to 8 weeks to work.

◆ Often the first drug the doctor prescribes will work well. If not, there are other choices. You may need to try several before you find the one that works best for you.

◆ The medicine may have side effects. Many of these are temporary and will go away as you get used to the medicine. If they continue, or if they bother you too much, talk to your doctor. You may need a different drug. To learn how to

manage side effects, go to the Web site on the back cover and enter **n429** in the search box.

◆ Make sure to tell your doctor if you take any other medicines or herbal products. Tell your doctor about any other health problems you have.

More

◆ Once you start to feel better, you will need to keep taking your medicine for 6 months or longer to help prevent a relapse. Keep taking your medicine as prescribed, even after symptoms go away.

Do not stop taking the medicine on your own unless you have chest pain, hives, trouble breathing, trouble swallowing, or swelling of your lips. Call your doctor immediately if you have any of these serious side effects.

While You Recover

Your mood will improve, but it takes time. In the meantime:

◆ Take your medicines as prescribed, and go to your counseling sessions. It may take several weeks before you notice a change.

◆ Take good care of yourself. Eat healthy meals. Get enough sleep. If you have problems sleeping, see the tips starting on page 237. Do not take sleeping pills unless your doctor has said it is okay.

◆ Stay active. Get outside and take walks. Go to a movie, concert, or ball game.

◆ Spend time with friends and family. Take part in social events or church.

◆ Do not drink alcohol or use illegal drugs. And don't take medicines that have not been prescribed for you.

◆ Break large tasks into smaller pieces that you can handle. Do what you can.

◆ If possible, put off major decisions like marriage, divorce, or a job change until you feel better. Talk over big changes with friends and loved ones who can offer other points of view.

◆ If you have another illness, like diabetes or heart disease, keep treating it.

Ask for help if you need it. And if you ever have thoughts of hurting yourself, call for help right away. You can call 911 or the national suicide hotline at 1-800-273-8255.

Depressed and Pregnant?

Some women get depressed during pregnancy. You are more likely to be depressed if you have had depression before. Your pregnancy can cause your symptoms to come back (relapse).

Managing your depression is important for your own health. It will also help you have a healthy baby. Work with your doctor to find a treatment you are comfortable with.

◆ If your depression is mild, your doctor may suggest that you try counseling first before you take medicine.

◆ If your depression is severe or counseling does not help enough, you may need medicine. You may also need medicine if you were depressed before and had a relapse when you stopped your medicine.

You may be worried about taking medicine while you're pregnant. But not treating your depression is also a risk to your baby. You may not take care of yourself as well if you're depressed. You may not bond well with your baby after birth. You may not eat or sleep well.

If you need an antidepressant, your doctor can prescribe one that's safest for you and your baby.

 To help decide if you should take antidepressants while you are pregnant, go to the Web site on the back cover and enter **p094** in the search box.

Feeling Better?

If you are feeling better, you may think it's okay to stop going to counseling or to quit taking your medicine.

Wait! Talk to your doctor before you do this. To keep depression from coming back, you may need treatment for 6 months or longer after you feel better. Some people need to take medicines for years.

 For help deciding whether medicines are still right for you, go to the Web site on the back cover and enter **k616** in the search box.

How to Prevent a Relapse

◆ Do not stop taking your medicine too early. It may help to keep taking it for another 6 to 12 months after you feel better (or longer in some cases). Some people need to take medicine for the rest of their lives to stay healthy.

◆ Do not stop taking your medicine suddenly. If you want to stop taking it, ask your doctor whether this is safe for you and how best to do it.

◆ Keep seeing your counselor after you stop the medicine. This helps some people avoid a relapse after they stop taking their medicine.

◆ Eat a healthy diet and get regular exercise. Stick to a regular sleep schedule.

◆ Avoid alcohol and illegal drugs.

◆ See your doctor right away if you have new symptoms or feel worse.

When to Call a Doctor

◆ You feel hopeless and cannot stop yourself from thinking about hurting yourself or someone else. **Call 911 or the national suicide hotline at 1-800-273-8255.**

◆ You hear voices.

◆ You think you are depressed, and you have not talked to your doctor about it.

◆ Your depression gets worse even with treatment.

◆ You have any problems with your medicine.

◆ You are taking antidepressants and think that you're pregnant.

Living Better With Diabetes

If you have diabetes, your body may not make enough of a hormone called **insulin** or may not use insulin properly. Insulin helps your body use sugar from your food as energy or store it for later use. When this doesn't happen, too much sugar stays in your blood.

Over time, high blood sugar can lead to serious problems.

◆ It can harm your eyes, nerves, and kidneys.

◆ It can damage your blood vessels, leading to heart disease and stroke.

◆ It can reduce blood flow to parts of your body, especially your feet. This can cause pain when you walk and slow healing.

How can you prevent these problems? The most important thing is to keep your blood sugar under control with these steps:

◆ Take your insulin or other medicine.

◆ Check your blood sugar.

◆ Eat healthy, balanced meals and snacks.

◆ Exercise throughout the week.

◆ See your doctor for checkups and tests on a regular schedule.

◆ If you have high blood pressure or high cholesterol, take medicines to control the problem.

Living with diabetes day after day can be a struggle. Watching what you eat, checking your blood sugar, taking your medicine on time—there will be times when you just can't do it all. Don't be too hard on yourself. Just try to get back on track.

And if you're already doing what you need to, keep it up!

Medicines for Diabetes

Some people with type 2 diabetes need medicine to help their bodies make more insulin or use insulin properly. Pills for type 2 diabetes can also slow down how the body digests sugar. This can help keep your blood sugar in a target range.

You may need to take one or more pills more than once a day. Some people need medicine for only a short time. Some have to take it for the rest of their lives. What you need will depend on how well your blood sugar stays in a target range.

People with type 1 diabetes have to take insulin to control their blood sugar. If you have type 2 diabetes, you may be able to avoid or delay the need for insulin with careful eating, regular exercise, and proper use of other diabetes medicines. Many people with type 2 diabetes do end up needing to take insulin at some point.

Cost tips for medicines

Your diabetes medicine helps keep you healthy and avoid more serious, costly problems. While the costs of the medicine can add up, there may be ways to get your diabetes medicine for less.

You can buy most diabetes medicines either by their brand names or as generic drugs. (For example, many people with diabetes take the drug metformin. You may know it by its brand name, Glucophage.) There can be a big cost difference between brand names and generics. If you are taking a brand-name drug, you might ask your doctor whether the generic one would work just as well for you.

See page 5 for other suggestions on how to save money on your medicines—like buying in bulk and using online drugstores.

What About Carbohydrate and Sugar?

When you have diabetes, you have to be careful about how much carbohydrate you eat at one time. If you eat too much at once, your blood sugar will quickly rise.

Carbohydrate is an important nutrient you get from food. It is a great source of energy for your body and helps your brain and nervous system work at their best.

It comes in two forms:

◆ Starch (complex carbohydrate). Starch is in foods such as breads, cereals, grains, pasta, rice, flour, beans, and vegetables.

◆ Sugar (simple carbohydrate). Sugar is in foods such as fruits, juices, milk, honey, desserts, and candy.

All forms of carbohydrate raise your blood sugar, depending on how much carbohydrate is in the food.

The goal is to keep your blood sugar steady and avoid high blood sugar after meals. You can help by spreading your carbohydrate throughout the day, rather than eating a lot at once. This will also keep you from getting too hungry. See Meal Planning: What Does Your Plate Look Like? on page 286 to learn more about this.

Unlike what you may have heard, you can eat foods that have sugar when you have diabetes. But if foods that are high in sugar make up a large part of your diet, you are probably not eating enough of other, healthier foods. And your blood sugar levels may be too unsteady.

Five Things to Do Today

1. Talk to your doctor about whether you should take low-dose aspirin. An aspirin a day may help you avoid a heart attack or stroke.

2. Order a medical alert bracelet or necklace online or at your local drugstore. If you have a health emergency and cannot speak, this ID will let medical staff know you have diabetes. This is even more important if you take insulin or often have problems with low blood sugar.

3. Check your feet every day for small cuts, sores, or toenail problems. Small problems can become big ones if you do not notice and take care of them. To learn how to take great care of your feet, go to the Web site on the back cover and enter **y813** in the search box.

4. Take a walk. Regular exercise can help you control your blood sugar and reduce your need for medicine. Make sure you wear sturdy shoes.

5. Call your local hospital and ask if it has a support group or education program for people with diabetes. Or visit the Web site of the American Diabetes Association, www.diabetes.org. It has recipes, exercise tips, and all kinds of information that can help you.

More

Meal Planning: What Does Your Plate Look Like?

Eating right helps keep your blood sugar in a target range. For some people, healthy eating and regular exercise are enough to keep their diabetes under control without medicines. If you take medicine, eating right can help the medicine work better.

Meal planning for diabetes includes eating certain amounts and kinds of foods at regular meals and snacks. For example, you may have heard about the need to count your carbohydrate grams.

It may seem overwhelming to have to watch what you eat. But there's an easy way to get started: the **plate format**. The plate format is a great way to learn about meal planning and get used to measuring how much you eat.

Using a plate format lets you picture what a meal should look like and how much space each food should take up on your plate. This can help you eat balanced meals. It also can stop you from eating too much carbohydrate at once.

8 oz milk (dairy, outside the plate)

½ cup peaches (fruit, outside the plate)

Carrots, asparagus, mushrooms (veggies, one-half plate)

Salmon (protein, one-fourth plate)

Brown rice (grain, one-fourth plate)

Sample plate for dinner

A typical healthy plate for lunch or dinner will have:

◆ Bread, starchy foods, or grain on one-fourth of the plate.

◆ Meat or another form of protein (like beans or an egg) on one-fourth of the plate.

◆ Vegetables on half the plate.

◆ 1 small piece of fruit outside the plate.

◆ 1 cup of milk or yogurt or ½ cup of no-sugar-added pudding or ice cream outside the plate.

Post a sample plate format on your refrigerator until you get used to what a healthy plate looks like. Once you can picture your plate, you can use the method anywhere, even when you eat out.

To learn how to use the plate format for all your meals and snacks, go to the Web site on the back cover and enter **f643** in the search box. And when you are ready to learn more about meal planning, talk with a dietitian or diabetes educator about other methods.

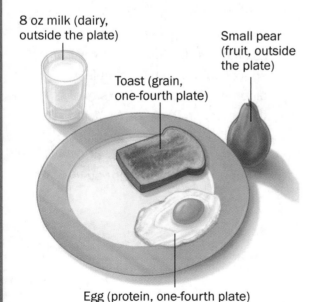

8 oz milk (dairy, outside the plate)

Small pear (fruit, outside the plate)

Toast (grain, one-fourth plate)

Egg (protein, one-fourth plate)

Sample plate for breakfast

If You Have Prediabetes

Prediabetes means that you are at risk for type 2 diabetes. Think of it as a wake-up call. Most people who get type 2 diabetes have prediabetes first.

If you have prediabetes, you may be able to avoid or delay type 2 diabetes (and the problems it can cause) by making some changes in your lifestyle.

◆ Eat a balanced, healthy diet. Try to eat an even amount of carbohydrate all through the day. This can help you avoid sudden peaks in blood sugar.

◆ Get a total of at least 2½ hours of exercise each week. For example, 30 minutes of exercise on most days of the week can help you reach this goal. Exercise helps control your blood sugar. It also helps you control your weight. Walking is a good choice for many people. You also may want to try swimming, cycling, or other activities. See page 311.

◆ Try to stay at a healthy weight. If you need to lose weight, keep in mind that even a small loss of 5 to 10 pounds can help. See page 300.

◆ If you smoke, quit. Smoking can make prediabetes worse. If you need help quitting, see page 316.

Check Your Blood Sugar

You may not like having to check your blood sugar and keep track of the results over time. But it can really help you keep your diabetes under control.

◆ Knowing how your blood sugar rises or falls in response to certain foods, exercise, and other things can help you reduce symptoms and prevent blood sugar emergencies.

◆ Having a record of your blood sugar over time can help you and your doctor know how well your treatment is working and whether you need to make any changes.

Simply put, you have a better chance of keeping your blood sugar in a target range if you know what it is from day to day. Controlling your blood sugar will help you feel better and will slow down the long-term damage to your eyes, kidneys, and heart that can result when your blood sugar is not controlled.

 Many people are able to do a good job of tracking their blood sugar once they get in the habit. It helps to:

◆ Know how and when to check your blood sugar.

◆ Have the right supplies and know how to use them.

◆ Have an easy way to keep track of your results.

For help setting up a routine that works for you, go to the Web site on the back cover and enter **p039** in the search box.

Safe Exercise

Exercise helps control your blood sugar. It also helps you stay at a healthy weight, reduce "bad" cholesterol, raise "good" cholesterol, and lower high blood pressure. These benefits help prevent heart disease, the main cause of death in people who have diabetes.

More

If Your Child Has Diabetes

If your child has diabetes, he or she needs your help to feel better and to avoid emergencies and long-term problems.

Healthy eating and safe exercise are vital to controlling your child's blood sugar. Some kids also need insulin or other diabetes medicines. There are lots of ways you can help them control their blood sugar:

◆ Make a plan for giving medicines on time and in the right amounts every day. Your doctor can help with this.

◆ Offer healthy choices for meals and snacks. A dietitian can help you design a meal plan that fits your child's needs. If your child eats the school lunch, find out what kinds of foods are offered.

◆ Cut down on junk food, especially soda. Soda has lots of sugar and calories and no health benefits.

◆ Take walks or bike rides with your child. Help your child find ways to be more active. (Check with your doctor if you're not sure whether an activity is safe for your child.)

◆ Set and enforce time limits on TV and video and computer games.

◆ Make sure your child's school knows he or she has diabetes. Meet with your child's teachers (including the gym teacher) to talk about what happens when your child's blood sugar drops. Give the school nurse special instructions for treating high or low blood sugar.

◆ Be a good role model. Your child will have the most success if the whole family chooses the same healthy foods and exercise habits.

◆ Make sure that your child always wears or carries ID showing that he or she has diabetes.

You will also need to help check and keep track of your child's blood sugar. Many older children and teens can do this on their own, but they still need support.

Talk to your doctor about what your child's blood sugar should be. And ask how to spot signs that your child's blood sugar is too low or too high before it becomes an emergency.

Try to get a total of at least 2½ hours of exercise each week. For example, 30 minutes of exercise on most days of the week can help you reach this goal. You may need to slowly work up to this if you are not used to being active. Even small amounts of exercise can help.

Walking, running, bike riding, and swimming are great for most people with diabetes. But some activities may not be safe. For instance, if you have diabetic eye disease (retinopathy), it may not be safe to lift weights. If you have nerve disease (neuropathy), running may cause foot problems.

Before you start a new exercise program, check with your doctor to find out what activities are best for you.

Here are some other safety tips:

◆ Check your blood sugar before you exercise, and be careful about what you eat. This is especially true if you take insulin or other medicines for diabetes.

   ❖ Do not exercise when your blood sugar is too low (less than 100 mg/dL, or the level your doctor told you). Some people need a snack before they exercise.

   ❖ Be careful when you exercise if your blood sugar is over 250 mg/dL. High blood sugar can make you dehydrated, causing your blood sugar levels to go even higher.

◆ Try to exercise at about the same time each day to keep your blood sugar steady. If you want to exercise more, slowly increase how hard or long you exercise.

◆ Have someone with you when you exercise, or exercise at a gym. You may need help if your blood sugar drops too low.

◆ Keep some quick-sugar food with you. You may get symptoms of low blood sugar during exercise or up to 24 hours later.

◆ Pay attention to your body. If you are used to exercise and notice that you cannot do as much as usual, talk to your doctor.

Schedule for Tests and Exams

Test	Why you need it	How often to get it
Hemoglobin A1c blood test Goal: below 7 percent (your doctor will set a goal for you)	Checks average blood sugar over past 2 to 3 months; best way to see how well treatment and self-care are working	Every 3 to 6 months
Blood pressure test Goal: less than 130/80 (your doctor will set a goal for you)	Need to monitor blood pressure; high blood pressure increases risk of heart disease, stroke, and damage to the eyes and kidneys	Every 3 to 6 months
Sensory foot exam	Reduced feeling in feet can be sign of nerve damage (neuropathy)	At least every year
Eye exam by an ophthalmologist or optometrist	Diabetes can cause glaucoma and can damage vision (retinopathy); does not cause symptoms until severe	Every year (may be less or more often depending on the results)
Fasting cholesterol test Goal: LDL below 100	Diabetes puts you at risk for high cholesterol and heart disease	Every year (more often if you take medicine for high cholesterol)
Urine test for protein	Protein in urine may be the only sign of early kidney damage (nephropathy)	Every year (may be more often depending on the results)
Dental exam and cleaning	Diabetes increases risk of gum problems and infection	Every 6 months

More ▶

Tests That Can Help You

Seeing your doctor and having certain tests on a regular schedule can help you watch for and avoid many of the problems caused by diabetes. Diabetes can damage many different parts of your body, but you may not have symptoms of the damage until it's too late to do much about it. Tests give you and your doctor a chance to find problems early, when they are easier to treat.

The table on page 289 lists some of the tests a typical person with diabetes may need. Ask your doctor which test schedule is best for you.

When to Call a Doctor

Call 911 if:

◆ Your blood sugar is low, and you are sleepy or confused.

◆ Your blood sugar is very high, you are becoming less alert, and your breathing is fast and deep.

◆ You have chest pain or pressure, especially if it occurs with other signs of a heart attack. See page 38.

Call your doctor if:

◆ You have problems with your blood sugar being too high or too low.

◆ You have burning pain, tingling, numbness, or swelling in your feet or hands.

◆ You have vision changes or pain in your eyes.

◆ A wound looks infected or will not heal.

◆ You often have a lot of bloating, belching, constipation, nausea and vomiting, or belly pain after you eat.

◆ You have a hard time knowing when your blood sugar is low.

Living Better With Heart Failure

When you have heart failure, your heart does not pump as much blood as your body needs. Failure does not mean your heart has stopped pumping. It means your heart is not pumping as well as it should.

Your body has an amazing ability to make up for heart failure. It may do such a good job at first that you may not feel like you have a disease.

But at some point, your body will not be able to keep up. Then fluid will slowly build up in your body and cause symptoms like weakness, shortness of breath, and swelling in your ankles, feet, and legs. This fluid buildup is called **congestion**.

What You Can Do

Heart failure usually gets worse over time. But there are many steps you can take to feel better and stay healthy longer. These are the most important:

- Take your medicines as prescribed. This gives them the best chance of helping you. See Take Your Medicines on this page.

- Limit salt (sodium). This helps keep fluid from building up and makes it easier for your heart to pump. See page 292.

- Watch for signs that your heart failure is getting worse so that your doctor can help you. Weighing yourself every day is one of the best ways to do this. Sudden weight gain may be a sign that your body is holding on to too much fluid. See page 292.

- Try to exercise throughout the week. Exercise makes your heart stronger and can help you avoid symptoms. See page 293.

- Find out what your triggers are, and learn to avoid them. Triggers are things that make your heart failure worse, often suddenly. A trigger may be eating too much salt, missing a dose of your medicine, or exercising too hard.

There are other things you can do to help too, like eating right, not smoking, not drinking much alcohol, controlling your blood pressure, and staying at a healthy weight. These things make it easier for your heart to keep pumping well. They will also reduce your risk for heart attack and stroke.

Take Your Medicines

You will probably take several medicines for heart failure. You may also need medicine to treat the problem that caused your heart failure, such as high blood pressure, heart disease, or a heart attack.

- Take your medicines exactly as your doctor tells you to. If you can't do this, or if you think you need to stop or change your medicine, talk to your doctor about it.

- If you have any problems with the medicines, tell your doctor. Ask your doctor what side effects you may have and what problems to watch for.

- See your doctor regularly so that he or she can check whether your medicine is working or needs to be changed.

- Always ask your doctor before you take any new medicines, including those you can buy without a prescription. Some medicines can make heart failure worse.

More

291

To get the best results from your medicines, be sure to take them properly. This can be tricky when you have to take more than one. For tips that can help, go to the Web site on the back cover and enter **m817** in the search box.

Cost tips for medicines

You will need medicine for the rest of your life to control your heart failure. This can get very expensive. But there may be ways you can reduce the cost—using generic instead of brand-name drugs and shopping for the best prices, for example. For help controlling costs, see page 5.

Cut the Salt

Eating less salt (sodium) can help you feel better and stay out of the hospital. Salt makes your body retain water, makes your legs swell, and makes it harder for your heart to pump.

Your doctor may want you to eat less than 2,000 mg (2 g) of sodium each day. That's less than 1 teaspoon. You can stay under this number by limiting the salt you eat at home and by watching for "hidden" sodium when you eat out or shop for food.

Write down what you eat and how much salt it has. That way you will know when you are close to (or over) your limit.

Five ways to reduce salt

◆ Read labels on food before you buy it. Buy foods labeled "unsalted" (no salt used to process), "sodium-free" (less than 5 mg per serving), or "low-sodium" (less than 140 mg per serving).

◆ Eat lots of fresh or frozen fruits and vegetables. They have very little salt, and they're good for you.

◆ If you use canned vegetables or beans, rinse them before you cook with them. They are very high in sodium unless you buy low-sodium or sodium-free kinds.

◆ Flavor your food with garlic, lemon juice, onion, vinegar, healthy oils (olive, walnut), herbs, and spices instead of salt. Do not use soy sauce, steak sauce, onion salt, garlic salt, mustard, or ketchup on your food. They all have a lot of salt.

◆ Eat fewer processed foods. These include anything that's not fresh, such as canned foods, packaged lunch meats and hot dogs, bottled sauces, boxed frozen meals, chips and pretzels, and pizza. Eat less often at restaurants, especially fast-food ones.

Eating less salt can be hard, but it has a big reward: feeling better and staying out of the hospital. The tips above can help you get started. If you are ready for even more ideas—or want an easy way to keep track of what you eat—go to the Web site on the back cover and enter **b532** in the search box.

Check Your Weight Every Day

Get in the habit of weighing yourself every day and writing down your weight. Sudden weight gain may mean that fluid is building up in your body and your heart failure is getting worse.

◆ Weigh yourself at the same time each day, using the same scale on a hard, flat surface. The best time is in the morning after you go to the bathroom and before you eat or drink anything.

◆ Wear the same thing each time you weigh yourself, or always wear nothing. Do not wear shoes.

◆ Keep a calendar by the scale. Write your weight on it each day, and take it with you when you see your doctor.

◆ Keep notes on how you feel each day. Is your shortness of breath worse? Are your feet and ankles swollen? Do your legs seem puffy?

Call your doctor if you gain 3 pounds or more over 2 to 3 days. (Or your doctor may tell you how much weight gain to watch for.) Also tell your doctor if you are gaining weight slowly.

Exercise Your Heart

If you are not active right now, starting to exercise may seem hard. But it's worth it. Regular exercise:

◆ Makes your heart stronger.

◆ Makes it easier to breathe.

◆ Helps you feel better and have more energy.

◆ Helps control your weight and blood pressure.

See your doctor before you start exercising. He or she may want to do a test to see how much activity your heart can handle so you don't push too hard.

Walking is a great way to get exercise. If your doctor says it's safe, start out with some short walks, then gradually make the walks a little bit longer. Swimming, cycling, or water aerobics might be other good choices. Your doctor can help you make a plan.

The important thing is to exercise throughout the week and not to overdo it. There are many ways you can exercise safely with heart failure. For some ideas that might work for you, go to the Web site on the back cover and enter **r291** in the search box.

What about cardiac rehab?

You might ask your doctor about joining a cardiac rehab program. In this type of program, a team of people, such as a doctor, a nurse specialist, a dietitian, and a physical therapist, works with you to help you learn how to stay healthier and feel better.

Many people with heart failure find cardiac rehab helpful. For help deciding whether this might be a good idea for you, go to the Web site on the back cover and enter **x867** in the search box.

If You Have to Limit Fluids

Your doctor may give you pills called diuretics to help get fluid out of your body. For many people, taking this medicine and reducing salt is enough.

If you have advanced heart failure, you may also need to limit how much fluid you drink. This can reduce symptoms and help you stay out of the hospital.

Your doctor will tell you how much fluid you can have each day. Usually, it will range from 4 to 8 cups (32 to 64 fl oz), which is about 1 to 2 liters. You will need to keep track of your fluids so you do not take in more than your body can handle.

More

293

◆ Find a method that works for you. You might simply write down how much you drink every time you do. Some people keep a container (like a pitcher or large plastic bottle) filled with the amount of fluid they can have for the day. If they drink from a source other than the container, then they pour out that amount. Once the container is empty, they stop drinking.

◆ Measure how much fluid your regular drinking glasses hold. Once you know this, you will not have to measure every time.

◆ Count any food that will melt or that has a lot of liquid as part of your fluid for the day. That means you need to measure and count ice cream, gelatin, ice, juicy fruits, and soup.

◆ If you feel thirsty, try chewing gum or sucking on hard candy, breath mints, or frozen grapes or berries. If your lips feel dry, use lip balm.

When to Call a Doctor

Call 911 if:

◆ You have chest pain or pressure, or a strange feeling in your chest that has not gone away with rest or within 5 minutes after you have taken one nitroglycerin, especially if these symptoms occur with shortness of breath, sweating, and nausea.

◆ You have symptoms of a stroke (see page 53). These may include:

   ❖ Sudden tingling, numbness, or weakness on one side of your body.

   ❖ Sudden, severe headache.

   ❖ Sudden changes in vision or speech.

   ❖ Stumbling or clumsiness.

◆ You have severe trouble breathing.

◆ You cough up foamy, pink mucus.

◆ Your heart suddenly starts to beat very fast or unevenly, and you feel dizzy, nauseated, or like you are going to faint.

Call your doctor if you have signs that your heart failure is getting worse. For example:

◆ You gain 3 pounds or more over 2 to 3 days. (Or your doctor may tell you how much weight gain to watch for.)

◆ You have new or worse swelling in your feet, ankles, or legs.

◆ Your breathing gets worse. Activities that did not make you short of breath before are now hard for you.

◆ Your breathing when you lie down is worse than usual, or you wake up at night needing to catch your breath.

Planning for the Future

Even if you are doing well now, it's a good idea to prepare for a time when your health might get worse. It can be hard to think and talk about these issues. But planning for the future while you are still active and able to communicate can:

◆ Bring you peace of mind.

◆ Help make sure your wishes are followed later.

◆ Save your loved ones the stress of making hard decisions for you.

Advance Directives

The best way to make sure your wishes are followed is to put them in writing. A written plan for your health care is called an advance care plan or **advance directive**. It is used only if you become so sick that you can't make choices for yourself.

There are two main types of advance directives.

◆ A **living will** tells what treatment you want at the end of your life. For example, it tells when you would or would not want to be on a breathing machine or be fed through a tube.

◆ A **durable power of attorney** lets you choose someone now who can make health care choices for you if a time comes when you can't make them yourself. This person is called your health care agent or health care proxy.

Do not assume that your doctor and family will know what you want if you don't have a written plan. Without one, choices about your care may be made by your family, who may not make the same choices you would. Or if you don't have family, a doctor who doesn't know you, or the courts, may have to decide. In some states, hospital staff must keep you alive as long as possible if they don't know your wishes. This may or may not be what you want.

How to Write an Advance Directive

1. Get living will and durable power of attorney forms for your state. You can usually get them from a doctor's office, hospital, law office, or senior center. You also can find them online at www.caringinfo.org.

2. Choose someone to be your health care agent, the person you want to speak for you if you can't speak for yourself.

3. Fill out the forms. If you don't understand them, ask a doctor, nurse, lawyer, or family member to help. Get them notarized or witnessed if your state requires it (many states don't).

4. Make sure your doctor, your family, and your health care agent have copies.

 For help writing an advance directive, go to the Web site on the back cover and enter **q652** in the search box.

Deciding About Life Support Treatment

When you create an advance directive, you can answer questions like:

◆ Do you want CPR if your heart stops?

◆ Do you want to be given liquids or food through a vein (IV) or stomach tube if you can no longer eat or drink?

More ▶

- Do you want to have a tube in your windpipe and use a breathing machine (ventilator) if you cannot breathe on your own?

- Do you want kidney dialysis if your kidneys stop working?

Think about what you would want, depending on things like how sick or hurt you were, how good your chances for recovery were, and what your life would be like if you chose treatment to keep you alive.

If you have an illness that can't be cured, a time may come when you decide not to have treatment that might keep you alive. This can be a hard decision. But if you are very ill, it may be the right choice for you and your family. Sometimes, using treatment to keep a dying person alive can cause unnecessary suffering.

 For many people, these are hard choices. If you want help thinking through them, go to the Web site on the back cover and enter **y609** in the search box.

Don't wait for your doctor to bring up the subject of an advance directive. Even if you are healthy right now, talk with your doctor about the kinds of treatment you would want or would not want. Try to get a clear idea of your wishes. And involve your family members so they know what you want.

Estate Planning

Along with planning for future health decisions, it's a good idea to get your business and personal affairs in order.

- Write or update your will. If you don't have a will, your state's laws may decide what happens to your money and property (your "estate") when you die. Consider naming a person to oversee your estate after your death. This person is called an executor.

- Appoint someone to make financial decisions for you in case a time comes when you can't make them for yourself.

- If you have young children (or someone else you take care of), choose someone to take care of them. This person is called a guardian.

- Make sure your will and other records (life insurance policies, pension and retirement account records, real estate deeds, stocks) are in a safe place. Close family members, the executor of your estate, and your lawyer should know how to access these records in case something happens to you.

A lawyer can advise you on how best to organize your estate so your family can handle your affairs after your death. A financial planner or social worker can also help. These resources may be available in your community or through a local hospital or hospice program.

If Your Health Gets Worse

Palliative Care

Palliative care is a kind of care for people who have illnesses that don't go away and often get worse over time. It is different than care to cure your illness. It focuses on improving your quality of life—not just your body, but also your mind and spirit.

Palliative care is not just for people who are near death. You can have palliative care at the same time that you are getting treatment for your health problem.

Palliative care can help reduce pain or treatment side effects. The doctors, nurses, and others on a palliative care team can help you and your loved ones talk more openly about your feelings and make future plans. They can also make sure the rest of your health care team and your family and friends understand your goals.

Many people like palliative care because it can focus on what's most important to them. If you think it could help you, talk to your doctor.

Hospice Care

Hospice provides medical care, emotional help, and spiritual support as you near the end of your life. It can also help your family and friends care for you and deal with their grief.

You can get hospice care when your doctor says that you have a limited time left to live. Medicare pays for hospice care when a person has 6 months or less to live if the disease runs its natural course. (Sometimes people getting hospice care wind up living much longer than 6 months.)

You may want to choose hospice care if:

◆ You are ready to stop treatment that tries to cure the disease or prolong your life, and you only want to receive care that makes you comfortable.

◆ You want to choose where to spend the time you have left (such as in your home).

◆ You want family and friends to be involved in your care.

The goals of hospice are to keep you comfortable and help you get the most out of life in the time you have left.

◆ Hospice focuses on relieving pain and other symptoms. It does not try to cure your illness.

◆ It does not speed up or lengthen dying.

◆ Hospice includes counseling and support for you and your loved ones; respite care, which gives some time off to those who take care of you; and help with things like meals and errands.

◆ Hospice programs can help in your own home or in a hospice center. Some hospices also go to nursing homes or hospitals.

Don't wait for your doctor or family to bring up your end-of-life care. Sometimes it's hard for a doctor to admit that a patient is nearing the final stages of an illness. And it can be hard for you and your family to accept.

For help working through your decisions about end-of-life care, go to the Web site on the back cover and enter **w249** in the search box.

Staying Healthy

Reaching a Healthy Weight

A healthy weight is a weight at which you feel good about yourself and have energy for work and play. It's also one that does not put you at risk for weight-related problems like heart disease, diabetes, stroke, arthritis, and cancer.

Many people are not at a healthy weight but want to get there. Does this describe you? If it does, there are things you can do today to move toward your goal.

Here are the big ideas to keep in mind as you get started:

◆ Focus on health first.

◆ Choose healthier foods.

◆ Be careful about how much you eat.

◆ Be more active.

◆ Decide not to gain any more weight.

◆ When you're ready, try to lose weight.

Focus on Health First

Eating healthier and being more active will probably help you lose weight. Even if you don't lose much weight, these changes can help you feel better, have more energy, and prevent disease.

Focus on these healthy changes rather than weight loss. Losing weight is very hard for most people. But you can take steps to start living healthier—and succeed—right now.

Eat Healthier Foods

The kinds of foods you eat have a big impact on both your weight and your health. Reaching and staying at a healthy weight is not about going on a diet. It's about making healthier food choices every day and changing your diet for good.

Pages 305 to 310 have information that can help you make healthier food choices at home and when you eat out. In general, fruits and vegetables, whole grains, lean protein (lean meats, fish, beans), and low-fat dairy foods should be most of what you eat. Planning your meals ahead of time can help you choose healthier foods from day to day.

But there's also room for a few sugary and high-fat foods in most people's diets. Most foods can be part of a healthy diet as long as you don't eat too much of them.

Watch How Much You Eat

Many people eat more than their bodies need. Part of controlling your weight means learning how much food you really need from day to day and not eating more than that. Even with healthy foods, eating too much can lead to weight gain.

◆ Eat meals at regular times so that you do not get too hungry between meals.

◆ Tune into how hungry or how full you are.

◆ Pay attention to how much food is on your plate.

◆ Read food labels to learn what a serving size is.

◆ Don't go back for seconds.

◆ If you eat out a lot, know that most restaurants serve much bigger portions than most people need.

With time, you can get used to knowing how hungry or full you are.

Start With Small Changes in Your Diet

Changing your diet is a big step. But you can break it into lots of small ones like these.

◆ Eat a healthy breakfast every day. Try whole-grain cereal with milk and fruit, or whole wheat toast with an egg and a small glass of juice or piece of fruit.

◆ Use a smaller dinner plate.

◆ Avoid buffets. If you go to a buffet, make one trip only. Forget about "getting your money's worth."

◆ Make a healthy lunch instead of eating out.

◆ Save money and calories when you eat out. Split an entrée with someone, or ask for half of it in a to-go box. Order a lunch portion instead of a dinner one.

◆ Bring a healthy snack to work: fruit, carrot or celery sticks with low-fat dip, or whole-grain crackers with string cheese. A good snack may keep you from overeating later.

◆ Drink water or nonfat milk with dinner instead of soda.

With time, these small changes may become routine. Look at every step you take as a success.

Be More Active

When people think of losing weight, they most often think of food or diets. But a big part of weight control is being active. When you change what you eat *and* you are more active, you increase your chances for success.

Exercise or just being active helps in three ways:

1. It burns calories. This makes it easier to lose weight and keep it off. To see how many calories you can burn when you exercise or are active, go to the Web site on the back cover and enter **q448** in the search box.

2. It reduces your risk for health problems like heart disease, high blood pressure, stroke, and diabetes.

3. It gives you more energy, makes you stronger, and lets you do more with less effort. For most people, the more active they are, the better they feel.

Pages 311 to 315 are all about how to be more active. For those who can't picture themselves "working out," there are tips on how to be more active that don't involve traditional exercise. You'll also find ideas for how to work around some of the things that may keep you from being active: having a busy schedule, feeling too out of shape, or not knowing how to get started.

Just being a little more active can make a difference. You can do it. Lots of people have.

Avoid Weight Gain

You may not be ready to try to lose weight. But if you are like many people, you can take a great step toward better health by making sure your weight stays right where it is.

Unlike losing weight, most people can gain weight without thinking much about it.

◆ They often do it so slowly that they don't even notice.

More ▶

◆ Most people tend to put on weight as they get older unless they are very careful. And as their weight creeps up, so does their risk for health problems.

How can you avoid this? Start by weighing yourself today. Use that as your weight limit, and then weigh yourself once a week to make sure you stay within a few pounds of that number.

If you start to put on weight, cut back on calories a bit or be a little more active so you can get back under your weight limit.

(Do not weigh yourself every day. Weight can go up and down a little from day to day without meaning that you are gaining or losing weight.)

Try to Lose Weight

Weight loss seems like it should be simple. Burn more calories than you eat, and you will lose weight. But for most people, it's not simple at all.

There is some good news, though:

◆ You don't have to reach an "ideal" weight to be healthier.

◆ Losing as little as 5 to 10 percent of your weight can make a difference. For someone who weighs 200 pounds, that's only 10 to 20 pounds.

You may want and need to lose more than that. But for most people, setting small goals and building on small successes is easier than trying to reach one big goal. Feel good about all your efforts, big and small, to take better care of yourself.

Which Diet Is Best?

By themselves, formal "diets" are not usually enough to lose weight and keep it off over the long run. The key is to make healthy food choices, not eat more than your body needs, and get regular exercise. If you follow this approach most of the time, you will have the best chance of reaching a healthy weight and staying there.

Formal diets may help some people get started. If you think this might work for you, be sure to choose a sensible, healthy one. Look for diets that:

◆ Rely on normal, everyday foods. If you have to eat special foods while you're on the diet, it may be hard to keep weight off once you go back to "regular" food.

◆ Do not cut out entire food groups. Most foods can be—and should be—part of a healthy eating plan, even when you are trying to lose weight.

◆ Work on changing your eating habits for good.

◆ Focus on slow, steady weight loss. Fast, extreme weight loss is not good for your body. And most people can't keep the weight off when they lose it that way.

 To make sure you are on a safe path to weight loss, go to the Web site on the back cover and enter **a895** in the search box.

Plan to Succeed

1. Think about what stops you, and look for solutions. Do you feel too busy to exercise or cook healthier meals? Are you afraid you are too out of shape and will feel foolish or hurt yourself? Do you not have the support you need? There are ways to get around all of these barriers.

2. Start small. For most people, it's easier to tackle a series of small changes than one or two big changes. Small successes add up. And if you don't succeed with a small change, it will be only a small setback—one that's easy to get past so you can try again.

3. Be specific. Simply planning to work out more and eat better is too general and too hard to follow. Instead, set specific goals you can measure (and reach). At the end of the day or the week or the month, you should be able to say "Yes, I met my goal" or "No, I did not meet my goal." For example:

- Make a plan to walk 2 days a week for 20 minutes each time.

- Replace your lunchtime soda with water or a low-calorie drink every day.

- Twice a week, bring a healthy lunch to work instead of eating out.

- Eat a piece of fruit in place of your regular dessert 3 nights each week.

Set goals like these that are right for you. When you have met them, set new ones.

4. Track your progress. It may help to write down what you eat and when and how long you exercise, at least in the beginning. This helps you do two things: feel good when you reach a goal, and know where you went wrong when you don't. Be sure to reward yourself when you succeed—perhaps with new clothes or new exercise gear.

5. Make new habits part of your daily life. Schedule exercise time on your calendar. Have your family eat the same healthy foods you do. It will be easier to make exercise and healthy eating a habit when you think of them as part of a normal day rather than as extras.

Controlling your weight takes daily effort. Some days you just won't feel like exercising. Some days you'll want a cheeseburger, not lean turkey on whole wheat. That's okay. Just don't let those days add up.

Why Weight Isn't the Only Thing That Matters

Weight is only one measure of your health.

- You can be a little overweight and still be healthy if you eat right and are active.

- If you do not eat right or exercise, you may not be healthy no matter what you weigh.

Healthy bodies come in lots of shapes and sizes. Everyone can get healthier by eating better and being more active. Most of us will never look like fashion models or world-class athletes. But when you treat your body well—feed it healthy food and move it in the ways it's built to move—you can feel good about it.

More

Are You at a Healthy Weight?

There are two measurements that can tell you whether your weight is healthy. Neither is perfect, but they can gauge whether your weight is putting you at risk for disease. They are:

◆ Your BMI (body mass index).

◆ Your waist size (circumference).

BMI

BMI is a measure of your weight compared to your height. Your risk of weight-related disease may be higher if you are above or below a healthy BMI range. For adults, the normal range is from 18.5 to 24.9.

Use the chart on this page to find your height and weight and find your BMI.

BMI is not always an accurate sign of your health risk. For example, athletes with a lot of muscle may have a high BMI but still be at a very healthy weight. A frail person with little muscle may have a low BMI but still have too much body fat.

But for the average person, BMI is a good guide, especially when you look at it with waist size.

	Underweight	Normal weight	Overweight	Obese
	A BMI below 18.5 is considered underweight.	A BMI from 18.5 to 24.9 is a normal weight.	A BMI from 25 to 29.9 is overweight.	A BMI of 30 and above is obese.

Waist Size: Apple or Pear?

Where you store fat in your body makes a difference.

◆ Some people store most of their fat around their hips; these folks are sometimes called "pear-shaped."

◆ Others store their fat around their belly, so they are "apple-shaped."

Of these two shapes, "apples" are more likely to have weight-related diseases.

One way to find out whether your body fat is putting you at risk is to measure the size of your waist. Place a tape measure around your body at the top of your hipbone. This is usually at the level of your belly button.

You have a higher risk of disease if you are:

◆ A man with a waist larger than 40 inches.

◆ A woman with a waist larger than 35 inches.

How to Use These Results

◆ If your BMI is from 18.5 to 24.9 and your waist size is lower than the cutoff (40 inches for men, 35 inches for women), you are probably at a healthy weight. Eat right and exercise so that your weight stays in a healthy range.

◆ If your BMI is over 25, or if your waist size is above the cutoff, you may need to lose some weight. Even a small weight loss can help.

Also talk to your doctor about any other risk factors for disease, such as smoking, high blood pressure, and high cholesterol. If you have these in addition to being overweight, you are at higher risk.

Eating Healthier

Eating healthy means eating a variety of foods from the basic food groups in reasonable amounts. It's not about "going on a diet." Food is one of life's great pleasures. All foods can be part of a healthy eating plan when eaten in sensible amounts.

There are lots of ways to eat healthier. Start with a few of the basics:

◆ Eat more fruits and vegetables.

◆ Learn which fats are good for you and which ones to avoid.

◆ Add whole grains and fiber to your diet.

◆ Choose lean sources of protein.

◆ Be careful about how much sugar you eat.

When you're ready to learn more, go to the Web site on the back cover and enter **h844** in the search box.

Eat More Fruits and Vegetables

A healthy diet includes plenty of fruits and vegetables. Nearly everyone could benefit from eating more of them. They're full of vitamins, minerals, and fiber, and most are very low in fat and calories. They also have substances that may help prevent heart disease, high blood pressure, and some types of cancer.

More ▶

Easy Ways to Add Fruits and Veggies to Your Diet

◆ Add fresh or frozen berries or a sliced banana to breakfast cereal or yogurt. Put apple slices in oatmeal.

◆ Have a glass of juice with breakfast. One 6-ounce glass is a serving. (Don't depend on juice for all of your fruit servings, though. Most juices have a lot more sugar and calories than plain fruits.)

◆ Add lettuce, tomato, cucumber, and bell peppers to sandwiches. Get pizza with veggies—try mushrooms, peppers, spinach, or broccoli.

◆ Add vegetables to soups, stews, and stir-fries. Puree them in a blender or food processor first if it makes them easier to use.

◆ Keep carrots, celery, and other veggies handy for snacks. Buy them already sliced and ready to eat if it makes you more likely to eat them.

◆ Have a salad with dinner every night. Make sure it's mostly vegetables, rather than mostly cheese, croutons, and salad dressing.

◆ Have fruit for dessert. If a piece of fruit doesn't seem like dessert to you, try baked apples or pears with cinnamon, or have fresh berries or melon with some vanilla yogurt.

◆ Make a fruit smoothie. Blend bananas, berries, or oranges with fat-free or low-fat yogurt or milk.

Healthy Ways to Cook

How you cook affects how you eat. For many people, "cooking" means frying. This often means using lard, shortening, butter, or lots of oil to make food taste good. But there are healthier methods you can use and still have great-tasting food.

Here are some low-fat ways to cook. Try one for your next meal.

◆ Bake in aluminum foil. This keeps food juicy and full of flavor. Wrap meat or fish in foil with some herbs for seasoning and even a little wine or broth. Add some vegetables too.

◆ Poach. Put chicken or fish in one layer in a pan. Cover it with water or broth, and add herbs or a little wine for flavor. Bring the liquid to a boil. Then lower the heat and simmer for 10 to 12 minutes until the food is done.

◆ Stir-fry. When you stir-fry, you cut meat, chicken, or vegetables into small pieces so they cook fast. Use a nonstick pan or a wok over medium-high heat. Add the food and constantly stir and turn it. If the food sticks, add a little canola, olive, or sesame oil; cooking spray; or water, wine, or broth.

◆ Try fat-free or low-fat yogurt, sour cream, or cottage cheese in place of full-fat cream and sour cream.

◆ Before you eat chicken or meat, cut off the fat. If you eat beef or pork, choose the leanest cuts. Lean cuts of beef usually have the word "round" or "loin" in them. Lean cuts of pork usually have the word "loin" or "leg" in them.

Understanding Fats

Type of fats	What foods are they in?
Healthy fats: monounsaturated, polyunsaturated	Fish (salmon, mackerel) Most nuts and seeds, soybeans Vegetable oils (canola, olive, peanut, corn, safflower, sunflower, walnut, flaxseed) Avocados, olives
Unhealthy fats: saturated fats, trans fats, cholesterol	**Saturated fats and cholesterol:** Whole milk, whole-milk cheese, whole-milk yogurt Butter, margarine, shortening, lard (and foods cooked in these) Meat (beef, pork) **Trans fats:** Packaged cookies, crackers, and chips Processed foods Nondairy whipped topping and creamer

Understanding Fats

Except for most fruits and vegetables, almost everything you eat has some kind of fat. Your body needs some fat to work properly. But there are healthy "good" fats and unhealthy "bad" ones. For many people, the least healthy types of fats—saturated and trans fats—make up too much of their diet.

A healthy eating plan can and should include good fats in reasonable amounts. They are high in calories, but they can help lower your cholesterol and may reduce your risk of some diseases.

It's best to avoid unhealthy fats as much as you can. Not only are they high in calories, but they also raise your cholesterol and increase your risk of heart disease.

Use the chart on this page to learn which fats to enjoy and which ones to avoid.

How much fat should you eat? If you're eating an average diet of about 2,000 calories a day:

◆ Aim for about 60 grams of fat each day. Most of that should be monounsaturated and polyunsaturated fats.

◆ Eat less than 20 grams of saturated fats a day.

◆ Eat as few trans fats as possible. Check food labels for trans fats.

Get More Whole Grains

Whole grains like whole wheat, oats, and brown rice are full of B vitamins, minerals, and fiber and are a great source of energy. They're also very filling. **Refined grains**, which include white flour, white rice, and pasta, have fewer vitamins and minerals. They're not as filling because they don't have much fiber.

More

How do you know if it's whole grain?

◆ Read the food label. The first ingredient should be whole wheat, whole grain, or whole oats. "Enriched wheat flour" is a refined grain, not a whole grain. Multi-grain breads and crackers are not always whole grains.

◆ Don't go by color alone. Brown bread does not equal whole-grain or whole wheat bread.

You can add whole grains to your diet by choosing whole wheat bread instead of white bread; whole-grain crackers and cereals; oatmeal; brown rice instead of white rice; and whole wheat pasta. Don't be afraid to try other whole grains like bulgur, barley, and quinoa.

Add Fiber to Your Diet

Fiber is the part of fruits, vegetables, and grains that your body cannot digest. It is found only in plants. Foods that come from animals (meats, milk and dairy foods, eggs) do not have fiber.

There are two types of fiber: insoluble and soluble.

Insoluble fiber helps keep your digestive tract healthy. If you are often constipated, eating more of this fiber will help. People who eat a lot of insoluble fiber have fewer problems with the colon (large intestine). Whole wheat bread, cabbage, beets, carrots, and apple skins are some foods high in insoluble fiber.

Soluble fiber may help keep your blood sugar steady, lower your cholesterol, and reduce your chance of heart disease. Oatmeal, beans, oranges, and apple pulp are some foods high in soluble fiber.

How to Get More Fiber

Most people need about 30 grams of fiber each day. To reach that amount:

◆ Choose whole-grain breads and cereals that have at least 2 grams of fiber in each serving. Read the label on the package.

High-Fiber Foods	
Type of food	**Examples**
Breads and grain products (especially whole-grain foods)	Bran (wheat bran, oat bran) Oatmeal Whole wheat breads, tortillas, cereals Brown rice Barley, bulgur, millet
Vegetables	Beans, peas Cabbage, brussels sprouts Broccoli, cauliflower Beets, turnips, carrots Baked potato skin
Fruits	Fruits with skin or seeds that you eat (apples, pears, strawberries, kiwifruit, figs, blueberries) Oranges, grapefruit

- Buy bread that lists whole wheat, stone-ground wheat, or cracked wheat first in the ingredient list.

- Eat brown rice, bulgur, or millet instead of white rice.

- Eat more fresh fruits every day. See the list of high-fiber fruits on page 308.

- Eat more raw or lightly cooked vegetables every day.

- Eat cooked beans, peas, and lentils in place of meat sometimes.

Choose Lean Protein

Protein is vital to your health. It helps keep your muscles, bones, skin, hair, blood, and internal organs healthy. But some forms of protein tend to have too much cholesterol and unhealthy fats. So it's best to choose lean sources of protein, such as:

- Fish, skinless chicken, and only the leanest cuts of beef and pork.

- Beans, peas, and lentils.

- Tofu and other soy products.

- Fat-free or low-fat dairy products.

- Eggs (in moderation).

- Nuts and seeds.

Most adults in North America get all the protein they need in their diets. If you eat animal products, your diet probably has plenty of protein. If you are a vegetarian, make sure you get protein from plant sources like beans, grains, and soy.

Don't Eat Too Much Sugar

A little sugar is fine. It tastes good, and it's not harmful for most people. But most sweets also have a lot of "empty" calories—that means they're high in calories but do not fill you up or have much nutritional

Using the USDA's Food Guide

ChooseMyPlate.gov

The USDA's food guide aims to help you make healthy food choices and be active every day. It is based on the idea that your calorie and nutrient needs depend on your age, sex, and activity level.

For example, a 40-year-old woman who gets more than 60 minutes of physical activity on most days may need about 2,200 calories a day. A 40-year-old woman who gets less than 30 minutes of daily exercise may need only about 1,800 calories a day. Both women need to eat a variety of healthy foods from all the food groups—grains, vegetables, fruits, dairy, and protein foods. But they don't need the same amounts of those foods.

Want to know what's right for you? Go to www.ChooseMyPlate.gov. There you can:

- Figure out what kinds and amounts of food you should eat each day.

- Get help with meal plans and serving sizes.

- Track your progress toward healthier eating.

MyPlate icon and Web address provided by the USDA.

More

value. If too many of your calories come from sugar, you may not be getting enough of the healthy foods you need. (You may also gain weight.)

Many people need to cut down on sugar. Here are a few things that can make a big difference:

◆ Drink fewer sugar-sweetened drinks, such as soft drinks, lemonade, and fruit juices. These are a major source of sugar for some people, especially kids. Try sparkling water or sugar-free soda instead. Or just drink plain water and milk.

◆ Make it a habit to eat fruit instead of sugary desserts and snacks most of the time. Have a bowl of strawberries instead of a bowl of ice cream. Grab an apple instead of a candy bar.

◆ Check the labels on food packages before you buy things. Yogurt, cereal, and canned fruits often have sugar added. Look for cereals that have 6 grams or less of sugar in each serving.

Nutrition for Your Family

Healthy eating habits are good for the whole family. If you're trying to eat healthier, it will be easier if the rest of the family eats healthier too. The same foods that are good for adults are good for children. A healthy diet can help your children feel good, stay at a healthy weight, and have lots of energy for school and play.

Get started by setting up a regular schedule for meals and snacks. Expect everyone to come to the table to eat. Offer healthy foods, but let your child decide how much to eat. This lets your child tune in to whether he or she is hungry. Meal times are important for learning about new foods and how to behave at the table. Make them a pleasant family time.

Childhood is a great time to learn healthy eating habits that can last a lifetime. Children learn by example: They will learn to eat the foods they see you eating, and they will learn what makes a good meal by what you serve them.

Should You Take Dietary Supplements?

For most people, the best way to get all the nutrients they need is to eat a healthy, balanced diet that includes a variety of foods.

Supplements can't make up for a poor diet. But they can help fill in the nutrition gap for people who have special needs or who limit their calories to 1,500 or less a day. For example, older adults tend to have trouble absorbing enough vitamin D and calcium from their diets, so they may need a supplement. Some women need to take calcium or folic acid.

Talk to your doctor or a dietitian about whether you need to take vitamin or mineral supplements. If you do:

◆ Unless your doctor recommends a specific vitamin or mineral, choose a balanced multivitamin-mineral supplement that has close to 100 percent of the Daily Values (DVs).

◆ Do not take a specific trace mineral unless your doctor recommends it. Taking some trace minerals as supplements can upset the way your body absorbs other minerals.

Exercise and Health

Being more active is one of the best things you can do to improve your health and your quality of life. It helps you to:

◆ Feel stronger and have more energy. (And you will look better too!)

◆ Lower your risk for heart disease, stroke, certain cancers, diabetes, and high blood pressure.

◆ Reach and stay at a healthy weight.

◆ Keep your bones, muscles, and joints strong, and relieve joint pain and stiffness.

◆ Better deal with stress, anxiety, and depression.

◆ Make daily tasks easier—moving around, carrying bags of groceries, climbing stairs, taking care of your children.

◆ Keep your mind sharp as you get older.

If you are already in good health, regular exercise can help you stay that way. But if you are not in good health, or if you have a long-term health problem, just a little more exercise every day can make a big difference.

It's never too late to become more active. And it's never too late to get the benefits that exercise can bring. No matter how old you are, how fit you are, or what health problems you have, there is a form of exercise that will work for you. You just have to find it.

Attitude Counts

Starting or changing an exercise routine doesn't have to be hard. Lots of people find ways to be more active that work for them. Success starts with the right attitude.

What if I Have a Long-Term Health Problem?

You may think that because you have a health problem like high blood pressure, arthritis, or diabetes, exercise is not for you. But exercise can help almost everyone. It may even be part of the treatment for your health problem.

You may not be able to do certain kinds of exercise. But there are dozens of ways to be more active. You only need to find a few. Talk to your doctor about what exercises are safe for you and how much exercise you should get.

"I know I can find time for a little more exercise."

Even the busiest people can find time. If you're worried about not having enough time:

◆ Focus on being more active. You don't have to do formal "exercise" to improve your fitness. You just need to move more.

◆ Spread your workout throughout the day. You don't have to do all your exercise at once. For example, walk for 10 minutes 3 times a day.

◆ Find a time in the day that works for you. Get up early to walk, do a workout video at lunchtime, or meet a friend at the health club in the evening. It may seem hard to find the time, but you'll get used to it. You might even start to like it.

◆ Look for ways to be more active in your everyday life. Take the stairs instead of the elevator. Park farther away from work

More

or the mall. Move faster through chores like cleaning, yard work, or vacuuming. You can get a good workout by doing daily tasks at a pace that gets your heart beating faster and gets you breathing harder.

◆ Be creative. Instead of emailing or phoning a coworker or neighbor, walk over. When meeting with someone, suggest that you take a walk instead of staying inside.

"I'll have more energy if I exercise."

At first, exercise may make you feel tired because you're not used to it. Start by doing a little bit at a time, and stick with it. You may be surprised at how much more energetic you'll start to feel.

"Exercise doesn't have to hurt."

Even gentle exercise can improve your health. If you are new to exercise, at first your muscles may ache and your lungs may "burn" a little when you are breathing hard. Start slowly, and your body will adapt. Talk with your doctor if you have chest pain or if your joints hurt.

"Exercise is for big people too."

No matter what your size, exercise can make you healthier and happier. At first you may get tired quickly and may not be able to move or bend very well if you are overweight. You might feel self-conscious. Just remember to take one small step at a time. Those steps will quickly start to add up.

"Exercise doesn't have to cost much."

You do not need to spend a lot of money to stay fit.

◆ Start walking. It's free.

◆ Get home workout videos from the library or a used bookstore.

◆ Apply for a reduced-cost membership at your local YMCA.

◆ Shop for used exercise equipment in the newspaper or at yard sales. Make sure it's in safe condition.

"I'll never be too old to exercise."

Exercise helps at any age. In fact, being active can help you avoid some of the problems that often come as we get older. Talk to your doctor about what kinds of activity might be best for you.

"Exercise can help me avoid a heart attack."

If you have a heart problem, you may worry that you could have a heart attack or stroke while exercising. You are probably more likely to have one if you do not exercise. There may be some limits on what you should do, but regular, safe workouts will strengthen your heart, blood vessels, and lungs. See your doctor before you get started.

"Exercise can be fun!"

◆ Look for something you enjoy. Try new things until you find something you like. If you like what you're doing, you are much more likely to stick with it. Ride a bike. Take a dance class. Go hiking.

◆ Don't do the same thing every day. Variety can keep you motivated, and it's good for your body. Swim one day, and take a walk the next. Try a yoga class.

◆ Get a partner, or join a group or class. For many people, the social aspect makes their workout more fun.

"It never hurts to try."

Don't worry about failing, no matter what your past experience with exercise has been. Just go slowly, and set small goals. When you meet them, set new ones. And if you don't meet a goal, think about what might have helped you meet it, and try again.

Make Your Heart Stronger

When exercise gets your heart beating faster and gets you breathing harder, it makes your heart stronger. Whether you call it aerobic exercise, cardio exercise, or just "exercising your heart," it all means the same thing. And just a little more every day can reduce your risk for heart attack, stroke, and other problems.

What kinds of workouts are good for your heart? Anything that raises your heart rate and keeps it there counts.

◆ Walking, hiking, and running

◆ Biking (outside or indoors)

◆ Swimming and water aerobics

◆ Dancing

◆ Doing household chores or yard work at a fast pace

◆ Climbing stairs

A simple way to tell if you are working your heart is the "talk-sing" test. If you are too short of breath to talk while you exercise, you may be pushing too hard. If you can sing while you exercise, you may do more for your heart by working just a bit harder. If you are in the "talking" range, your heart is getting a good workout no matter what you're doing.

Go to Web Getting started can be as simple as taking a walk a few times a week. If you want more help planning an exercise routine, go to the Web site on the back cover and enter **a481** in the search box.

Walking Works

Want to start making your heart stronger today? Take a walk. Walking is one of the easiest ways to be more active and improve your health.

◆ Start with small, short-term goals you can reach. For example, if you have not been active in a long time, start with 15-minute walks 3 times a week. The next week, increase your walks to 20 minutes.

◆ Start each walk with a warm-up. Pick up your pace in the middle of the walk, and then slow down at the end.

◆ Walk fast enough to raise your heart rate and make you breathe harder. But do not walk so fast that you can't talk.

◆ Wear comfortable shoes with good arch support.

There are three tips that have helped lots of people stick to their walking routines. They can help you too.

◆ Find a friend, family member, or coworker to walk with. You will be less likely to skip your walk if you know someone is expecting you.

◆ Get a pedometer, a small device that counts your steps. Set a daily step goal, and wear your pedometer all day. You may be surprised how fast the steps add up when you park your car a little farther away, use the stairs instead of the elevator, or walk to the store instead of driving there.

◆ Get a dog. Dogs love to walk, and taking your dog for a walk once or twice a day is a great way to fit walking into your life.

More

Make Your Body Stronger

You do not have to lift heavy weights or grow big, bulky muscles to get stronger. Doing a few simple strength exercises twice a week can make a difference.

◆ You can do push-ups or sit-ups, use weights, or use machines. You can even do strength exercises with a piece of rubber tubing. For a guide to some basic exercises, go to the Web site on the back cover and enter **s462** in the search box.

◆ Do exercises that include all of the different muscle groups: chest, arms, stomach, back, and legs.

◆ Give muscles at least a full day's rest between strength workouts.

Your goal may be to strengthen your knees or back or to be able to get around better. You may want to reduce body fat and stay trim. Or you may want to protect your bones as you get older. Strength training helps with all of these.

Stretch Your Muscles

Stretching keeps you flexible and helps with sore or tense muscles. It improves your balance and posture and can also be a great way to relax. And you can do it for free.

There are lots of ways to bring stretching into your life.

◆ Stretch at home when you first get up in the morning or before you go to bed (or both). If you need help, get a video you can follow, or find a good fitness book or magazine that explains some stretches.

◆ Take a stretching class at a gym or health club.

◆ Try yoga or tai chi. These are great ways to stay flexible and reduce stress.

Basic stretches are easy to learn. The pictures on the next page show some simple stretches you can do on your own. The shaded area in each shows where you should feel the stretch. Here are a few tips to get you started:

◆ Ease into each stretch. Stretching is not about going fast or making sudden movements.

◆ Hold each stretch for at least 15 to 30 seconds. You should feel a pull in the area you are stretching, but you should not feel sharp pain.

◆ Do not hold your breath or bounce during a stretch.

Should I See My Doctor Before I Get Started?

Talk with your doctor before you start an exercise program if:

◆ You have heart trouble, frequent chest pain or pressure, or high blood pressure.

◆ You often feel faint or dizzy.

◆ You have arthritis or other bone or joint problems.

◆ You have diabetes (you may need to adjust your medicine).

◆ You are older than 65 and are not used to exercise.

◆ You have two or more risk factors for heart disease. These include diabetes, high cholesterol, high blood pressure, smoking, obesity, an inactive lifestyle, and a family history of heart disease.

Quadriceps stretch

Triceps stretch

Calf stretch

Groin stretch

Latissimus stretch

Hip, buttocks, and hamstring stretch

Quitting Smoking

Millions of people have quit smoking. Some have quit on their own. Some have quit with the help of stop-smoking programs or support groups. Some used medicines.

The point is that people find ways to quit for good. So can you.

It's best to get ready. Giving up tobacco is a big change, and the process of deciding that you will quit may take time. If you aren't sure whether you're ready, go to the Web site on the back cover and enter **b373** in the search box. The quiz there can help you figure out where you are in the process.

Thinking About Quitting?

If you're thinking about quitting, you're already on your way. It may help to know that you don't have to quit smoking through willpower alone. There are:

◆ Treatments that can help with the physical effects of giving up smoking and nicotine.

◆ Resources that can help with the emotional side of quitting smoking.

These approaches have helped many people stop smoking for good. They can help you too.

Nicotine Replacement and Medicines

When you try to stop smoking, you may have trouble sleeping, strongly crave nicotine, or feel grumpy, depressed, or restless. These symptoms of withdrawal are at their worst during the first week or so after you quit, but they may last up to a few weeks.

Treatment can reduce withdrawal symptoms and help you quit. You can try:

◆ Nicotine replacement products, such as gums, patches, inhalers, sprays, and lozenges. They help your body slowly get used to less nicotine until you do not need it at all. You can buy these products without a prescription.

◆ Medicines, such as bupropion (Zyban) or varenicline (Chantix). These medicines do not have nicotine but can help you cope with cravings and mood swings. Your doctor can prescribe them for you.

 For help in deciding whether to try these approaches, go to the Web site on the back cover and enter **b169** in the search box.

It's Not Just the Nicotine

If you are like many smokers, smoking is part of your daily routine. You enjoy it. It's relaxing. When you quit smoking, you have to give all that up (or at least find something to replace it).

It's Never Too Late

Anyone who smokes has good reason to stop—even if you have smoked for decades. No matter how long you've smoked, your risk of a heart attack and other health problems will start to go down once you quit. You will start to feel better and breathe easier.

It can be hard to break a long-time habit. But you can do it, just like thousands of other smokers who have quit.

The good news is that you don't have to do it alone. Lots of ex-smokers have found support in:

◆ Stop-smoking programs. Call your health plan, your local hospital, or the American Lung Association to find out what programs are offered in your area.

◆ Telephone "quitlines," such as 1-800-QUIT-NOW (1-800-784-8669). These connect you to trained counselors who can help you make a plan for how to quit.

◆ Online quit groups. Like quitlines, these are convenient for lots of people since you can get help from home at nearly any hour.

◆ Support groups, such as Nicotine Anonymous.

◆ Counseling from doctors, nurses, or therapists.

This kind of support can help you change your habits. Think about whether any of these options appeal to you, and give one a try. If it's not for you, try something else.

Once You've Decided to Quit

No one approach works for every smoker, but for many people it helps to:

◆ **Set a quit date.** Pick a date within the next month. Give yourself time to get ready (but not too much time).

10 Reasons to Quit

1. Live longer and better. On average, people who smoke die more than 10 years earlier than people who do not smoke. But it is not as simple as just dying younger. Smoking can affect the quality of your life as well. Having chronic lung disease is not an easy or pleasant way to live or die.

2. Cut your risk of heart attack in half within 2 years. Five years after quitting, your risk will be about the same as that of someone who never smoked.

3. Set a good example. Children whose parents do not smoke are less likely to use tobacco than those whose parents are smokers.

4. Stop having to find places to smoke at work or in public, and stop exposing others to secondhand smoke.

5. Breathe easier and cough less. You may have more energy and stamina after you stop smoking.

6. Reduce your risk of erection problems. Smoking can damage your blood vessels, including those that bring blood to the penis.

7. Reduce your risk for lung cancer, mouth and throat cancer, gum disease, and dental problems.

8. Get fewer colds and be less likely to get the flu or pneumonia. If you have asthma, you will have fewer and less severe asthma attacks.

9. Have a brighter smile, better sense of taste and smell, and fewer wrinkles.

10. Save money by not buying cigarettes. (Also, as a nonsmoker, you may pay less for health insurance.)

More

◆ **Plan.** Will you go to a class, join a support group, or use nicotine replacement? Make sure you have low-calorie snacks on hand. Clean your clothes, carpet, furniture, and car to get rid of the smoke smell. If you know you tend to smoke in certain situations, plan for ways to avoid them.

◆ **Quit!** Stick to your quit date. That day, get rid of cigarettes, ashtrays, and lighters.

 For more tips and techniques that can help you get ready to quit and then stop smoking for good, go to the Web site on the back cover and enter **p811** in the search box.

Started Smoking Again?

You're not alone. Many people who have quit smoking had to try several times before they were able to quit for good. The good news is that each time you try to quit—whether it's your second attempt or your tenth—you can get closer to quitting for good.

Think about why you started smoking again. Was it stress? Were you with a certain group of people or in a certain situation? What might have triggered you to smoke? Learn from what worked for you and what didn't.

Knowing what went wrong can help you when you are ready to quit again. The important thing is to keep trying.

Dealing With Stress

Some stress is normal and even healthy. Stress releases hormones that speed up your heart, make you breathe faster, and give you a burst of energy. This can be useful when you need to focus or act quickly. It can help you win a race, finish a big job, or get to the airport on time.

But too much stress or being under stress for too long is not good for you.

◆ It can make you moody, anxious, and depressed. You may find it hard to concentrate, and you may lose your temper more easily.

◆ It can cause headaches, back pain, and muscle tension.

◆ It can make health problems like heart disease, diabetes, and asthma worse.

◆ It can hurt your relationships. You may not do as well at work or school.

You may not have these problems right away. Most people can get through short periods of stress without long-term effects. But over time, continued stress will take its toll on you.

The good news is that you can learn ways to reduce and cope with stress that will help you avoid stress-related health problems.

Ways to Reduce Stress

1. Decide what is most important and what can wait. (Maybe there are things you don't need to do at all.) At work, ask your boss if you're not sure what the priorities are.

2. Learn to say no. Don't commit to things that don't matter to you.

3. Do one thing at a time. When you try to do too many things at once, each usually takes more time than it would if you focused on it alone.

4. Get organized. Make lists, or use an appointment book. Keep track of deadlines.

5. Don't put things off. Use a schedule planner to plan your day or week. Just seeing on paper that there is a time to get each task done can help you get to work. Break a large project into small pieces, and set a deadline for each one.

6. Save some time for yourself. Leave your job at the office, even if your office is a room in your home. If you give up free time to get more work done, you may pay for it with stress-related symptoms. If your employer offers a flexible work schedule, use it to fit your work style. Come in earlier so you have time for a longer lunch or a workout.

7. "Unplug" when you leave work. Leave your work cell phone behind or turn it off. Don't check work email at home.

8. Get enough sleep. Stress can seem worse than it is when you're tired all the time. And you may not get as much done when you're too tired.

How to Cope Better With Stress

For most people, there's just no way to totally avoid stress. It's part of life. But you can control how you react to stress.

People don't always realize that they feel bad because of stress. Classic signs of stress include headache, stiff neck, or a nagging backache. You may lose your temper more

often. You may feel jumpy or exhausted all the time.

 Just knowing why you're feeling the way you do may help you cope with the problem. For a tool that can help you gauge your stress level now or anytime, go to the Web site on the back cover and enter **r030** in the search box.

Healthy Ways to De-Stress
Listen to music
Exercise
Go outdoors
Play with a pet
Laugh or cry
Spend time with someone you love
Write, draw, or paint
Pray or go to church
Take a bath or shower
Work in the yard or do home repairs
Do yoga, meditation, or muscle relaxation

Unhealthy Ways to De-Stress
Drive fast
Eat too much or too little
Bite your fingernails
Drink too much coffee
Criticize yourself
Avoid people
Yell at your spouse, children, or friends
Smoke
Drink alcohol
Use illegal drugs
Get violent or aggressive

Are You Stress-Hardy?

Some people seem to stand up to or bounce back from stress better than others. They adjust to change more easily. They are more "stress-hardy."

More

How stress-hardy are you? There is a short quiz that can tell you. Go to the Web site on the back cover and enter **d856** in the search box.

If you would like to be more stress-hardy, here are a few things that may help:

◆ Know what's important to you, whether it's your family, your work, or something else. When you are under a lot of stress, try to remember what matters most.

◆ Try to have a sense of control over your life. You cannot control every detail, but look for areas where you can make a difference. Not everything is out of your hands.

◆ Try to look at change as a challenge or opportunity rather than a threat.

◆ Do things that let you be creative and let you be yourself. Some people can do this through their work. But sometimes activities outside of your job—hobbies, sports, social groups, volunteer work, travel—are better chances to "do your own thing."

◆ Stay in touch with friends and family. Knowing that you are not alone in the world makes stress easier to bear.

Learn to Relax

There are many techniques you can learn to help you relax. Progressive muscle relaxation and the relaxation response are two that seem to work well.

To learn these skills, practice them in a time and place where nothing will interrupt you. Do them once or twice a day until you can do them easily.

Progressive Muscle Relaxation

Relaxing your muscles can reduce tension and anxiety. It can help reduce stress-related health problems and often helps people sleep better.

You can buy a tape or CD that takes you through all the muscle groups, or you can do it by just tensing and relaxing each muscle group on your own.

◆ Choose a place where you can lie down on your back and stretch out.

◆ Tense each muscle group (hard, but not to the point of cramping) for 4 to 10 seconds. Then give yourself 10 to 20 seconds to release it and relax.

◆ At various points, check the muscle groups you've already done and relax each one a little more each time.

Muscle Groups

Remember to relax between each muscle group.

Hands: Clench them.

Wrists and forearms: Extend them and bend the hands back at the wrist.

Biceps and upper arms: Clench your hands into fists, bend your arms at the elbows, and flex your biceps (the muscles in your upper arms).

Shoulders: Shrug them. Check your arms and shoulders for tension.

Forehead: Wrinkle it into a deep frown.

Around the eyes and bridge of the nose: Close your eyes as tightly as you can. (Take out your contact lenses before you do this.)

Cheeks and jaws: Grin from ear to ear.

Around the mouth: Press your lips together tightly. (Check your face for tension.)

Back of the neck: Press the back of your head against the floor.

Front of the neck: Touch your chin to your chest. (Check your neck and head for tension.)

Chest: Take a deep breath and hold it. Then let it go.

Back: Arch your back up and away from the floor.

Belly: Suck it into a tight knot. (Check your chest and belly for tension.)

Hips and buttocks: Squeeze your buttocks together tightly.

Thighs: Clench them.

Lower legs: Point your toes toward your face, as if trying to bring your toes up to touch your shins. Then point your toes away and curl them under at the same time. (Check the area from your waist down for tension.)

When you are finished, return to alertness by counting backward from 5 to 1.

Relaxation Response

The relaxation response is the opposite of the stress response. It slows your heart rate and breathing, lowers your blood pressure, and helps relieve muscle tension.

1. Lie down in a place where you can stretch out. Close your eyes.

2. Begin progressive muscle relaxation. See page 320.

3. Tune in to your breathing for 10 to 20 minutes. Focus on breathing from your belly, not from your chest. Each time you breathe out, say the word "one" (or any other word) silently or out loud. Or instead of saying a word, fix your gaze on an object in the room. As thoughts enter your mind, don't dwell on them. Let them drift away.

4. Sit quietly for several minutes, until you're ready to open your eyes.

5. Notice the difference in your breathing and your pulse.

Don't worry about trying to become deeply relaxed. The key to this exercise is to stay passive and let distracting thoughts go without thinking about them.

(Technique adapted from Herbert Benson, MD)

Safe Sex

Safe sex is all about avoiding sexually transmitted infections (STIs), also called sexually transmitted diseases. STIs can cause a lot of problems in your body. Some of them can even kill you. It's up to you to protect yourself and your sex partner from them. The good news is that you can.

To learn about the symptoms of STIs and what to do if you think you have one, see page 229.

Who Gets STIs?

Anyone who has sex can get an STI. It does not matter how old you are, whether you're male or female, what race you are, or whether you're gay, straight, or bisexual.

You can get an STI from any kind of sexual contact, not just intercourse. STIs are spread through skin-to-skin contact between the genitals and through contact with body

More

fluids such as semen, vaginal fluids, and blood (including menstrual blood). This means you can get an STI from:

◆ Vaginal sex.

◆ Anal sex.

◆ Oral sex.

How You Can Stay Safer

Only two things completely get rid of the risk of STIs and HIV infection:

1. Not having sex at all (abstinence). This means not having vaginal, anal, or oral sex.

2. Total monogamy between uninfected partners. This means you and your partner have sex only with each other, and you are absolutely sure that neither of you has an infection.

If you do not choose one of those two options, you can still greatly reduce your risk if you follow the guidelines below.

◆ Have safe sex every time you have sex. This means using condoms correctly every time. Use latex condoms from the beginning to the end of sexual contact. "Natural" or lambskin condoms do not protect against HIV infection or other STIs. If you or your partner is allergic to latex, use polyurethane ones instead.

◆ Do not rely on spermicides or a diaphragm to protect against STIs. If spermicide irritates your genital area, it may increase your risk of infection.

◆ Before you have sex with a new partner, ask about his or her sexual history. Keep in mind that a person can have HIV or an STI and not know it.

◆ Do not have sex without a condom with anyone who has symptoms of an STI or whose behavior puts him or her at risk for HIV infection or an STI.

◆ Agree with your partner that neither of you will have sex with anyone else.

◆ Do not have sex if you or your partner has symptoms of an STI, such as sores on the genitals or mouth.

◆ Do not have sex while you or your partner is being treated for an STI.

◆ If you or your partner has genital herpes, do not have sex when either of you has a blister or an open sore or feels tingling or pain in the genital area. These may be signs of an outbreak. At other times, use latex condoms. You can spread genital herpes even when no sores are present.

How to Use a Condom

Condoms work best if you follow these steps:

◆ Use a new condom each time you have sex.

◆ When you open the wrapper, be careful not to poke a hole in the condom with your nails, teeth, or other sharp objects.

◆ Put the condom on as soon as your penis is hard (erect) and before any sexual contact.

◆ Before putting the condom on, hold the tip of it and squeeze out the air to leave room for the semen.

◆ If you are not circumcised, pull down the loose skin from the head of the penis (foreskin) before you put on the condom.

◆ While holding onto the tip, unroll the condom all the way down to the base of your penis.

◆ If you want to use a lubricant, never use petroleum jelly (such as Vaseline), grease, hand lotion, baby oil, or anything with oil in it. Oil or petroleum can make the condom break. Instead, use a personal lubricant such as Astroglide or K-Y Jelly.

◆ After you ejaculate, hold onto the condom at the base of your penis and pull out from your partner while your penis is still hard. This will keep semen from spilling out of the condom.

◆ Wash your hands after handling a used condom.

Buy condoms that meet strict safety standards. These are less likely to break or leak.

Keep the condom in its original package until you are ready to use it. Store it in a cool, dry place out of direct sun. Do not keep it in your wallet, car, or other hot places for a long time. The heat weakens the latex.

Allergic to Latex?

Some people are allergic to latex. If you have a skin reaction after using a latex condom, think about whether it could have been something else (lubricant, spermicide) that caused the problem. If you are sure it was the latex, do not use latex condoms again. Use polyurethane ones instead.

Polyurethane condoms may not prevent STIs as well as latex condoms do. But they are much safer than not using a condom at all.

Get Immunized

Immunizations help protect the body from diseases. When you get a vaccine, your body learns to find and attack the bacteria or virus that causes the disease before it can cause problems.

Immunizations save lives. They help prevent serious illness in children as well as adults. They cost less than treating the diseases they protect against. And the risk of serious side effects from the vaccines is much lower than the risk of serious illness if you do not get the vaccines.

 Make sure to get your child (and yourself) immunized. If you need more information than you find here, go to the Web site on the back cover and enter **w921** in the search box.

Keep good records. You may need to show proof of immunizations when you enroll your child in day care or school. You may need them for travel too.

More

Immunizations for Children

The chart on page 325 is a basic guide to which vaccines children need and when. Talk to your doctor about what schedule is best for your child.

◆ If your child is at higher risk because of a long-term (chronic) illness or weak immune system or because of where you live or travel, he or she may need a different schedule.

◆ If your child has missed any vaccines, he or she may need a "catch-up" schedule.

◆ If there is a disease outbreak (such as measles) and your child has not been vaccinated yet, call your doctor or health department to see if your child should get the vaccine early.

◆ Even the basic schedule changes from time to time. Make sure you have the most current information.

You do not need to delay immunizations because your child has a cold or other minor illness. If you have concerns, talk with your doctor.

Reactions to Immunizations

Brief, mild reactions are common.

◆ If your child gets a slight fever, acetaminophen (Tylenol) or ibuprofen (Advil, Motrin) can help. Do not give aspirin to anyone younger than 20. Also see Fever on pages 158 and 160.

◆ The area around the shot may swell, be mildly red, and hurt a little. Put ice or a cold pack on it for 10 to 15 minutes.

◆ A mild skin rash may appear a week or two after the MMR or chickenpox vaccine. The rash does not need treatment and should go away within a few days.

Call your doctor right away if your child has more than just a mild reaction.

Immunizations for Teens and Adults

The need for immunizations does not end with childhood.

◆ Thousands of adults are hospitalized, and many die, because of flu and other diseases that vaccines can prevent.

◆ Illnesses like chickenpox and measles can be quite serious if you get them as a teen or adult. They are especially dangerous for pregnant women.

◆ Having rubella or chickenpox while you are pregnant increases the risk of miscarriage, stillbirth, and severe birth defects.

◆ Hepatitis B can lead to serious, sometimes fatal liver disease.

If you are in any of the groups for whom a vaccine is recommended, make sure you get immunized. Use the chart on page 326 as a guide, and then talk to your doctor. The recommendations change from time to time.

Other Immunizations

If you are in close contact with people who have contagious diseases or you plan to travel to places where malaria, typhoid, cholera, yellow fever, or other illnesses are common, call your local health department. You may need other shots.

Childhood Immunizations

Immunization	Who should have it?	Comments
Diphtheria, tetanus, pertussis (whooping cough) vaccine (DTaP)	All children	5 shots: First shot at age 2 months, last at age 4–6 years Booster shots for tetanus, diphtheria, and/or whooping cough are needed throughout life, starting at age 11–12 years.
Rotavirus vaccine	All children	2 or 3 doses: First dose at age 2 months, last at age 4–6 months
Polio vaccine (IPV)	All children	4 shots: First shot at age 2 months, last at age 4–6 years
Pneumococcal vaccine (PCV)	All children under 2 years	4 shots: First shot at age 2 months, last at age 12–15 months
Haemophilus influenzae type b (Hib) vaccine	All children	3 or 4 shots: First shot at age 2 months, last at age 12–15 months
Measles, mumps, rubella vaccine (MMR)	All children	2 shots: First shot at age 12–15 months, second at age 4–6 years
Hepatitis B vaccine (HBV)	All children	3 shots: First shot at birth, last by age 6–18 months
Flu vaccine	All children	1 dose each year; children under 9 years may need 2 doses. Vaccine cannot be given before age 6 months
Chickenpox vaccine	All children 12 months and older who haven't had chickenpox	2 shots: First shot at age 12–15 months, second at age 4–6 years
Hepatitis A vaccine (HAV)	All children 12 months and older	2 shots: First shot at age 12 months, second at least 6 months later
Meningococcal vaccine	All children 11 years and older	2 shots: First shot at age 11–12 years, second at age 16 Children who have a weak immune system, a damaged or missing spleen, or who live in or travel to areas where the disease is common need at least 2 shots before age 11, plus they may need booster doses throughout life.
Human papillomavirus vaccine (HPV)	All children ages 11–12	3 shots over a period of 6 months

More

Teen and Adult Immunizations	
Immunization	**Who should have it (if not already immunized)?**
Flu vaccine	◆ All teens and adults
Chickenpox vaccine	◆ All teens and adults who haven't had chickenpox or the vaccine
Meningococcal vaccine	◆ All teens (First shot advised at age 11–12; second at age 16.) ◆ All college freshmen living in dorms ◆ People who live in or travel to areas where the disease is common ◆ People with weak immune systems (HIV, damaged or missing spleen)
Hepatitis A vaccine (HAV)	◆ Anyone who lives in or travels to areas where outbreaks have occurred ◆ Anyone who will be in close contact with an adopted child from a country where the rate of hepatitis A is high ◆ People who inject illegal drugs ◆ Men who have sex with men ◆ People with chronic liver disease or blood-clotting problems
Hepatitis B vaccine (HBV)	◆ Anyone 18 years or younger who hasn't been vaccinated ◆ Adults whose travel or work puts them at risk ◆ Health care and public safety workers ◆ People who inject illegal drugs ◆ Men who have sex with men ◆ People who have had more than one sex partner in the past 6 months or who have a history of sexually transmitted infection ◆ Household contacts and sex partners of hepatitis B carriers ◆ People with chronic liver disease or diabetes ◆ Prison inmates
Measles, mumps, and rubella vaccine (MMR)	◆ Teens and adults who haven't had measles, mumps, or rubella, or the vaccine, and who were born after 1956
Pneumococcal vaccine	◆ All adults 65 and older ◆ Anyone under 65 who has a chronic disease (such as heart or lung disease), who has a damaged or missing spleen, or who smokes
Polio vaccine (IPV)	◆ People whose travel or work puts them at risk
Tetanus, diphtheria vaccine (Td)	◆ All adults, every 10 years throughout life ◆ Anyone who gets a deep, dirty wound and hasn't had a booster in the past 5 years
Tetanus, diphtheria, and pertussis vaccine (Tdap)	◆ All teens and adults who haven't had the Tdap vaccine before
Human papillomavirus vaccine (HPV)	◆ Females ages 13–26 and males ages 13–21 who didn't get the vaccine when they were younger ◆ Men ages 22–26 who have a weak immune system or who have sex with men
Note: If you are pregnant or have a weak immune system, you may not be able to get some of these vaccines. Talk to your doctor about which ones are safe for you.	

Wellness Exams and Screening Tests

One way to protect your health is to watch for changes in your body and find problems early, when they may be easier to treat.

Preventive health care can help you do this. This type of care includes:

◆ Wellness exams. These are checkups you have when you are healthy. They are focused on your overall health.

◆ Screening tests. These tests look for signs of disease before you have symptoms. Pap tests, mammograms, and PSA (prostate-specific antigen) tests are examples of screening tests for cancer.

◆ Immunizations. See page 323.

The recommendations for wellness exams and screening tests here are for mostly healthy people at average risk for health problems. Some things that affect your level of risk are your overall health, family history (whether close relatives had certain diseases), and lifestyle factors such as tobacco use, exercise habits, and sexual history.

People with a chronic illness or other problems may need checkups and tests more often. Work with your doctor to decide on the best schedule for you.

For Children

Younger than 3 years:

◆ Well-baby visits: A good schedule for visits is at age 2 weeks and at 2, 4, 6, 9, 12, 15, 18, 24, and 30 months. Your doctor may suggest a slightly different schedule. The point is that babies need regular checkups.

◆ Hearing tests: All babies should be tested for hearing problems by age 3 months.

Three years and older:

◆ Well-child visits: Starting at age 3, children usually come in for a visit one time a year. It's important to check the height, weight, blood pressure, and other measures of your child's growth and health.

◆ Vision tests: Have your child's vision checked starting around age 3.

Don't forget immunizations! See page 324. These can be done at regular checkups.

For Adults

The right schedule of wellness exams and screenings is one you and your doctor agree on, based on your age, your risk factors for disease, how healthy you are, and how important preventive care is to you.

The schedule on page 328 lists common screening tests. Most adults need some or all of these tests. Or take a short quiz to find out which screenings you need. Go to the Web site on the back cover and enter **v233** in the search box.

For Women: Pelvic Exams and Pap Tests

A pelvic exam looks for early signs of problems in the reproductive organs. The exam usually includes:

◆ An external genital exam. The doctor looks at the genital area for skin changes, sores, or other problems.

◆ A manual exam. The doctor inserts two gloved fingers into your vagina and presses on your lower belly with the other hand to check the shape and size of your ovaries and uterus.

◆ A Pap test.

More

Sample Health Screening Schedule

Screening	Who should have it?	How often?
Blood pressure	All adults	Every 1 to 2 years. More often if you are at risk for high blood pressure. See page 191.
Cholesterol	All adults	Talk to your doctor.
Type 2 diabetes (fasting blood sugar)	All adults whose blood pressure is higher than 135/80 (your doctor may suggest testing if you have other risks)	Every 3 years. More often if you are at high risk. Talk to your doctor.
Vision problems, especially glaucoma (see page 172)	All adults	Talk to your doctor. Need for exams increases with age.
Colorectal cancer (colonoscopy, flexible sigmoidoscopy, fecal occult blood test, or other tests)	All adults ages 50 to 75. Sooner if you are at increased risk.	Depends on which tests you have. See Colorectal Cancer on page 127.
Breast cancer (mammogram and clinical breast exam)	All women	**Mammogram** Age 50 and older: Every 1 to 2 years Younger than 50: Talk to your doctor **Clinical breast exam** Talk to your doctor.
Pap test for cervical cancer	All women starting at age 21	Every 2 to 5 years for women at average risk. Talk to your doctor about the best schedule for you. See page 329.
Chlamydia (see page 230)	All sexually active females 24 and younger All females over 24 who are at risk	Whenever you have a pelvic exam and Pap test. See page 327.
Prostate cancer (PSA test or digital rectal exam)	Some men. See Should You Be Tested? on page 221.	Talk to your doctor.

Other things you and your doctor may want to keep track of: height and weight; hearing; thyroid level; HIV status (if you are at risk); and skin changes that could be cancerous.

Pap tests

The Pap test is a screening test for cancer of the cervix, which is the lower part of the uterus that opens into the vagina. The test looks for early changes in the cells that could lead to cancer. When done regularly, Pap tests can find most cervical cancers.

To do the test, the doctor inserts an instrument called a speculum into your vagina to spread apart the vaginal walls. He or she then collects cell samples from your cervix with a wooden or plastic device that gently scrapes some cells off the surface. The cells are sent to a lab.

Your doctor should let you know the results of your Pap test when they come back from the lab. If your results are abnormal, you may need to return for more tests. You may need another Pap test, or you may need a test called a colposcopy, which provides a more complete view of the cervix.

Abnormal Pap results can mean many things. Most of them are not cancer.

Women should have their first Pap test at age 21. After that, Pap tests are recommended every 2 to 5 years for women at average risk for cervical cancer. Some women are at higher risk and may need to have Pap tests more often. Talk to your doctor about the best schedule for you.

It may be okay to stop having Pap tests if:

◆ You are 65 or older and have had recent normal Pap tests or recent normal combination HPV (human papillomavirus) and Pap tests.

◆ You have had a hysterectomy for a reason other than cancer.

You and your doctor can decide on the right age to stop being tested, based on your health history.

Arrange to have the Pap test 1 to 2 weeks after your period ends. Do not douche, have sex, or use feminine hygiene products for at least 24 hours before a Pap test, because it may affect the test results.

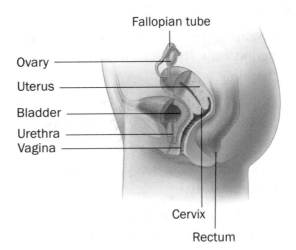

The female pelvic organs (front and side views)

More

For Women: Mammograms and Clinical Breast Exams

Breast cancer can often be cured if it is found early. There are two ways to screen for early breast cancer: mammograms and clinical breast exams.

A **mammogram** is a breast X-ray that can find tumors while they are still too small to be felt in a breast exam.

Mammograms save lives. If you are not at high risk for breast cancer and you are:

◆ Age 50 or older, have a mammogram every 1 to 2 years.

◆ Younger than 50, talk to your doctor about mammograms for routine screening.

If your mother, a sister, or another close female relative had breast cancer before menopause, you may need to start having mammograms sooner and have them more often. Talk to your doctor. Women who have already had breast cancer need to have mammograms every year.

To prepare for a mammogram:

◆ Arrange to have it 1 to 2 weeks after your period ends. (It will be least painful at that time.)

◆ Do not wear deodorant, perfume, powder, or lotion. They can affect the quality of the X-ray.

◆ Wear clothing that lets you easily undress from the waist up.

◆ If your last mammogram was at a different facility, have the original X-ray sent before your test, or pick it up and take it with you.

During a **clinical breast exam**, a doctor or nurse looks at your breasts and gently feels them for lumps or other changes. Ask your doctor if you should have this exam.

No matter what your age, talk to your doctor if you find a lump or have a problem with your breasts. See Breast Problems on page 103. You may need a breast exam or a mammogram to help find the cause.

What about breast self-exams?

Breast self-exams are a good way for you to learn what your breasts normally look and feel like. Once you know what's normal for you, you'll be better able to notice changes and know when to get help early instead of waiting for your next checkup. A self-exam is not a substitute for a mammogram.

A breast self-exam is easy to do. It includes looking for changes in the shape of your breasts or nipples as you stand in front of a mirror and move your arms in different ways. For the second part of the test, you use your hands to examine all areas of each breast, nipple, and armpit.

If you do not know how to do a breast self-exam, ask your doctor or nurse for help. Your doctor's office may have the instructions printed on a sheet or card that you can take with you.

Self-Exams

Watching for changes in your own body is an easy thing you can do to find problems early. Self-exams help you better understand your own body and what is normal for you.

Some of the self-exams you can do include:

◆ Breast self-exam for women. See page 330.

◆ Testicular self-exam for men. See page 246.

◆ Skin self-exam. Every month or so, look for changes in moles (changing color, size, or shape), sores that won't heal, or any other changes in your skin that could be early signs of skin cancer. See page 235.

In general, try to be a good observer of your body. If you notice a change from what's normal for you and the change does not go away, it may be a good idea to talk to your doctor about it.

Dental Checkups

Regular visits to the dentist are an important part of your preventive care.

◆ Most experts recommend that your child see a dentist either by age 1 or within 6 months after the first tooth comes in.

◆ Children and adults should see the dentist once or twice a year. During a checkup:

❖ The dentist will examine your teeth and gums for cavities, tooth decay, and gum disease.

❖ You may have X-rays of your teeth (usually once a year).

❖ A dentist or dental hygienist will scrape hard buildup (tartar) off your teeth with a metal tool, floss your teeth well, and clean and polish your teeth.

For people who go to the dentist regularly and take good care of their teeth, cleanings are usually not painful. If you have not been to the dentist in a long time, or if you have problems with your teeth or gums, cleanings may be a little uncomfortable.

Tuberculin Skin Test

A tuberculin test is done to find out if you have been infected with the bacteria that cause tuberculosis (TB). TB is a lung infection that spreads among people easily. It can be very serious in children and in people who have weak immune systems.

Whether you need to be tested depends on how common TB is in your area and how likely you are to come in contact with TB. If you think you may have been exposed to TB and want to be tested, call your doctor or the local health department.

Be Safe

Ten Steps to a Safer Home

1. Install smoke detectors. Check the batteries once a month, and replace them every year.

2. Keep a working fire extinguisher in your home. Make sure everyone in the house knows where it is and how to use it.

3. Have an emergency plan in case of a fire. Include how everyone will get out of the house and where to meet outside. Practice the plan with your family. Don't forget your pets.

4. Set your water heater to 120°F or lower to prevent burns. When you are cooking, turn pot handles toward the back of the stove. Never smoke in bed.

5. Keep appliances away from water. Turn off or unplug appliances when you are done with them. Replace frayed electrical cords. Unplug appliances (including your computer) when you need to clean or repair them. Turn off power at the circuit breaker if you need to work on wall or ceiling fixtures.

6. If you have children, put plastic safety caps into electrical outlets that are not in use. Keep electrical cords out of the reach of small children and pets.

7. Have your heating and cooling system checked at least once a year. Keep fireplaces and stoves in good working order. Think about installing a carbon monoxide detector.

8. Store firearms unloaded and with the safety on in a secure, locked place. Lock ammunition in a separate place.

9. Keep medicines, cleaning products, plant food, and other poisonous products (see page 44) where kids and pets cannot reach them. Keep products in their original containers. Never store poisons in food containers. Use childproof latches on your cabinets.

10. Make your home fall-proof. Use good lighting inside and out. Keep stairs and walking paths clear of electrical cords and clutter. Make sure carpets are firmly attached to the floor. Remove snow and ice from porches and sidewalks promptly.

Prevent Serious Injuries

◆ Wear your seat belt every time you get in a car. Teach your children to do the same. Children younger than 13 should ride in the backseat. Use car seats for babies and small children (see pages 333 to 334).

◆ Never drink and drive, and don't ride in a car with a drunk driver. Do not drive if you are taking medicine that makes you sleepy.

◆ Wear a helmet and other protective gear whenever you are biking, motorcycling, skating, kayaking, horseback riding, skiing, snowboarding, or rock climbing.

◆ If you keep a gun in your home:

❖ Make sure you know how to use the gun properly. Take a safety course.

❖ If there are children living in your home, store the gun unloaded, with the safety on, and locked in a secure spot. Do not store the ammunition with the gun.

- Do not dive into shallow or unfamiliar waters.

- Do not let young children play near water without a responsible person watching them.

- Wear safety glasses whenever you mow the lawn, use power tools, or work with chemicals. Closely follow the instructions on the label when you work with pesticides, fertilizers, strong cleaning products, and other chemicals. If it says to wear a mask and gloves, wear them.

- Use a sturdy step stool or ladder to reach objects that are up high. Do not stand on chairs or countertops. And be extra careful when you are up high on a ladder or on a roof. Don't take chances.

Use Child Car Seats

Infant and child car seats save lives. Children who are not in car seats can be hurt or killed during crashes or even by sudden stops at low speeds.

Most states require car seats for all children younger than 4 and those who weigh less than 40 pounds. Find out what the laws are where you live.

Use a car seat every time your child rides in the car. The safest place for your child is in the back middle seat.

Make sure the car seat is the right fit for your child's current age, weight, and height. For safety, it's very important to have a car seat that fits your child. Be sure to follow the car seat maker's recommendations. They should include weight and height guidelines. They should also tell you how to install the seat and how to secure your child in it.

The following guidelines come from the National Highway Traffic Safety Administration:

Ages Birth to 12 months

Your child under age 1 should always ride in a car seat that faces the back of the car (called rear-facing). There are different types of rear-facing car seats: Infant-only seats can only be used rear-facing. Convertible and 3-in-1 car seats typically have higher height and weight limits for the rear-facing position, allowing you to keep your child rear-facing for a longer period of time.

A rear-facing car seat

Ages 1 to 3 years

Keep your child rear-facing as long as possible. It's the best way to keep him or her safe. Your child should remain in a rear-facing car seat until he or she reaches the top height or weight limit allowed by your car seat's maker. Once your child outgrows the rear-facing car seat, your child is ready to travel in a car seat that faces the front (called forward-facing) and that has a harness.

More

Ages 4 to 7 years

Keep your child in a forward-facing car seat with a harness until he or she reaches the top height or weight limit allowed by your car seat's maker. Once your child outgrows the forward-facing car seat with a harness, your child can travel in a booster seat, but still in the backseat.

A booster seat

A forward-facing car seat

Ages 8 to 12 years

Keep your child in a booster seat until he or she is big enough to fit in a seat belt properly. For a seat belt to fit properly the lap belt must lie snugly across the upper thighs, not the stomach. The shoulder belt should lie snug across the shoulder and chest and not cross the neck or face. Remember: your child should still ride in the backseat because it's safer there.

If you have questions about your car seat, call the National Highway Traffic Safety Administration at 1-888-327-4236 or visit its Web site at www.nhtsa.gov.

Be Prepared for Emergencies

Natural disasters, chemical spills, disease outbreaks—these are dangers of modern life. They can affect air quality, cause shortages of safe water and food, and cut off access to electricity, gas, phones, and other services. Family members may be separated. Hospitals and clinics may not be able to handle everyone who needs help.

While these events are scary to think about, there are things you can do to be better prepared:

◆ Have a plan for you and your family. This can help in almost any kind of disaster.

◆ Keep an emergency kit with water, food, first aid supplies, and other essentials. It's also a good idea to know how to purify water (see page 336).

◆ Learn what to do if you are exposed to chemicals (see page 27) or other hazards.

◆ Always follow the advice of local authorities and public health officials.

❖ During an emergency, tune in to a local radio or TV station. Don't try to call for instructions. Phone lines may be busy or out of order.

❖ If you are told to evacuate, do it. Follow the schedule and route for your area.

❖ If there is an outbreak of a contagious disease in your area, don't leave your community unless authorities tell you to. If you are already infected, you could spread the disease or miss getting treatment you need.

❖ For major public health crises, you can rely on information from the Centers for Disease Control and Prevention (www.cdc.gov) and the World Health Organization (www.who.int/en).

Your Emergency Plan

It's easy to put together an emergency plan.

◆ Choose a contact person for family members to call or email if they get separated. A friend or relative who lives out of state is best. Make sure everyone has the contact's phone number and email address.

◆ Pick a place to meet outside your neighborhood in case you can't go home. Make sure everyone has the address and phone number.

◆ Pick a place to meet just outside your home, like a neighbor's front yard, in case there's a fire in your home.

◆ Write down where and how to turn off water, gas, and power. Make sure you have any tools this requires.

◆ Talk about what you would do if you had to leave. Include your pets in your plans. Shelters and health facilities may not let you bring your pets.

You may have other things you want to include in your plan, especially if you have children in school or if anyone in your household has special needs.

Review your plan once a year. Make sure that phone numbers, email addresses, and other items are still correct.

Your Emergency Supplies Kit

You need the same basic supplies no matter what the situation:

◆ Water. Store 1 gallon (4 quarts) for each person for each day. Most people need to drink about 2 quarts a day. Count on another 2 quarts for hygiene and cooking.

For example, a family of four that wanted to keep a 3-day supply of water on hand would need to store 12 gallons. That's 4 gallons a day (1 for each person) times 3 days. A 7-day supply for four people would be 28 gallons.

◆ Foods that you don't have to cook or keep cold, such as canned foods, peanut butter, crackers, granola bars, powdered milk, and staples like sugar, salt, and pepper. (Don't forget a manual can opener or utility knife.)

◆ First aid supplies and medicines

◆ Blankets and clothing

◆ Soap, toilet paper, and other personal hygiene items

◆ Special needs items (such as baby formula, diapers, and contact lens supplies)

◆ Certain tools and household items, such as a battery-powered radio, a flashlight, extra batteries, matches, and tools needed to shut off the water, power, or gas.

◆ Cash or traveler's checks. ATM machines may not be working.

More

For a complete checklist to help you build your emergency kit, go to www.redcross.org.

Store everything in one place. Somewhere cool and dark is best. You also might want to keep a small version of your emergency kit on hand in case you ever have to leave your home.

Once you have your supplies, remember to check them from time to time. Replace water, food, batteries, expired medicines, outgrown clothing, and other items as needed. Even bottled water and "nonperishable" foods need to be replaced after a while.

You should also know where your important documents are so that you can gather them quickly if you need to. These are things like passports, social security cards, wills, insurance policies, bank account and credit card information, and health records.

Safe Drinking Water

Knowing how to purify water can help you if:

◆ Your normal water supply becomes unsafe. Never ignore a "boil order" issued by local officials.

◆ You are in a place where there is no clean water.

◆ You run out of the clean water you have stored for an emergency.

Purifying water can greatly reduce your chance of getting sick from the water. You can purify water with one of these methods:

◆ Boil the water for 3 to 5 minutes. This method works the best but may not be practical if you need a lot of water. It also requires a stove, fire, or other heat source, which you may not have.

◆ Use an eyedropper to add 16 drops of liquid bleach to a gallon of water. Stir, and let it stand for 30 minutes. If the water does not smell slightly like bleach after 30 minutes, add 16 more drops of bleach and let it stand for another 15 minutes. There should be a bleach smell.

◆ Use iodine or chlorine tablets or drops. You can buy these at stores that sell camping equipment and at some drugstores. Do what the label says. Tablets and drops don't work as well as boiling or bleach, but they do kill some types of organisms.

◆ Use a water filter. Filters can get rid of some harmful things in the water and can improve the taste. Some filters work better than others.

Index